Neurotic and Psychotic Language Behaviour

Multilingual Matters

"Bilingualism: Basic Principles" (Second edition)
HUGO BAETENS BEARDSMORE
"Evaluating Bilingual Education: A Canadian Case Study"
MERRILL SWAIN AND SHARON LAPKIN
"Bilingual Children: Guidance for the Family"
GEORGE SAUNDERS
"Language Attitudes Among Arabic-French Bilinguals in Morocco"
ABDELÂLI BENTAHILA
"Conflict and Language Planning in Quebec"
RICHARD Y. BOURHIS (ed.)
"Bilingualism and Special Education"
JIM CUMMINS
"Bilingualism or Not: The Education of Minorities"
TOVE SKUTNABB-KANGAS
"An Ethnographic/Sociolinguistic Approach to Language Proficiency Assessment"
CHARLENE RIVERA (ed.)
"Communicative Competence Approaches to Language Proficiency Assessment: Research and Application"
CHARLENE RIVERA (ed.)
"Language Proficiency and Academic Achievement"
CHARLENE RIVERA (ed.)
"Pluralism: Cultural Maintenance and Evolution"
BRIAN BULLIVANT
"Placement Procedures in Bilingual Education: Education and Policy Issues"
CHARLENE RIVERA (ed.)
"The Education of Linguistic and Cultural Minorities in the OECD Countries"
STACY CHURCHILL
"Learner Language and Language Learning"
CLAUS FAERCH, KIRSTEN HAASTRUP AND ROBERT PHILLIPSON
"Bilingual and Multicultural Education: Canadian Perspectives"
STAN SHAPSON AND VINCENT D'OYLEY (eds.)
"Multiculturalism: The Changing Australian Paradigm"
LOIS FOSTER AND DAVID STOCKLEY
"Language Acquisition of a Bilingual Child"
ALVINO FANTINI
"Modelling and Assessing Second Language Acquisition"
KENNETH HYLTENSTAM AND MANFRED PIENEMANN (eds.)
"Aspects of Bilingualism in Wales"
COLIN BAKER
"Minority Education and Ethnic Survival"
MICHAEL BYRAM
"Age in Second Language Acquisition"
BIRGIT HARLEY
"Language in a Black Community
VIV EDWARDS
"Language and Education in Multilingual Settings"
BERNARD SPOLSKY (ed.)
"The Interdisciplinary Study of Urban Bilingualism in Brussels"
ELS WITTE and HUGO BAETENS BEARDSMORE (eds.)
"Introspection in Second Language Research"
CLAUS FAERCH and GABRIELE KASPER (eds.)
"Talk and Social Organization"
GRAHAM BUTTON and JOHN R. E. LEE

Please contact us for the latest information:
Multilingual Matters, Bank House, 8a Hill Road,
Clevedon, Avon BS21 7HH, England.

Neurotic and Psychotic Language Behaviour

Edited by

Ruth Wodak and
Pete Van de Craen

MULTILINGUAL MATTERS LTD
Clevedon · Philadelphia

British Library Cataloguing in Publication Data
1. Mentally ill——Language
2. Psycholinguistics
I. Wodak, Ruth II. Van de Craen, Peter
401′.9 RC455.4.P78
ISBN 0–905028–77–5
ISBN 0–905028–76–7 Pbk

Library of Congress Cataloging-in-Publication Data
Neurotic and psychotic language behaviour.
Includes index.
1. Mentally ill——Language. 2. Schizophrenics——Language. 3. Psycholinguistics. I. Wodak, Ruth, 1950– . II. Craen, Pete Van de. [DNLM: 1. Neurotic Disorders. 2. Psycholinguistics. 3. Schizophrenic Language. 4. Verbal Behavior. WM 170 N4935]
RC455.4.P78N48 1987 616.89 87–7744
ISBN 905028–76–7 (pbk.)
ISBN 905028–77–5

Multilingual Matters Ltd,
Bank House, 8a Hill Road,
Clevedon, Avon BS21 7HH,
England.

Typeset by Photo·graphics, Honiton, Devon, UK.
Cover designed by Jussi Nurmi
Printed and bound in Great Britain by
Short Run Press Ltd, Exeter EX2 7LW.

For Jakob and Ilse

Contents

Introduction

Pete Van de Craen

What is offered here is a collection of essays studying aspects of neurotic and schizophrenic language behaviour using various methodological approaches. In this introduction I would like to make a few comments on this field in general, since the study of deviant language behaviour is characterized by at least two striking features. First, it is generally considered to be interdisciplinary in the sense that there is a common ground for (social) psychologists, psychiatrists, sociolinguists and psycholinguists, philosophers and sociologists. Second, it is also considered to lack any methodological uniformity. Let me expand on these observations.

If we look back at the development of social scientific thought during, let us say, the past fifteen years, the term 'interdisciplinary' may well figure in the top ten of a scientific vocabulary frequency list — 'interdisciplinary' then meaning the study of the same problem or object by a group of scholars, each of whom is a specialist in his own field. However, this kind of interdisciplinary work did not guarantee better results or deeper insights into the matters studied. It soon became clear that each researcher had to be, in one way or another, interdisciplinary herself or himself, if new insights were to be produced. One of the interesting features of the present collection of papers is that they reflect this development. With a few exceptions, each contributor has thoroughly studied more than one discipline. The result can therefore be called 'interdisciplinary' in the new sense.

Let us now turn to methodological aspects, since these are closely linked with the interdisciplinary approach as understood here. Almost simultaneously with the rise of the term 'interdisciplinary', another term gained considerable importance, with perhaps even more impact than the former. I am referring to the paradigmatic approach to understanding the evolution of scientific thought. The notion of paradigm was introduced by the physicist Kuhn (1962) in an attempt to describe the evolutions of patterns of thinking in the natural sciences. According to Kuhn, 'a paradigm is what members of a scientific community, and they alone, share' (Kuhn 1977: 294); this is one of the many definitions that have been put forward. What we have been witnessing with respect to the social sciences is that Kuhn's notion of paradigm was — and still is — often interpreted as, first, a yardstick with which to measure the degree of scientific objectivity of any one discipline, and secondly, the justification for a monolithic methodology. Although it is fairly easy to agree with Kuhn's (1977) definition of the term paradigm, these interpretations of that definition are much more difficult to accept. They seem to be grounded in a rather narrow view of scientific research in general and of the social sciences in particular. Let me illustrate by referring to the study of deviant language behaviour as it is to be understood in the present volume.

The study of deviant language behaviour is the study of communication patterns of and/or with people suffering from some kind of breakdown in 'normal' interaction patterns due to some kind of communicative stress, as PEUSER* writes. With respect to schizophrenia this is clearly not the generally accepted view, at least not in medical circles. The medical paradigm — to consider schizophrenia as some kind of a disease — has been much more popular. It is only recently that the interactive and psychotherapeutic approaches towards neurotics and schizophrenics have raised some interest in medical circles. We are thus confronted with two competing paradigms, but this should not necessarily be a disadvantage. As DE DECKER and VAN DE CRAEN, along with others, suggest, the paradigm clash could well lead to an entirely new way of looking at schizophrenia: the interactional and (at least some part of) the medical paradigm need not be contradictory. If this is true, the whole idea of the paradigm as some kind of scientific standard and of a monolithic methodology is seriously challenged, since it is precisely the combined methodologies of different approaches which have provoked new insights into origins and therapies of certain forms of deviant (language) behaviour.

A further important point needs to be made regarding the social sciences in general. Linguistics can be taken as an example, since we are after all dealing with language behaviour; moreover, the recent evolution in linguistics exemplifies the argument perfectly. Structural linguistics has been called an example for all social sciences (cf. Lévi-Strauss 1963), and the enormous popularity enjoyed by transformational grammar from the beginning of the 1960s until the mid-1970s has certainly strengthened this conviction among many social scientists. But the rigidly formal approach

* capital letters refer to authors in this volume.

of transformational grammar, together with the bold philosophical claims about innateness and the way language is acquired by young children, completely neglected any form of interactionism. After all, the transformational paradigm continued structural linguistic thinking and did not put forward any new insights apart from syntactic description. Its popularity, however, resulted in the fact that interactional ideas put forward in earlier decades by linguists, psychologists, sociologists and other students of the humanities became a completely forgotten undercurrent in the 1950s and 1960s. Indeed, in the first decades of the twentieth century scholars such as Bühler (1934), Vygotsky (1934; English translation 1962) and Mead (1934) had started to look at language, behaviour and human development from an angle entirely divergent from the static Cartesian approach, which had until then prevailed, and which had re-emerged in the 1960s. By the time sociolinguistics appeared, it had to turn to the interactionists' work for philosophical and methodological support. This was especially true for those sociolinguists who were trying to develop their discipline into a social science capable of accounting for intricate social interaction patterns as a means of explaining human behaviour in general (cf. Hymes 1974).

It is within the forgotten interactionist tradition that the present volume should be placed. And it is no accident that both editors of this work have been constructing approaches echoing interactional and multimethodological ideas. Outlining these views will clarify the underlying theoretical position of most articles presented here. Wodak (1981; 1984) has been looking at language and behaviour from what she calls a sociopsycholinguistic approach. This framework is based on a three-level mode, and aims at relating (language) behaviour to a number of sociological and psychological variables. With reference to verbal behaviour she has put forward a socio-psychological theory of text planning (SPTT), a dynamic approach capable of examining subtle strategies in communicative behaviour between therapist and client, but equally valid for other interaction patterns. In Wodak's view, any sharp distinction between psycholinguistics and sociolinguistics would misrepresent the underlying reality (see also WODAK). These ideas are shared by Van de Craen (1982; 1986), who also emphasizes the influence of the nature of interactions upon the development of cognitive structures. He has named this approach 'social linguistics', in an attempt to distinguish this line of thought from traditional — especially correlational — sociolinguistics. In his view, human development is considered to be greatly influenced by communicative experience and some communicative experiences are more likely to provoke deviancies than others (see Bateson 1972 and VON BLOCK). On a less dramatic level, this means that communicative behaviour intervenes, not only in socialization processes, but also in cognitive development.

Both Wodak's and Van de Craen's views could be summarized as follows. In some way or other behaviour is greatly influenced by experience, as psychoanalysis and other developmental theories have suggested. This means that it should be possible to find traces of the communicative experience in the overall (language) behaviour patterns of individuals, but also in their degree of anxiety, in their emotional state, etc. In cases of deviancy such as neuroticism or schizophrenia, evidence for all this should present itself even more clearly.

With respect to deviant language behaviour, Wodak's and Van de Craen's approach not only echoes that of the scholars already mentioned, such as Bühler, Vygotsky and Mead, but also the work of those who, perhaps more than anybody else, could be considered the founding fathers of the interactionistic approach for the social sciences, namely Sullivan and Sapir. In what became his intellectual testament, *The Interpersonal Theory of Schizophrenia* (1952), Sullivan states that looking at psychiatry as the study of interpersonal interaction is in fact a tautology. There is simply no other way of approaching psychiatry which 'must be concerned only with the human living which is in, or can be converted into, the public mode' (Sullivan 1953: 20). What is needed, therefore, is a developmental theory of personality based on the study of interpersonal relations. Since each person is an undeniable social construct, it must be in the study of personality that the answers lie, not only for the psychiatrist but also for the social scientist in general. All behaviour is social behaviour because, as Sapir writes, 'To say that the human being behaves individually at one moment and socially at another is as absurd as to declare that matter follows the laws of chemistry at a certain time and succumbs to the supposedly different laws of atomic physics at another, for matter is always obeying certain mechanical laws which are at one and the same time both physical and chemical according to the manner in which we choose to define its organization' (Sapir (1927), in Mandelbaum 1949: 545). Neither Sullivan nor Sapir had the opportunity to develop their research programmes, since both scholars died prematurely. But their ingenious approach to the inherent social aspects of man, which can merely be mentioned here, still contrasts sharply today with the seemingly indestructible notion of mental disease.

The chapters in the present volume reflect many of the developments described above. The first six chapters deal with the problems of neurotic language behaviour. Together they form the first part of this volume; and the authors of all six chapters have studied therapeutic communication from various angles. The second part consists of studies of schizophrenic language behaviour. FISHER and VON BLOCK offer theoretical views of this type of language use by comparing schizophrenic language respectively with the Wittgensteinian concept of language game and/or with everyday language and the language of science. PEUSER and DE DECKER and VAN DE CRAEN refer to aphasia and lateralization problems; while the conversationalist approach is represented by KAESERMANN, VAN BIJSTERVELD and VAN BELLE. SCHONAUER and BUCHKREMER have studied written material, while WROBEL has looked more closely at semantic aspects of the term 'father' in observed conversations, as well as in reports in the literature. Finally, the cognitive approach is treated by BUHLER and VOGT, with an interesting experiment connected with the idea of over-inclusive thinking.

I do not think that it is too optimistic to predict the growing importance of the interactional approach in the future. As is demonstrated in the first part of this collection, therapy with neurotic patients has already benefited considerably from interactional research. As yet we are not so far on with schizophrenics; but it is clear that the approach is very promising, because communicative strategies not only 'represent the underlying concepts of surface futures of social meaning', as Dittmar (1983: 251) has argued, but, even more importantly, these strategies mould the meanings. Eventually this must lead to an entirely new way of thinking in the social sciences.

Acknowledgement

The articles in this volume were first presented at the special symposium on neurotic and psychotic language behaviour during the VIIth World Congress of Applied Linguistics, held at the Vrije Universiteit Brussel in August 1984. The editors are grateful to Professor Nivette, organizer and chairman of AILA Brussels 84 and currently AILA President, and to the organizing committee for having consented to the publication of this symposium.

Ruth Wodak
Pete Van de Craen

References

Bateson, G. 1972: *Steps to an Ecology of Mind*. New York: Ballantine.
Bühler, K. 1934: *Sprachtheorie*. Stuttgart: Fischer; second edition 1965.

Dittmar, N. 1983: Descriptive and explanatory power of rules in Sociolinguistics. In B. Bain (ed.), *The Sociogenesis of Language and Human Conduct*. New York: Plenum.

Hymes, D. 1974: *Foundations in Sociolinguistics*. Philadelphia: University of Pennsylvania Press.

Kuhn, T. 1962: *The Structure of Scientific Revolutions*. Chicago: Chicago University Press.

— 1977: Second thoughts on paradigms. In T. Kuhn, *The Essential Tension*. London: University of Chicago Press.

Lévi-Strauss, C. 1963: *Structural Anthropology*. Harmondsworth: Penguin.

Mandelbaum, D. (ed.), 1949: *Selected Writings of Edward Sapir*. Berkeley: University of California Press.

Mead, G. 1934: *Mind, Self and Society*. Chicago: University of Chicago Press.

Sullivan, H. 1953: *The Interpersonal Theory of Schizophrenia*. New York: Norton.

Van de Craen, P. 1982: Sociale linguïstiek. Dissertation, University of Brussels (VUB).

— 1986: The status of sociolinguistics as a science. *Sociolinguistics Newsletter*.

Vygotsky, L. 1962: *Thought and Language*. Cambridge, Mass.: MIT.

Wodak, R. 1981: *Das Wort in der Gruppe*. Vienna: Verlag der Österreichischen Akademie der Wissenschaften.

— 1984: Wege der Soziolinguistik. *Journal für Sozialforschung* 24(3).

Part 1

Neurotic language behaviour

1 'At last I know . . .': Sociolinguistic and psycholinguistic aspects of the therapeutic process and its effect

Ruth Wodak

Introduction: The aim of socio-psycholinguistics in the study of institutionalized discourse

The study of institutionalized discourse, such as interaction at court or in therapy, can be motivated by different intentions and has several goals:

1. Every restricted and explicitly defined speech situation (Leodolter 1975a; Wodak 1981a; Labov and Fanshel 1977) allows the linguist to arrive at constitutive rules of interaction, of language behaviour and discourse, that are never found so clearly in everyday conversation. Turn-taking and the roles of the participants are defined from the beginning, norms are explicitly stated. The goal of the interaction is known. For example, it may be necessary to ascertain the truth — or at least a plausible 'truth' which can be defined in legal terms in court — or to be 'healed' in therapy.
2. Sociolinguists and psycholinguists have goals that go beyond the linguistic and ethnographic description of the therapeutic process. Their main interest is to find typical (language) behaviour corresponding to certain sociological (class, age, sex) or psychological (concentration, emotionality) variables using an interdisciplinary framework such as the 'three-level model' or a 'sociopsychological theory of text planning' (Wodak 1983; 1984; 1986; Wodak & Schulz 1986). What consequences do the different types of behaviour have on the therapeutic process: who 'succeeds' in establishing a 'good' image for him/herself (Wodak 1981b; 1981c)? What kind of language barriers exist (not only

between therapeutic and everyday language, but also between different styles and strategies in everyday speech, between therapist and patient)?

3 This kind of research leads us to a third interest: to be able to explain certain types of behaviour at a theoretical level in terms of different cultural and class- or sex-specific socialization processes (Wodak 1983; 1984). On the other hand, at a practical level, it would be useful to draw conclusions about the training of therapists, perhaps with a view to changing the therapeutic technique.

1 Linguistics and psychotherapy

The interest of linguistics in therapeutic communication has greatly increased in recent years, and has indeed only now begun. The reasons for this lie on the one hand in the development of pragmatics and speech act theory, and on the other in the aim actually to deal with empirical material; owing to the precisely defined setting and the familiarity of the institution and its rules, the material from therapeutic situations makes it possible to explain important fundamental conditions of human communication. From a logical research viewpoint, it is always meaningful and useful to use material from 'extreme' communication situations, as it is easier to grasp everyday communication in relation to such interactions. This interest must be regarded as fundamental research. On the other hand is the scientific and historical development that led from rigid structuralism and transformational grammar to pragmatics, which deals with the 'significance' and 'intention' of speech acts (pragmalinguistics). The tendency has therefore been to follow in the footsteps of Wittgenstein (1967), Schütz (1960) and symbolic interactionism (Goffman 1959). This was of prime importance in studying a speech situation in which explanation, scenic comprehension and hermeneutic interpretation are actively integrated as immanent action schemata, and are not presented merely as methodological concepts. These methodologies can therefore be subjected to realistic examination. Thirdly, the language game 'therapy' is a speech situation in which the action is almost exclusively verbal, with the consequence of intended self-reflection and alteration: it thus involves speaking in direct connection with human practice. There is one further motive that can be mentioned, and that is an interest in the processes of socialization and the acquisition of language and behaviour. As, on the one hand, psychoanalysis provides a concept of socialization and, on the other, it is clear from previous investigations that language is the means of socialization and is acquired through socialization, psycholinguistic and sociolinguistic fundamental research is the obvious choice (Wodak 1981a; 71). We know that neurotic symptoms have their roots in childhood and can be traced back to certain communicative mechanisms; on the other hand, such pathogenic mechanisms are repeated in the transference situation. It is therefore possible to gather experience of disturbed family interactions and develop guidelines and postulates for 'alternative pedagogics'.

Several approaches will subsequently be mentioned by way of example, particularly from the methodical viewpoints of the interpretative techniques used and of the guiding interest. It is by no means possible to list here all the investigations of therapeutic communication; although this would provide bibliographical information, it would serve to confuse rather than to illuminate the points which seem important to us, and might possibly bore the reader. Similarly, we are less interested in the scientific and historical aspect than in the actual level of research (Flader and Wodak-Leodolter 1979: v-x).

1.1 'Speech act oriented' analyses

Initial attempts in the direction of a speech act oriented analysis were made by Goeppert and Goeppert (1973; 1975). Transcribed psychotherapeutic discourses have been examined according to various criteria, such as person used, temporal and spatial reference, intention, speech acts, and provided with a psychoanalytical commentary and interpretation.

Although the categories used in these investigations were fairly undifferentiated, more recent case studies such as those of Frankenberg (1979) and Klann (1979) already contain an expanded and diversified range of devices, but without offering a theory of meaning or pragmalinguistic theory of therapeutic communication as a background. The choice of indicators and the study and interpretation of speech acts thus remain unfounded and left solely to subjective decision, making it impossible to reproduce them. The problem of allocating individual expressions to categories within the theory of speech acts was also dealt with recently (Wunderlich 1979).

Apart from these methodological objections, an essential principle must be taken into consideration: if we start with the assumption that speech acts (both direct and indirect) are always the result of intentional, deliberate action (Searle 1975), then for obvious reasons therapeutic communication in particular is unsuitable for such analysis. After all, it involves spontaneous, often subconscious action, and 'neurotic' speech acts in particular cannot be regarded as planned and intentional, but as the result of resistance, clichés, social compulsion and transference phenomena (Habermas 1969; Lorenzer 1973; Wodak 1981a: 59ff.). The text thus resists analysis using the devices of the speech act theory, a fact that unfortunately is not taken into consideration!

1.2 The expansion model

In their detailed analysis of psychotherapeutic discourse, Labov and Fanshel (1977) demonstrated how it is possible to interpret tiny sections of text using a variety of different methods, thus gaining an insight into the therapeutic process, the patient, her illness and life history. However, I have already described the methods and procedures of these two authors in detail elsewhere (Wodak 1981a: 39ff.), and will therefore confine myself here to criticism of the text analysis used.

'Expansion' is an essential feature of the text analysis carried out by Labov and Fanshel (1977: 49ff.): each sequence is expanded into a complete text using the background knowledge of the authors, i.e. incomplete sentences and expressions are expanded, indirect and implicit meanings made explicit for concrete analysis. However, this knowledge does not form the basis of the text as a second, latent level of meaning, but the text as such is subjected to analysis after expansion in this manner (a sort of 'repaired' text). The criteria and categories for this expansion are not defined, and psychoanalytical and linguistic precepts are mixed in such a way as to make reconstruction impossible, a procedure which — in my opinion — is inadmissible. If the expansion were only of an interpretative nature (and even then psychotherapeutic categories would have been suitable), it cannot be taken as an object of the text analysis itself, as it would then have a metafunction. The diversity of language in the therapeutic situation is not therefore adequately apprehended; methodologically speaking, content and metalevel have been mixed.

To this extent — although this is an extremely differentiated analysis and description of the situation — there is no theory of therapeutic communication! The question also remains unanswered as to whether the devices developed can be transferred to other therapeutic processes, or whether they are suitable only to describe the individual case.

Despite these critical considerations, such work has made a considerable contribution to the interest in linguistic therapy research and certainly also provides the most detailed analysis of psychotherapeutic discourse to date. Although my own investigation (Wodak 1981a; Wodak & Schulz 1986) contains methods from both the approaches described above, it also offers a theoretical background (of an interdisciplinary nature) and combines therapeutic discourse with elements of the theory of 'cognitive planning procedures' (Wodak 1981a: 127ff.; Wodak 1983). The advantages of this procedure will be demonstrated later.

1.3 Conversational analysis

Conversational analysis — the scientific description of extremely small speech units ('turns') — represents an approach which sets out to explicate the processes controlling dialogue in everyday life, and in some cases even formally to record them. It is not therefore surprising that an attempt should be made to investigate psychoanalytical therapy more closely as a specific, institutionally organized form of discourse with the aid of these devices (Flader 1979: 25ff.; Trömel-Plötz 1979: 56ff.).

The interesting thing about this approach — which is allied to the tradition of ethnomethodology — is the attempt to reconstruct the therapeutic dialogue without explicit categorical knowledge of psychotherapy. What, then — from the viewpoint of textual immanence — is the nature of the interpretative routines and active habits of the patient, which reflect his everyday knowledge, and how is the gradual reorganization of this everyday knowledge, the elimination of systematic distortion effected by the analyst? The advantage of such an analysis is its text orientation: every individual utterance, every sequence is minutely examined for implicit ambiguities, the doctor's procedure — his often intuitive choice of a meaning — made explicit as a communicative strategy. Communication conflicts are therefore due to non-reciprocity of utterance patterns, which often occurs, particularly in the case of constructions on the part of the doctor and when the patient's resistance is encountered.

In spite of the precision of such a method, 'it deceives itself': the text is central; all communicative interactions that occur are supposed to be explained from the text; typical features of the therapeutic discourse are elaborated. However, the knowledge of therapy and technique which the investigator possesses is naturally included in the interpretation; he knows, of course, that this is a therapeutic discourse. This circle, which as a 'hermeneutic circle' is valid for every social scientific text interpretation, might possibly be offset if the investigator were uninformed about text type and institutional frame; however, he would then be unable to register manifest and latent meaning.

The corpus of this investigation is also too limited; the levels of interaction within the therapy are not considered. Nevertheless, due to their detailed treatment of the empirical corpus, such studies form a preliminary stage on the way to theoretically oriented investigations and approaches to interdisciplinary research.[1]

2 Therapeutic communication in groups

2.1 The investigation

In my own longitudinal investigation of therapeutic communication in groups at the crisis intervention centre in Vienna, I recorded therapy sessions on tape over a period of three years and examined them from various aspects[2] (Figure 1.1 shows the course of the investigation).

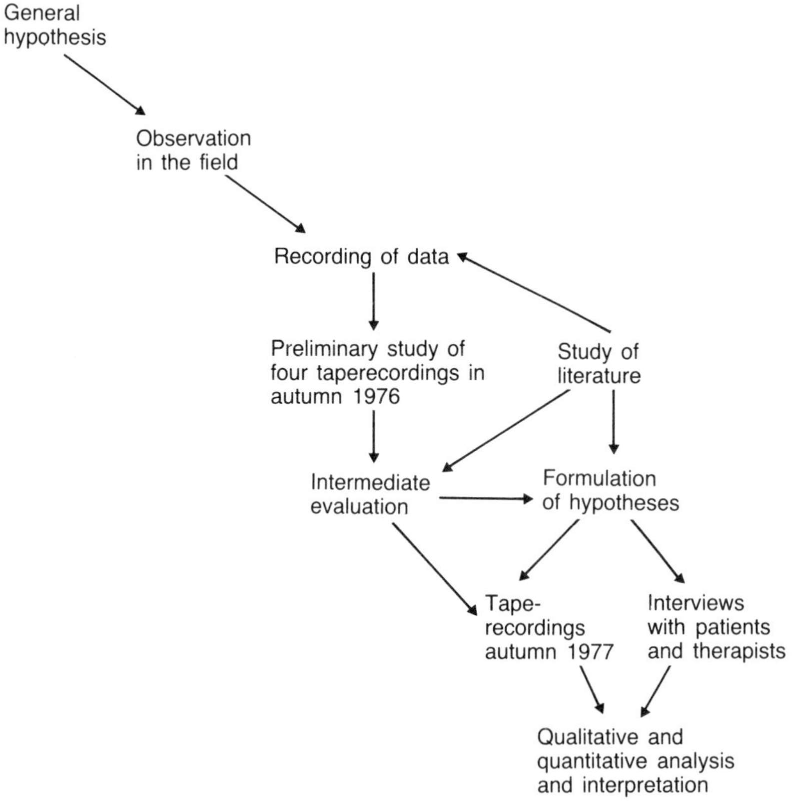

FIGURE 1.1 *The course of the investigation.*

1 The aim was to determine theoretically and empirically the difference between therapeutic and everyday communication.
2 I was interested too in the quality and quantity of class-specific speech behaviour (Wodak 1981a; 1981c).[3]
3 At the same time I investigated the question of whether there were sex-specific behaviour patterns in the group and, if so, the extent to which they altered the course of the therapy[4] (Wodak 1981a: 80ff.; 1981b).
4 Finally, the therapeutic effect was examined in the light of stylistic and linguistic factors (Wodak 1981c).

This was all based on a comprehensive language concept, embracing not only verbal behaviour but also cognitive and emotional aspects (Wittgenstein 1967; Habermas 1977).

I shall continue by outlining the pragmalinguistic model, which allows us to record the diversity of therapeutic communication in groups. I shall then examine the therapeutic effect by means of an illustrative text analysis of two passages spoken by the same female patient at the beginning and at the end of the therapy. I shall investigate these in the light of a single indicator: 'narrative structure'. Further information, a description of other methods and categories used, and the results of an analysis of class- and sex-specific speech behaviour can be found in Wodak (1981a, 1981b; Wodak & Schulz 1986).

2.2 The 'three-level model' of therapeutic communication in groups

2.2.1 A new conception of 'meaning' Therapeutic discourse in groups is a complex phenomenon. Its diversity is the result of three factors: the actual communication and group dynamics that take place (the 'here and now'), the 'family transference', and the expectations and life history of the individual. It therefore follows that verbal interaction and communication reflect these three factors.

As a result, verbal expressions and texts in a therapeutic situation are made up of three significant components: colloquial meaning, which is based on membership of a speech community; group meaning, which relates the value of what is said to the latent transference level in the group; and finally, personal semantics, the expression of the individual's life history, psychogenesis and pathogenesis, and the position of the patient in the social structure of society.

A threefold interpretation frame by itself, therefore, offers a satisfactory means of recording and interpreting the complete significance of therapeutic discourse. The concept of meaning such as that used in linguistics recently (Wittgenstein 1967; Searle 1971: 68ff.) therefore has to be expanded by two dimensions that certainly also have an effect on everyday communication (Klann 1979), but which are only tangible in a clearly defined therapeutic setting.

It is a well known fact that linguistics and linguistic schools have by no means reached agreement on a serviceable definition of 'meaning', at least since the revolutionary work of Bühler (1934), Morris (1938) and Ogden and Richards (1972).

The 'usage theory' (Wittgenstein 1967; Searle 1971), which — according to Brekle (1972: 60) — has considerable advantages compared to a narrower term (above all its closeness to reality), is contrasted with transformational-generative concepts (Katz 1970: 142), with structural hypotheses (Brekle 1972; Schifko 1975) and with the integrative approach of Mel'čuk (1974; 1976). Nevertheless, the champions of the 'utilization theory' do not reach the emotional and unconscious levels of spoken texts, although Cavell (1976: 72) draws an analogy between Freud and Wittgenstein and sums up the basic assumptions as follows (Cavell 1976: 52):

> We learn and teach words in certain contexts, and then we are expected, and expect others to be able to project them into further contexts. Nothing assures that this projection will take place . . ., just as nothing insures that we will make, and understand, the same projections. That on the whole we do is a matter of our sharing routes of interests and feeling, modes of response, senses of humor . . . — all the whirl of organism Wittgenstein calls 'forms of life'.

It is above all the microanalysis of therapeutic discourse (in groups) that can enable us to find more precise interpretations of the spoken word, as the verification of the interpretation is often explicity contained in the text. However, in my opinion the concept of the 'usage theory' (of which I am a traditional supporter) should be expanded by the dimensions of emotion and unconscious meanings.

It remains to be said that even in individual therapy — as in the model presented here — communication is determined by three perspectives: the working relationship of the analyst with the patient (i.e. the healthy 'I') represents the colloquial level; regression to earlier communicative strategies (re-enactment of scenes in the relationship and transference to the therapist), the transference level; and, finally, the real personal and social characteristics of doctor and patient also exist (individual level) (Schröter 1979: 180ff.). Figure 1.2 shows the 'three-level model', the dimensions necessary to analyse and understand therapeutic discourse.

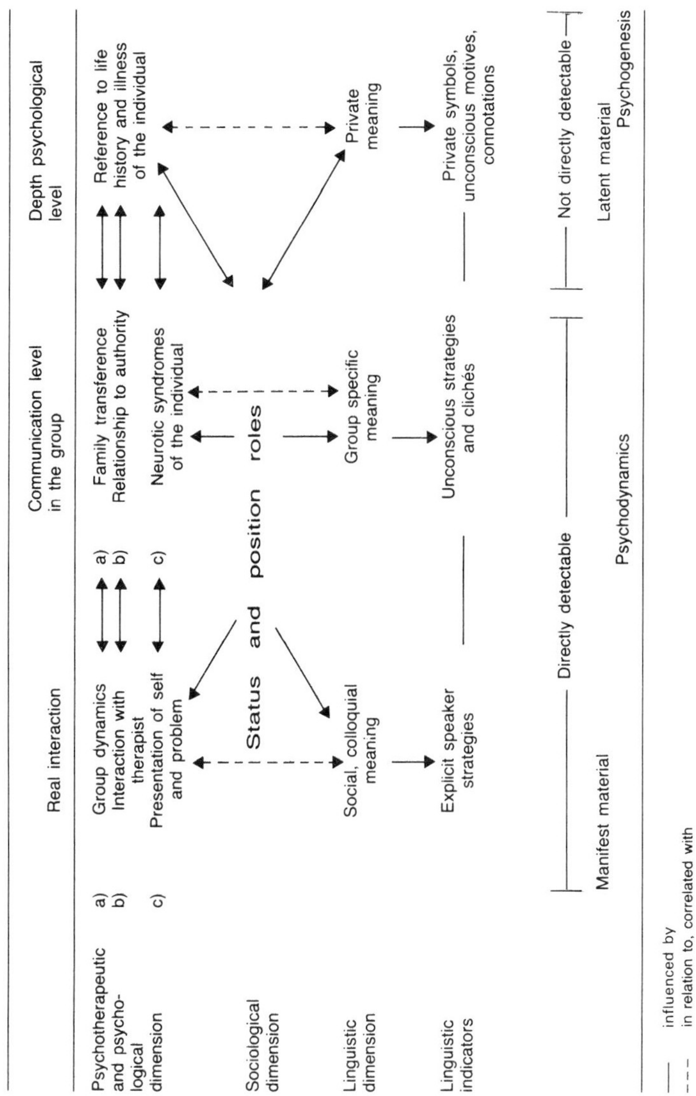

FIGURE 1.2 *Interaction levels in group therapy: 'three-level model'.*

2.2.2 The colloquial level This level involves expressions in a group therapy situation that can be explicitly apprehended in their everyday colloquial meaning. Patients describe their problems, discuss the activities of the group, discuss relationships, settle conflicts (Wodak 1981a: 113ff.). Although everything that occurs in a therapeutic situation has a particular significance for the group process and the individual (latent meanings), attention is focused initially on the text as such, without further analysis or interpretation. As the technique of the 'open group' for suicide candidates aims initially to treat real problems, the use of colloquial meaning for analysis is necessary and legitimate. Figure 1.3 shows the taxonomic system that allows the 'speaker strategies' used in therapeutic discourse to be distinguished (cf. Halliday 1976: 3ff.).

2.2.3 The level of group language In order to avoid possible misunderstanding, it should be emphasized from the start that we are dealing here not with a completely different language or with another dialogue that has taken place simultaneously, but with a second dimension of meaning that allows us to interpret the meaning of each expression with reference to the dynamics of the group. A second set of categories obtained from the theories of group processes, of 'family transference', is applied to the text (Bion 1961; Kutter 1971; Grumiller 1975; Finger 1976; Slater 1978). Owing to the peculiarities of the therapeutic setting, many of the transference factors of individual patients are manifest in the group situation, in their relationships to one another and to the therapist. Typical group structures and processes, hierarchies and conflicts take their course, normally unnoticed and initially unconscious. Every utterance made by the individual participant must therefore be analysed not only with respect to its colloquial meaning, but also with regard to its value and its function in a group context. What did the speaker intend to achieve by his utterance? Why did he address a particular member of the group? Why does a conflict occur between two people? Finger (1976: 91) attempts to integrate the various group concepts; all the phenomena mentioned here manifest themselves in typical verbal expressions (whether these be symbols or clichés):

> To the extent that the process of integration within the group is also a process of eliminating linguistic subversion, it is more than a formal repetition of the infantile process of socialization. With the reconstruction of language a process begins that allows the private language of each individual to become gradually incorporated in the linguistic community. To an increasing extent this would be equivalent to a contextually new process of socialization that makes it

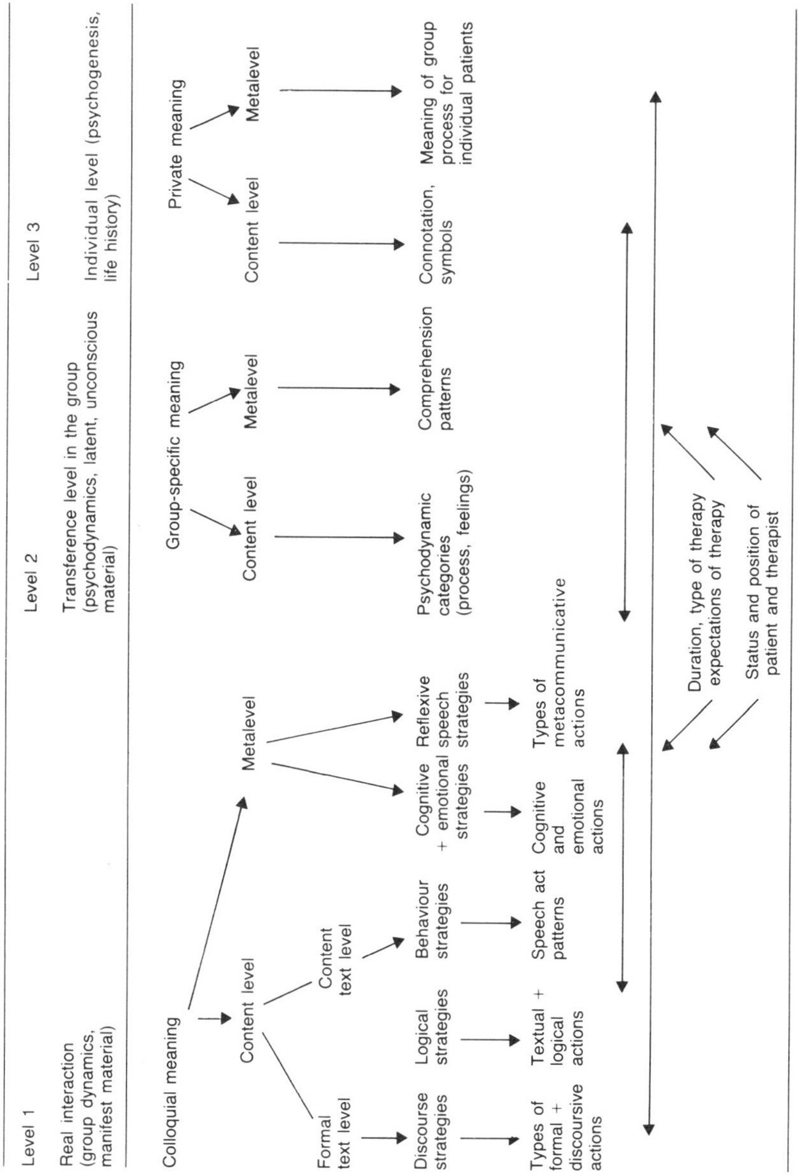

FIGURE 1.3 *Structure of therapeutic communication in the group.*

possible to transform old interactive forms into new ones and allows old methods of solving conflicts to be replaced by new and better ones. (Finger 1976: 91).

2.2.4 The level of private language Communication in a group conceals yet another aspect besides that of manifestly apprehensible verbal language and group meanings. Each individual always subconsciously associates specific meanings with his verbal utterances, his own connotations that can only be understood in the context of his life history and expectations.

The small child learns linguistic behaviour through specific interaction with his primary parental figure. The experience gained in these first interactions has a cognitive and emotional effect on the small child. Although in the course of time the child learns to abstract the interactions experienced with the primary parental figure, the emotional component of these first experiences remains, and is passed on. Colloquial speech games therefore have a private component.

Private meanings and private language are quite clearly apparent in psychotic patients, particularly schizophrenics (Leodolter 1975a). In my own investigation of schizophrenic speech behaviour, I found that the so-called 'disturbed' speech of these patients had quite different structures that bear many similarities to the mechanisms of dream texts, or in other words unconscious material. This private language can be translated back into colloquial language using psychotherapeutic methods (Green 1974). As a result, neurotic people — and even normal people — always add their private symbols and connotations to everyday speech acts, though they are not as apparent as in the case described above.

In group behaviour it is not only group dynamics that plays a decisive role, but also the psychogenesis and pathogenesis of the individual, the expectations of the individual, his/her experiences and knowledge. When comprehended in a broader sense, the private linguistic elements are only apparent against the background of each life history and the history of individual object relationships that are not accessible from observation of the group situation alone. The most one can do, therefore, is to establish hypotheses that can then be verified with the help of individual therapy. Detailed discussion of the linguistic analysis of connotations would exceed the limits of this paper (Wodak 1981a: 69ff.).

3 Qualitative test analysis: the therapeutic effect

3.1 Problem presentation in group therapy

Like therapeutic discourse, the type of text in which we are chiefly interested — 'problem presentation in group therapy' — involves several levels of meaning. Not only the manifest content is significant, but also the context (when, or at what time during the session, a problem is discussed) and, finally, the motives that induce the individual patient to describe a problem in a certain manner.

Problem presentation in group therapy involves lengthy sections of monologue during which a patient expresses a personal problem. The passages of text subjected to analysis also extend to the immediate reaction of the group and/or therapist, and to the patient's answer (we are thus dealing with an interaction unit). Three types of text serve the implementation of this speaker strategy: 'scene', 'narration' and 'circumstance', which according to the 'sociopsychological theory of text planning'[5] must be derived from a common thematic deep structure (Wodak 1983). The questions and hypotheses elaborated were tested in the light of a quantitative analysis of 1,134 problems presented in group therapy.

3.2 The 'narrative structure'

This category is used to describe the text structure (of a discourse strategy). Typical forms of problem presentation in group therapy can be placed into three subcategories: 'scene', 'narration' and 'circumstance'. The theoretical basis for these categories, and for their relationship to class- and sex-specific hypotheses, has already been provided (Wodak 1981a: 127ff.), and it is therefore only necessary here to specify the criteria for their application.

The indicators selected are 'speaker's perspective' (Werlich 1975: 46ff.), the presence (or absence) of metacommunicative speaker strategies, the narrative tense used (Werlich 1975: 51ff.), and the coherence of the text (Kallmeyer *et al.* 1974: 57ff.), of certain utterances which

> . . . contain a number of constituents that all indicate and limit the root of the viewpoint from which the speaker speaks in a communicative situation and to which all objects, changes and facts described in the text refer. Text constituents that fulfil this function clarify various aspects of the speaker's perspective. — (Werlich 1975: 46).

The speaker's perspective is determined by 'person' (that is, the choice of the impersonal 'one' or 'you' in contrast to the personal 'I', 'presentation' as a selective speaker's attitude to situational factors, 'focus', 'aspect', 'genus' and 'modus' (Leodolter 1975b: 88ff.).

A difference is made between an 'opening' and a 'closing' focus. The former means temporal sequences that gradually become more comprehensive, while the latter comprises local and temporal sequential forms that become less and less comprehensive (Werlich 1975: 50).

> The choice of an aspect . . . indicates how the speaker sees changes and circumstances with reference to segments in the temporal continuum, or how he would like them to be seen. The speaker's perspective of the aspect is thus always closely linked to the choice of tenses. — (Werlich 1975: 52).

Although in German the aspect is expressed lexically, rather than directly in the form of a verb, the marked and continuous aspect can nevertheless be differentiated. 'Genus' refers to the choice of the aspect 'active' or 'passive', and indicates whether the speaker wishes to view changes and circumstances of phenomena as an agent, or as happening to them (Werlich 1975: 53).

> The choice of modus . . . provides information about the entity attributed by the speaker to persons, objects and facts. There are three main modi from which the speaker can choose: the factual modus, the negative modus and the probable modus. — (Werlich 1975: 54).

As will be shown, it is precisely the combinations of these elements that constitutes an important criterion in differentiating the three types of text.

The choice of the 'narrative tense' is also an important indicator:

> The choice of the tense of a verb indicates how the speaker views objects and facts with relation to an axis of orientation formed by his momentary situation, i.e., by the speech act at any moment in time within the temporal continuum. — (Werlich 1975: 51).

Finally the coherence of the text affects the textual structure as a whole (Beaugrande and Dressler 1981: 88ff.). Can the speaker realize his intentions; does the planned strategy secure its objective, the desired reaction from the listener? Is the subject consistently pursued? Are references clear and understandable? Kallmeyer *et al.* (1974: 58) define 'coherence' as follows:

> The coherence of dialogistic text results from the connective elements, the thematic definition and the interactive context.

This also naturally applies to longer monologic sections, such as problem presentation in group therapy, in a wider interactive context. Accordingly, against the background of the established indicators, 'scene' is characterized by the absence of metacommunicative speaker strategies. It is a defined, personalized speaker's perspective (use of 'I'), the presentation is very selective (one event), the focus closes (unique experience), the aspect is marked (description of events), the genus active, the modus factual.

'Scenes' take place in the narrative present, with a lot of direct speech. Although there is coherence, the great degree of complication coupled with the absence of metacommunicative signals make understanding difficult.

'Narration' means the classical narrative form of Labov and Waletzky (1967: 23). Orientation, complication, evaluation, resolution and code are present, and ensure the coherence of the text. The orientation and evaluation provide the metacommunicative frame. The definite, personalized speaker's perspective comes to the fore, the focus closes (generalizations are normally only possible in connection with problem solution). The aspect is marked, the genus active or passive ('it happened to me' and 'I have done'), the modus factual. There is coherence, and — if the other patients allow — a story will be related from beginning to end, normally without being able to establish a direct connection to the problem.

'Circumstance' means the description of a symptom, of the circumstance in which the speaker suffers. In this case there is no metacommunicative frame at all. The speaker's perspective is impersonal (use of *one* or *you*), the focus opens, problem presentation in group therapy is kept very verbal and formal, the presentation is not selective, the aspect unmarked (circumstance, continuity), the genus is passive and the modus finally 'probable'; (*perhaps it could . . .*). The text is superficially coherent; a circumstance is described coherently, but much remains unclear to the listener owing to defence mechanisms; and, above all, the reference to the causes of the patient's case history is missing completely, or is only intimated.

3.3 Summary hypothesis concerning the therapeutic effect

Psychic symptoms manifest themselves linguistically, and at the same time psychotherapy claims to be able to treat symptoms and problems, or to recreate 'subverted language games'. I therefore assume that the language used by patients at the start of therapy will be different from that used at the end of therapy. This will apply to both cognitive and emotional spheres (Wodak 1981a: 147ff., 191ff., 234ff.). In the following passage the therapeutic effect is illustrated in the light of one category — the 'narrative structure' (eleven main categories are used in the overall analysis: cf. Wodak 1981a: 127ff.).

There should typically be a predictable, significant difference between the text types of problem presentation in group therapy used for solved and unsolved problems (by the same patient for the same topic).[6] However, it should be mentioned here that only simultaneous alteration at a verbal, cognitive and an *emotional* level (expression of feelings, defence) indicate the positive effect of the therapy.

3.4 Technical aspects

The description of the nonverbal level is only an outline, and is based on the impressions of the session, which were noted down. Comments provide additional important information during the verbalization of the text (actions of members of the group, tone of voice). The texts were transliterated using the method of Gumperz and Herasimschuk (1972) and also that of Ehlich and Switalla (1976: 89ff.)[7] Each contribution is defined as a unit ('turn') with the change of speaker. The latent level of meaning is not recorded using linguistic categories (such as 'indirect speech act'). The inability of speech act analysis to describe this level has already been mentioned elsewhere. The subject of both texts is one and the same problem encountered by a female patient: it is the patient's extremely difficult and disturbed relationship with her parents, and with her father in particular. The second presentation of this problem in group therapy was recorded exactly a year after the first, and shows the change in the patient particularly well. The qualitative analysis is therefore intended not only to illustrate the technique of interpretation and discuss the difficulties and limits of quantification, but also — and above all — to prove the hypothesis of the therapeutic effect.

4 Text A: The problem is acute

1 F: Wenn irgendein, eben so ein Problem in einem steckt, da geht's am
(If there's some, well if you have a problem, you feel)
2 so, dass man, dass ma so beinander ist, dass man gar net glaubt
(*door opens, a woman enters, sound of chairs being moved*)
(so awful, you just wouldn't believe it)

3 und dass man mit dem Problem z.B. net fertig geworden ist,
(and that you haven't managed to cope with the problem, for example,)
4 z.B. ja — ich hab g'sagt, es geht ma gut — letztes Mal — dass es so, also
(for example, yes — I already said, everything's fine — last time — that it was)
5 ich bin wieder zu ruhig, obwohl — aber, das Problem, was in einem Menschen
(I am too calm again, although — but the problem of what is inside you,)
6 drinnen steckt, dass was ma mit der Geburt mitkriegt, oder wie einen
(what you have in you from birth on, or how)
7 die Eltern erzogen haben oder — I wass net, wie ich da heute sagen soll, aber —
(your parents bring you up or — I don't know how I should say this today, but —)
8 bled, dass das gerade heute aufgenommen wird —; i hab mit meinem Vater
(silly, that this is being recorded, today of all days — I talked to my father,)
9 gesprochen, also er gibt mir immer die Schuld, also, dass ich (cough)
(and he always blames me, and after all)
10 schliesslich und endlich erst 33 Jahre alt bin; — i kann —, es geht heut
(I am only 33 years old; — I can — I can't do it)
11 net.
(today.)
12 M: No redens aus!
(No, finish what you were saying!)
13 F: I red a viel—
(I talk a lot, too!)
15 F: Na, aber — na i wass schon, dass i net a Stunde jetzt red — aber aber — dass
(No, well — I know I haven't been talking for hours, but, but —)
16 i halt net so viel mitgemacht hab, wie er; — dass i net im Krieg war, dafür
(I haven't been through as much as him; — it's not my fault that)
17 kann i ja nix, i kann ja nix dafür, dass i erst so alt bin und dass i
(I wasn't in the war, I can't help being as old as I am and that I —)
18 bis jetzt — no ka Krieg war, na? Oder, bei uns ist es so, wir haben einen
(that there's been no war so far. In our case we had a)
19 Familienbetrieb und er hält mir eben vor, dass er — also gestern hab'ma
(family business and he reproaches me that he — only yesterday we)
20 G'sprochen — i möcht das nur zu Ende bringen noch — telefoniert hab'ma
(talked — I'd just like to get this over with — we spoke on the phone —)
21 ganz nett, ruhig ang'rufen — und dann ist das immer — und also, er hält
(quite nicely, all calm — and then it is always — and so he accuses me,)
22 mir vor, er mant, er hätte vor 10 Jahren in Pension gehen können,
(he says he could have retired 10 years ago,)
23 konnte aber nicht gehen, weil ich krank war, also seit 12 Jahren die
(but couldn't because I was ill, as for 12 years I've had)
24 Depressionen hab und i man, des halt er mir immer vor. Er sagt 'Ja, wenn
(depressions and he never lets me forget it. He says 'Yes, if)

25 Du net krank gewesen wärst, da waret i schon in Pension und kriegert
(you hadn't been ill, I would already have retired and would get my)
26 jedes Monat mei' — also — was er halt von der Pension kreigt, net —
(— you know, whatever he gets from his pension insurance — every month.)
27 vielleicht wirkt das gar nicht so, wenn ich das so erzähle, aber in
(Perhaps that doesn't sound much, as I tell it to you, but inside)
28 mir, also — kann gar net reden drüber — so hab i mi aufg'regt, den
(me, — I can't even talk about it — I got so excited that I)
29 Hörer hab i hing'haut, also, und da sagt er 'ja, die Bekannten, die
(threw down the receiver and then he said, 'yes, our friends, the one)
30 ma haben, der is schon 10 Jahr, der is scho 22 Jahr' — sag i — 'erzähl
(has already been retired 10 years, the other 22 years', — and I say 'don't)
31 ma kan Blödsinn, der is — wass i — 68 Jahr and kann net jetzt schon
(talk rubbish, he's only —I don't know — 68 years old and can't have)
32 22 Jahr in Penison — kann nicht sein'. Aber i mein, i hab des schon
(been retired for 22 years'. But I think I have already)
33 abgebaut, in mir ja, so wie Sie das letzte Mal erklärt haben, Ihr Vater
(got rid of that, as you said last time, your father)
34 net — i wass net — i glaub, Sie waren das, ja? Sie sollen so viel
(yes — I don't know — I think it was you? They say you smoke such a lot)
35 rauchen und die Diät, net, also — er immer wieder an mich heran — also,
(and the diet, and so on — he always comes to me, you see)
36 mit, wie er halt mant, also und so; i kann ihn nit amal mehr sehen, obwohl
(and as he says, and so; I can't stand the sight of him any more, although)
37 er net schlecht is, ja — er tut alles für mich, er war immer für mi
(he's not bad, — he does everything for me, he has always been there for me)
38 da und — i hab schon amal g'sagt, i bin net 12 Jahr zum Arzt'gangen und
(— and I said to him once, I haven't been going to the doctor for 12 years and)
39 wenn i eing'stellt wäre, i bringert meinen Vater um, i halt des nimmer
(if I had a job, I'd kill my father, I just can't stand it any more,)
40 aus, das Seelische, i hab so drüber nach'denkt, hab i von ihm — Jahrzehnte
(this mental — I thought about it, he drilled it into me for decades)
41 des eindrillt 'kriegt; 'Zuerst denken, na zuerst schalten — zuerst denken schalten
('First think, then act — first think, then act,)
42 dann sprechen' also, so ha i des immer — wenn i den Mund aufg'macht hab,
(then speak', that's what I always got — whenever I opened my mouth,)
43 hab i immer 'zuerst denken, dann schalten, dann sprechen'. I man, so
(I heard 'first think, then act, then speak'. I mean, I'm)
44 dumm bin i sicher net, aber aber — des is — voriges jahr hab i des
(certainly not so stupid, but, but — that is — last year I was)

45 Glück g'habt, also Gott sei Dank, dass i an die Klinik 'kommen bin, $2\frac{1}{2}$
(lucky, thank heavens, that I came to the clinic, $2\frac{1}{2}$)
46 Monat, und drüber war i dann so selig, und die haben mich g'sund g'macht,
(months, and I was so happy about it then, and they made me healthy,)
47 mit Medikamenten und da hab i 'glaubt, i hab das abgebaut, also es ist weg
(with medicaments and I thought I had got rid of it, that it was gone)
48 von mir und seit — wass i — a paar Monat oder paar Wochen schleichen
(and since a couple of months or a couple of weeks — I don't know how long,)
49 sich langsam diese Depressionen an und jetzt — na, des halt i net durch,
(these depressions have been creeping up, and now — well, I can't stand it,)
50 war beim Herrn Dr . . ., hab — hat er mir a anderes Mittel geben und des
(I went to Dr . . ., and he gave me another medicine and that)
51 is ja eh gut, aber — Man sollte so sagen: Mit dem Menschen, der einen
(was fine, but — perhaps I should put it like this: the person who)
52 immer wieder in das hineintreibt, warum man ja die Depressonen hat, dass
(repeatedly forces you into that, why you have depressions, that)
53 man mit dem nie wieder in Kontakt gehen soll. — Wie kann man denn das, wann
(you don't want to see him again. — How can you do that if)
54 das so a Mensch in der Familie is — na der Vater?
(such a person is a member of your family — your own father?)
55 M: Na, habens durch eahm die Depressionen 'kriegt, oder hat er?
(Was it because of him that you got depressions, or did he?)
56 F: Na ja, 'des kannst net, des wirst nie können, für des bist zu bled', —
(Well, 'you'll never be able to do that, because you're too stupid',—)
57 bin immer schon so gehemmt gewesen, dass i — wann ma so — wass i — mit der
(I've always had such inhibitions, that I — if we — I mean — when we)
58 Firma von meinem Mann fort'gangen san, hab i kein Wort gesprochen,
(went out with my husband's firm, I never said a word)
59 weil i mi net 'traut hab, den Mund aufzumachen, dass ich vielleicht
(because I was afraid to open my mouth, in case I)
60 irgenwas sag, was blöd wär.
(said something stupid.)

4.1 Context of the session

The patient presents her problem shortly after the commencement of the session. One has the feeling that she literally explodes, the problem breaks out, although she has many inhibitions about talking, particularly as the taperecorder was placed within sight for the first time. It is immediately obvious that the presence of the taperecorder is not subsequently a hindrance: she speaks openly and honestly, in a very excited and emotional manner, about her problem. The problem is subsequently discussed almost until the end of the session, and many new aspects become apparent (cf. Wodak 1981a: 123ff.). The interventions come mainly from a young working-class man who described his problem with his father in the previous session and also opened this session with a description of his dreams. The group is very emotionally involved. When the tape was played back with the therapist, the latter explained that he had allowed the problem to be discussed in such detail because many patients had troubled relationships with their parents, and could therefore benefit from the discussion.

4.2 Colloquial level: narrative structure

The limits of quantitative evaluation are reached even in the first category (which is dealt with exclusively here). Although this is certainly a true story, the narration of a telephone call and the resulting conflicts (an 'event' in the narrative past with interspersed direct speech, in the definite personal speaker's perspective), it also includes both scenic moments (lines 41–3) and descriptions of symptoms (32, 45–51). Classification with the aid of Labov and Waletzky's categories is fairly obvious: orientation (1–19), complication (19–32) and scenic element (40–3), evaluation (33–40), coda (resolution incorporating description of symptoms: 45–54).

Orientation: The patient begins with a description of how difficult it is to talk about her problem. She withdraws (10, 11) and continues only after encouragement (12–14), beginning with a part of the conflict: reproaches of her father (16, 17), in the face of which she justifies her actions, and a further assurance that she will not speak for too long. It is particularly interesting to note the change from the impersonal 'one' in the introduction (1, 2, 3, 5, 6), with the personal interjection in 4, to the definite personal speaker's perspective in the remainder of her problem presentation.

Complication: The event (20) of the telephone call is not described coherently, but in brief, chopped sentences, repeatedly interrupted by the scenic description of the conflict in direct speech (reproaches of her father, justifications) and the description of her feelings (28).

Evaluation: Evaluation and self reflection begin with the speech act *ich mein* (32). Initially she addresses the working class patient from whose account she appears to have learnt something. Anger and aggression then come to light, explicitly, with restrictions (37). The primary scene — her memory of the 'drill' — is also interwoven in the narration (41–3).

Resolution: The resolution in this case is very brief, and coincides partly with the evaluation and the coda. It is condensed (between 44 and 46) and changes into evaluative speech acts, disappointments, as in the coda.

Coda: She describes the conclusion of her therapeutic 'career' and again mentions the main problem: namely that it is impossible to avoid one's own father; that a solution to the conflict must be found (51–5), although this is a person who always hurts her. Part of the coda remains a description of the symptoms by the use of the descriptive present. Her explicit addressing of the therapist (50) — a sort of cry for help — is also typical.

There is a striking difference in style between complication on the one hand, and evaluation and coda on the other, from very excited, hurried and emotional speech (socio-phonological style 1: Feldstein *et al.* 1963; Leodolter 1975b: 260) to the assessment, which is relatively consistent in explicit, evaluative speech acts, and to the descriptive coda. This is reminiscent of Labov and Fanshel's description of 'frame shifts' (1977: 35ff.) (cf. *so hab'i mi aufg'regt, den Hörer hab i hing'haut, hab so drüber nach'denkt, hab ich von eahm des eindrillt 'kriegt und 'da hab ich 'glaubt, ich hab das abgebaut, also es ist weg von mir* . . . 'I got so excited, I threw down the receiver, and thought about it, he drilled it into me, and then I thought I had got rid of it, that it had left me . . .').

4.3 The level of the group meaning

Text A has several functions and meanings in the transference within the group. It is not by chance that precisely this problem is verbalized in the session. As mentioned above, the patient continues from the previous session, during which the working-class patient spoke about his relationship with his father. At the same time, she attaches her verbalization to a dream described by the same patient, and addresses him explicity (34, 35), and is supported (12, 14) and interpreted (55) by him. There is therefore identification, solidarity, a brother/sister relationship between them.

The content of the father problem — the problem of authority — is not a matter of chance either. In reality the entire problem presentation should be interpreted as a censure of the therapist's authority, as disappointment that the therapy has not yet helped her to solve her problem.

This is conclusively apparent from the coda (44ff.), particularly in her direct address of the therapist (49, 50). She still suffers from depression, although he has prescribed medicines for her (if she didn't take them, she would kill her father (39)). Her massive feelings of guilt for taking up too much time stem on the one hand from her father's aggression towards her (8, 9, 36, 37, 53, 54), and on the other from her — unconscious — censure of the therapist. For this reason the coda also contains rationalizations (*es wird schon gut gehen* (51), *die Therapie muss ja wirken*) ('it will work out alright', 'the therapy must work'.)

The group gives the patient the opportunity of settling ambivalencies; to begin with, she assumes both roles in the dialogue (those of her internalized father and of herself). These functions are subsequently assumed by members of the group; the conflict with authority is acted out, but not directly against the therapist. The patient's mention of an extremely authoritarian upbringing in a scenic recollection (41, 42, 56), and the frequent repetition of reproaches (16, 17) brings out similar associations in many members of the group. The patient's explicit mention of the precepts opens her to interrogation; only several sessions later does the group discuss the sense of the therapy, certainly initiated in part by the latent disappointment of this patient.

4.4 The individual private linguistic level

This problem presentation in group therapy is the patient's first large outbreak in the group. She has been receiving treatment for some time, partly as an in-patient, and has been calmed by medicaments. The patient's central conflict with her parents comes to light here, the difficulty of breaking away due to her massive feelings of guilt vis-à-vis her parents. (Only her father is mentioned in the current problem presentation. However, it subsequently becomes apparent that her mother has exemplified for her the suffering, self-sacrificing woman's role, and is also involved, and perhaps plays an even more important role — for example, with respect to sex identification.) Important scenes are verbalized, together with the relevant feelings and connotations, and the first steps are taken towards understanding her symptoms. In spite of her inhibitions (58, 60), the patient manages to describe her problem in detail, but she needs help, which she implicitly asks for (11- 15). Addressing other members of the group, particularly males, is typical and quite understandable as a result of her relationship with her father. Only relatively late in the course of the therapy does she also deal with women. In spite of her feelings of guilt and 'attacks on her own person', this outbreak in the group represents a great step forward. For the first time, she admits her aggressions, her fantasies, her recollections of her strict father (not an unusual problem for women, though certainly the experience is always different and individual for each person). There is much that conforms with recent psychoanalytical concepts of women (Windoff-Héritier 1976): the bond with the therapist is very strong, and not only in this text. Her father's drill has driven her to depression; in this context she also shows a strong urge to work; she 'rushes herself', is a perfectionist (all this is subsequently mentioned in the discussion). The scenic recollection, the 'repressed language games', are very clear in this problem presentation. 43 and 56 certainly have quite specific connotations in connection with the patient's father. It is only through assimilation of her past history that she can come to terms with the present, and find a solution to the conflict. I cannot go any further into the patient's life history without endangering her anonymity. The text is self-explanatory!

5 Text B: The problem is solved

Subtext 1

1 F1: Na ja gut. I wass ja, jetzt . . . und i wollt eh mit
(Alright, I know now, . . . and I wanted to make)
2 Herrn Dr . . . an Termin ausmachen. Da red i nur über mein Vater.
(an appointment with Dr . . . Then I only talk about my father.)
3 Jetzt wass i a, was is und was is und wieso, der Grund is und warum er des
(Now I know what's what, and what the reason is, and why he)
4 immer macht, was er da g'macht hat. — Lang hat's ja 'dauert.
(always does that, what he has done. — It's taken a long time, though.)
5 F2: I bewunder Dich eigentlich immer, dass Du immer no bei Deine Eltern
(I always think it's great, actually, that you will work)
6 arbeit'st, also
(with your parents.)

Subtext 2

7 F1: Na ja, na wo soll i hingehn, was anders, weil i ma ja doch irgendwie im
(Well, where should I go, something different, because somehow inside me, I)
8 Innersten do net zutrau, dass i wo acht Stunden den ganzen Tag beschäftigt
(don't really dare, because if I were employed for eight hours, the whole day,)
9 bin, ununterbrochen steh und und doch, net, i man, halb tags täglich
(and had to stand the whole time, and, well, I mean, half days)

10 sicher, aber den ganzen Tag is ja doch, dass i wass, ich a Stund, dass i nix
(of course, but the whole day is rather, I know, an hour during which I)
11 tu oder so. Aber dafür hol i des dann wieder auf, dass i oft halt ka
(don't do anything. But I make up for it later, as I often don't have)
12 Pause hab oder oft halt — so halt; aber aber wohin gehen und — sag ma — dort ar —
(a break, or often — that's it; but going somewhere and — say — working)
13 beiten, des wass i net, ob i — aber um des gehts ja jetzt gar net. I
(there, I'm not sure whether I — but that's not the problem. I)
14 wass, warum mei Vater immer so war.
(know why my father was always like that.)
15 M1: Du, entschuldigen, i weiss net, ob's Dir so unangenehm is, aber mich würd
(I'm sorry, I don't know whether it's so unpleasant for you, but I would)
16 des aus dem Grund interessieren, weil ja so ähnlich die Lage is viel-
(like to know about it, because my situation may be simi-)
17 leicht bei mir und wen Du auf was draufkommst, hätt i a gern g'wusst, was
(lar and if you realise something, I'd also like to know what)
18 Du da machst.
(you do then.)
19 F1: Auf was i drauf'kommen bin?
(What I realized?)
20 M1: Ja.
(Yes.)

Subtext 3

21 F1: Auf eh ganz was Harmloses. Also mei Vater is furchtbar eifersüchtig auf
(Something quite harmless. You see, my father is terribly jealous)
22 mi, und dass er halt nur in der Werkstatt is und sunst nix tut und i ei-
(of me, as he's only in the workshop and doesn't do anything else and I)
23 gentlich mit der Mutter eigentlich alles mach, net, das G'schäft und des
(and mother actually do everything, you see, the business and every-)
24 alles, net. Des is halt a, is halt a Pech, wann der Chef nimmermehr halt
(thing, you know. That's bad luck, when the boss is no longer)
25 so kann. I man, i sehs ja ein. Er is 70, er hat halt in seinen früheren
(able to do everything. I mean, I accept it. He is 70, he produced his achieve-)
26 Jahren des geleistet, und jetzt gehts halt nimmer, net und wann er in die
(ments when he was young, and now he can't manage any more, and when he)
27 Werkstatt kommt, sagt er, 'da, scho wieder 1,500,— S Reparatur,
(comes into the workshop, he says 'there now, another repair for S 1,500,)
28 scho wieder 3,000,—', und wann das zählst, sans drei Reparaturen um 90,— S
(another S 3,000', and if you count it up, that makes three repairs for S 90)

29 net, und sagen tut er 1,500,— net. Na, da redst halt nix und, weil er
(you know, and he says S 1,500. Well, you don't say anything and because he)
30 hat die Kunden . . . und so. Die Mutti erzählt immer
(has got the customers . . . and so on. Mother always tells me)
31 'na Jessasna', s'is ihr scho zuviel und des tuts and des machts and jetzt, san
('my word', it's too much for her and this and that and now)
32 da, seit Tagen hat er so einen Zorn und eine Wut und eine Aggression auf
(for days he has been so angry and so cross and so aggressive towards)
33 mich g'habt und die hat er mir dann halt vorigen Freitag wieder spüren
(me and he let me feel that again last Friday,)
34 lassen, net; aber es is, Gott sei Dank, nimmermehr so tief gegangen, dass i
(you see; but, thank heavens it wasn't so bad that I)
35 im Betrieb umg'fallen bin, net. I war nur a bissl halt, war i unsicher,
(collapsed at work, you see. I was just a bit, I was unsteady,)
36 hab i ma 'denkt, 'Jesas-Maria, wenn i jetzt wieder tiefer g'falln bin, wie
(and I thought 'My God, if I fall so low again, how will I ever)
37 komm i da wieder auf', net. Aber i bin — nach drei Tag wars wieder vorbei
(get up again', you see. But I did — three days later it was all over)
38 und vergessen, net. Und er hat auf d'Nacht scho wieder g'lacht und hat
(and forgotten, you see. And that night he laughed again and said)
39 g'sagt, 'schau, weh tuts ja mir, weil i schrei mit Dir und i reg mi auf,
('Look, it hurts me, because I shout at you and get excited,)
40 Dir tut ja des gar net so weh, i leid ja und net Du'. (laughs) Also müsste
(it doesn't hurt you so much, I suffer, not you'. So)
41 ich
(I'd have to)
42 M2: I glaub, beide leiden bei so an Streit.
(I think both parties suffer in such a quarrel!)
43 F1: Ja, des is ma ja eh jetzt scho egal.
(Yes, well it's all the same to me now.)
44 M1: Es is angenehm, wenn ma's weiss, net, die Zusammenhänge.
(But it's nice if you know the relationships.)
45 F1: Na ja sicher, wenn ma einmal weiss.
(Yes, of course, once you know.)

5.1 Context of the session

This session focuses on the job problem. Several patients describe their difficulties in detail, in particular a male middle-class patient, a civil servant. Even the therapist intervenes, pointing out how the latter always goes round in circles. All the other patients in the group are bored, we notice that our female middle-class patient — (this session was recorded exactly a year later) — wants to say something. She begins by addressing the therapist directly initially, and announces that she has actually discovered the solution to a problem.

5.2 Selection of the text

A problematical text has deliberately been chosen here: it actually consists of three problem presentations (by formal definition) that together make up one problem presentation, in view of the fact that subtexts 1 and 2 can be regarded as introductions to subtext 3, which contains both an account and a problem solution. This is the knowledge acquired by the patient, which has enabled her to see things in their proper perspective. This type of immanently coherent problem presentation in group therapy must be regarded as something of an exception, and was selected for interpretation with this in mind. Most problem presentations in group therapy — as the many published examples show (Wodak 1981a) — are complete, even if the problem continues to be dealt with after verbalization.

The limits of quantification are thus particularly clear in this instance. Three problem presentations have to be classified from the necessarily restrictive definition of the contribution to the discussion (determined by change of speaker), although intrinsically and thematically the texts belong together. It is thus very difficult to assign them to categories, because all three types of text occur. Subtexts 1 and 2 are descriptions of circumstances; in subtext 3 an 'event' with scenic elements is interwoven in the problem solution. However, in text 3 in particular, the value of the story is of secondary importance.

Subtext 1 (1–6) can be assigned to the category of 'circumstance', although it contains a definite speaker's perspective, an active genus and factual mode, which point rather to 'scene' and 'narration'.

Subtext 2 (7–20) in this instance can definitely be assigned to the category of 'circumstance'. The description of everyday life at work is passive. However, it must be regarded as a strategy of justification, as an answer to the implicit reproach in 5, 6. (The fact that every typology involves abstraction and idealization is discussed in Wodak 1981a: 144.)

As far as interpretation is concerned, subtext 3 is a 'parable': a little story illustrates the nature of the problem solution, representing this and the newly acquired strategies for coping with the conflict.

It must therefore be assumed that this is a mixed type (with regard to narrative structure). Circumstance (problem solution) and narration are interwoven and occur simultaneously (Wodak 1981d).

The success of the therapy is thus manifest not only in the content of the successful problem solution, but also in the form, in a new type of text which contains elements of all three basic types: circumstantial, scenic and narrative elements occur without special priority being given to any one component, *a mixed type*.

In the context of the session and group dynamics, subtexts 1 and 2 pave the way for subtext 3 (and can be interpreted as strategies for awakening curiosity). Subtext 3 is therefore mainly used in the qualitative analysis, as an example of the *effect of therapy* on the *form of problem presentation in group therapy*.

5.3 Colloquial level: narrative structure

The problematics of this classification have already been mentioned: firstly, subtext 2 contains an introduction to a circumstantial description, which is abruptly interrupted in 13. Secondly, the core of the problem presentation is the problem solution (21–31), with a narration inserted by way of illustration. The text was classified as a 'mixed type' mainly for psychoanalytical reasons, after a playback with the therapist. The patient is naturally very concerned about the renewed conflict with her father, but she is now in a position to relate it differently, against the background of a problem solution.

Psychoanalytically, the question remains as to whether the suggested problem solution can be considered as a rationalization, as a purely intellectual solution of the problem. This interpretation is strengthened by the patient's subsequent reluctance to admit that she suffers in the conflict, though she certainly must. On the other hand, the validity of the problem solution is strongly supported by other factors, by the patient's distance — both verbally and emotionally — and by her quite different and new manner of coping with the conflict. An interpretation as rationalization is also refuted by the strong emotional involvement. As is so often the case in therapeutic communication, various motives and interpretations can be applied, many of them conflicting.

Introduction: The Introduction is very long (1–4, 7–14, 21). The patient begins twice, mainly because intervention 5 forces her briefly into a circumstantial description, which is also related in another linguistic style. Conflict and ambivalence can be felt here (short, incomplete sentences, pauses, hesitations, expletives). She announces her knowlege of her problem, makes the group curious as she says that she only wants to tell the therapist about her insight. Text 2 is thus a renewed description of everyday life at work, presented as a justification of the internalized (and not explicitly verbalized) reproach of her father that she does not work enough. However, it follows the intervention, which she obviously misinterprets (perceiving it as reproach instead of praise). Only the intervention (15–18) induces the patient to describe her solution.

Problem solution: 21–32 must be classified as an evaluation, a metacommunicative, reflexive speech act (strategies for problem solution are metacommunicative acts:) see Figure 1.3. The patient interprets the conflict and sets the frame in which the 'event', the complication, must be seen. It is this consistent, calmly presented evaluation in particular that indicates the speaker's new perspective. The linguistic style is significantly different from that used in subtext 2 and text A. She outlines her father, and has seen through him.

Narration: The actual incident only comes to light in 32–7, an incident (she almost collapsed) which is dealt with very briefly. The speaker merely mentions the incident in a subordinate clause (35, *daß i im Betrieb umg'fallen bin)*. The speaker relates feelings and reactions, and how she copes with the conflict (35–7): this is again evaluative. Although the incident was certainly subjectively terrible, her language is also consistent here (there is a definite personal speaker's perspective — she is excited — but significantly different from that in text A).

Resolution: The summary of the problem presentation is partly narrative, partly evaluative and reflective. She describes her strategy for coping with the conflict, and at the same time assesses her condition, expressing pleasure at her successful strategy. A scenic moment is also woven in, as a sort of conclusion (39–41). This is her father's realization (and her own) that he is actually the one who suffers most from this conflict.

5.4 The level of the group meaning

This problem presentation is extremely interesting with regard to group dynamics. The patient wishes to describe her success to the group, and to be praised (the kind of expectations that are otherwise directed at the family). At the same time, she wants to make the group particularly curious, and even jealous, by initially addressing the therapist directly (2). She has 'made it', while the others have not. The group immediately takes its revenge in intervention 5: the hidden problem which the patient did not want to mention at all comes to light. The group reproaches her with not always having solved her job problem — so she need not think she is any better, or possibly loved. One can feel the terrible dread that somebody could be better off than oneself, could be more advanced in the therapy. The competition, even for the therapist (the female patient who intervenes is very dependent on the therapist (7–13)) can therefore be regarded as a justification, laden with feelings of guilt even vis-à-vis the group. Intervention 15 shows interest, helps the patient to drop the unpleasant subject, showing solidarity and a willingness to learn. This patient in particular is very pleased to have his problem dealt with by others, so that he can act as a listener and interpreter, a role which he also assumes here. Praise for the account is not immediately forthcoming, whereupon the patient withdraws, disappointed. She has not received what she wanted: the group has not behaved in the way in which she unrealistically expected it to. Nobody likes to see success. It is obvious that the mechanisms in the group are similar to those in everyday life. The patient subsequently assimilates her disappointment, and in doing so acquires a slightly more realistic viewpoint.

5.5 The individual private linguistic level

For the first time the patient is able to feel pleasure, to feel pleased at her success. The terrible ambivalence and conflict situation have been cleared up; she can now see things in perspective and is better able to cope with any conflicts that may occur. She also dares to admit her pleasure publicly, something which she was previously unable to do, in keeping with her socially imposed, suffering female role. The fact that she is still instable is shown by her rapid retreat after intervention 5, her regressive tendencies (30, 31) and her great disappointment (43) when praise is not forthcoming. She can now tackle other problems, above all her job problem and her relationship with her mother, on the basis of her new perspective, her first resolution of a conflict. The entire narrative mode has changed (as shown by the linguistic indicators): she describes the strategy used to solve her problem self-confidently and coherently. There is also a far higher degree of explicit, verbalized self-reflection. She is no longer torn between different evaluations: she has found her own standard, establishes her own evaluative frame, puts forward arguments and explanations. The difference from text A is obvious, providing evidence of the effect of the therapy, which is linguistically apparent ('mixed type'). This patient can by no means be regarded as cured, but her progress is unmistakable, her renewed pleasure in life which is finally expressed in this 'joyous outcry':

> Man freut sich so, dass man es schon geschafft hat, dass man, dass man sieht, dass man glücklich ist, und ich muss sagen, mein Gott, der schöne, also der Tag ist schön und — entschuldigen, dass i

des no g'schwind dazu sag, — i hab so ein' herrlichen Blick vom Wohnzimmer, i siech im Wald rauf and jetzt — und wie i grad so glücklich war und mei Vater sagt drauf — 'nichts zu arbeiten' —. Also momentan hab i ma — hab i des gar net so mit'kriegt, weil i so in die Gegend 'schaut hab. Mein Mann hat mi sofort ang'schaut, 'bitte sag nix, bitte, sonst is wieder was' — Aber in mir drinnen, des hab i wieder notwendig g'habt, so Sachen; das Leben, wie schön, das Leben ist lebenswert!

('You're so glad you've made it, that you, that you realize how happy you are, and I have to say, my God, the beautiful, well, the day is beautiful and — excuse me if I just say this quickly — I have such a wonderful view from my living room, I look out into the woods and now — when I was just feeling so happy and my father says — 'nothing to do' —. Well, just for a moment I — I didn't quite realize what he had said, I was so intent on the view. My husband immediately looked at me, 'Please don't say anything, please, otherwise there'll be trouble again' — But inside me, I really needed that, such things; life is wonderful, life is worth living!')

6 Final remarks

Although a single qualitative text analysis can only succeed in illustrating the hypotheses, I believe this proves the sense of applying linguistic indicators to an investigation of the therapeutic effect. This positive impression was strengthened and further evidenced by case studies and interviews carried out in the course of the overall investigation (Wodak 1981a: 263; 1981d).

This is not a 'superficial' change (a new type of text being introduced, as it were), but a lasting, far-reaching alteration of personality. To this extent it can be said that the occurrence of the 'mixed type', coupled with changes at the emotional and cognitive level, can be regarded as an indicator of the positive effect of therapy. Institutions that carry out basic research and psychiatric practice should not overlook the relevance of such investigations.

Notes to Chapter 1

1 The approaches presented here are dealt with in detail in Wodak 1981a; Wodak & Schulz 1986. In particular, this work refers to generative-transformational theories and methods and research in the USSR.

2 The overall investigation is dealt with in detail in Wodak 1981a; Wodak & Schulz 1986. Here too, I should like to express my thanks to the team of the crisis intervention centre, who made it possible for me to carry out this project.
3 Quantitative and qualitative analysis of the material showed that members of the working class can cope very well with the therapeutic situation in a group, and that a lot can be done to help them. This contradicts prevalent prejudices and opens up new perspectives for psychiatric practice (e.g. Wodak 1981c).
4 Analysis of sex-specific speech behaviour showed significant differences in speaker strategies between men and women, which also correlated with the factor of 'class'. To this extent I am of the opinion that both variables (class and sex) should always be considered, as they are strongly linked. See Wodak 1981b on the theory of 'balancing identity' and individual results.
5 We can postulate a 'socio-psychological theory of text planning' on the basis of our results. In other words, depending on the class and sex of the speaker, another text type will normally be selected to deal with the same topic in problem presentation in group therapy. One must therefore assume a principal text sort (class) (frame) from which the individual 'schemes' can be derived (see also Freedle 1977; 1979; Kintsch and van Dijk 1978; Wodak 1981a; 1983; 1984).
6 Forecasts were produced with the aid of Goodman's log-linear model. We predicted the probability with which a patient of a certain class and sex, at a specific phase in the therapy, and with a given topic would select a certain text type (Wodak 1981a: 234ff.). Here too, weightings were produced between individual variables such as topic, class, sex, defence mechanisms and expression of feelings.
7 See Wodak 1981a: 108 on the 'Quasi-orthographic' transliteration of Viennese dialect. The English translation of these texts is a standard translation which makes no attempt to reproduce the Viennese dialect.

References

Beaugrande R. de and Dressler, W. 1981: *Introduction to Linguistics*. London: Longman.

Bion, W. R. 1961: *Experiences in Groups*. London: Tavistock.

Brekle, H. E. 1972: *Semantik*. Munich: UTB.

Bühler, K. 1934: *Sprachtheorie: Die Darstellungsfunktion der Sprache*. Jena: Gustav Fischer.

Cavell, S. 1976: *Must We Mean What We Say?* Cambridge: Cambridge University Press.

Ehlich, K and Switalla, B. 1976: Transkriptionssysteme — eine exemplarische Übersicht. *Studium Linguistik* 2.

Feldstein, S., Brenner, M. and Jaffe, J. 1963: The effect of subject, sex, verbal interaction and topical focus on speech disruption. *Language and Speech* 6.

Finger, U. D. 1976: *Sprachzerstörung in Gruppen*. Frankfurt/Main: Suhrkamp.

Flader, D. 1979: Techniken der Verhaltenssteuerung im psychoanalytischen Diskurs. In D. Flader and R. Wodak-Leodolter (eds), *Therapeutische Kommunikation*.

Flader, D. and Wodak-Leodolter, R. (eds.) 1979: *Therapeutische Kommunikation*. Königstein/Ts: Scriptor.

Frankenberg, H. 1979: Gestörte Kommunikation als Reproduktion einer Beziehungsstörung in der Ehetherapie. In D. Flader and R. Wodak-Leodolter (eds), *Therapeutische Kommunikation*.
Freedle, R. (ed.) 1977: *Discourse Production and Comprehension*. Norwood, NJ: Ablex.
— (ed.) 1979: *New Directions in Discourse Processing*. Norwood, NJ: Ablex.
Goeppert, H. and Goeppert, S. 1973: *Sprache und Psychoanalyse*. Hamburg: Fischer.
— 1975: *Redeverhalten und Neurose*. Hamburg: Fischer.
Goffman, E. 1959: *The Presentation of Self in Everyday Life*. New York: Harcourt.
Green, H. 1974: *Ich habe dir nie einen Rosengarten versprochen*. Stuttgart: Klett.
Grewendorf, G. (ed.) 1979: *Sprechakttheorie und Semantik*. Frankfurt/Main: Suhrkamp.
Grumiller, I. 1975: Therapeutische Gruppenkonzepte. In H. Strotzka (ed.), *Psychotherapie: Gundlagen, verfahren, Indikationen*.
Gumperz, J. J. and Herasimchuk, E. 1972: *The Conversational Analysis of Social Meaning: A Study in Class-Room Interaction*. Unpublished MS.
Gunderson, K. (ed.) 1975: *Language, Mind and Knowledge*, vol. 7. Minneapolis.
Habermas, J. 1969: *Systematisch verzerrte Kommunikation*. Unpublished MS.
— 1977: *Erkenntnis und Interesse*. Frankfurt/Main: Suhrkamp.
Halliday, M. A. K. 1976: System and function. In G. Kress (ed.), *Halliday: System and Function in Language.*.
Helm, J. (ed.) 1967: *Essays on the Verbal and Visual Arts*. Oxford: Pergamon.
Kallmeyer, W. *et al.* 1974: *Lektürekolleg zur Textlinguistik*, vol. 1. Frankfurt/Main: Athenäum.
Katz, J. J. 1970: *Philosophie der Sprache*. Frankfurt/Main: Suhrkamp.
Kintsch, W. and van Dijk, T. 1978: Toward a model of text comprehension and production. *Psychological Review* 85.
Klann, G. 1979: Die Rolle affektiver Prozesse in der Dialogstrukturierung. In D. Flader and R. Wodak-Leodolter (eds), *Therapeutische Kommunikation*.
Kress, G. (ed.) 1976: *Halliday: System and Function in Language*. Oxford: Oxford University Press.
Kutter, P. 1971: Übertragung und Prozeß in der psychoanalytischen Gruppentherapie. *Psyche* 1.
Labov, W. and Fanshel, D. 1977: *Therapeutic Discourse*. New York: Academic Press.
Labov, W. and Waletzky, J. 1967: Narrative analysis: oral versions of personal experience. In J. Helm (ed.), *Essays on the Verbal and Visual Arts*.
Leodolter, R. (Wodak) 1975a: Gestörte Sprache oder Privatsprache: Kommunikation bei Schizophrenen. *Wiener Linguistische Gazette* 10/11.
— 1975b: *Das Sprachverhalten von Angeklagten bei Gericht*. Kronberg/Ts: Scriptor.
Lorenzer, A. 1973: *Sprachzerstörung und Rekonstruktion*. Frankfurt/Main: Suhrkamp.
Mel'čuk, I. A. 1974: *Opyt Teorii Lingvestičeskich Modelej 'Smysltekst'*. Moscow: Akademičeskij.
— (ed.) 1976: *Das Wort: Zwischen Inhalt und Ausdruck*. Munich: Fink.
Morris, C. 1938: *Foundations of a Theory of Signs*. Chicago: Chicago University Press.
Ogden, C. K. and Richards, I. A. 1972: *The Meaning of Meaning*. Cambridge:

Cambridge University Press.
Schifko, P. 1975: *Bedeutungstheorie: Einführung in die linguistische Semantik*. Stuttgart: Klett.
Schröter, K. 1979: Einige formale Aspekte des Psychoanalytischen Dialogs. In D. Flader and R. Wodak-Leodolter (eds), *Therapeutische Kommunikation*.
Schütz, A. 1960: *Der sinnhafte Aufbau der sozialen Welt*. Vienna: Herder.
Searle, J. 1971: *Sprechakte*. Frankfurt/Main: Suhrkamp.
— 1975: A taxonomy of illocutionary acts. In K. Gunderson (ed.), *Language, Mind and Knowledge*, Vol. 7.
Slater, P. E. 1978: *Mikrokosmos: Eine Studie über Gruppendynamik*. Frankfurt/Main: Suhrkamp.
Strotzka, H. (ed.) 1975: *Psychotherapie: Grundlagen, Verfahren, Indikationen*. Munich: Urban & Schwarzenberg.
Trömel-Plötz, S. 1979: 'She is just not an open person': Linguistische Analyse einer restrukturierenden Intervention in der Familientherapie. In D. Flader and R. Wodak-Leodolter (eds), *Therapeutische Kommunikation*.
Werlich, E. 1975: *Typologie der Texte*. Heidelberg: UTB.
Windhoff-Héritier, A. 1976: *Sind Frauen so, wie Freud sie sah?* Hamburg: Fischer.
Wittgenstein, L. 1967: *Philosophische Untersuchungen*. Frankfurt/Main: Suhrkamp.
Wodak, R. 1981a: *Das Wort in der Gruppe: Linguistische Studien zur therapeutischen Kommunikation*. Vienna: Verlag der Akademie der Wissenschaft. Translated as *Language Behavior in Therapy Groups*. Los Angeles: University of California Press, 1986.
— 1981b: Women relate, men report: sex differences in language behavior in a therapeutic group. *Journal of Pragmatics* 5.
— 1981c: *Speech, power and psychotherapy: can members of the working class speak?* Unpublished MS.
— 1981d: How do I put my problem? *Text* 1.
— 1983: Arguments in favour of a socio-psychological theory of text planning. *Klagenfurter Beiträge zur Sprachwissenschaft* 9.
— 1984: *Hillflose Nähe? — Mütter und Töchter erzählen*. Vienna: Bundesverlag.
Wodak, R. and Schulz, Muriel, 1986: *The Language of Love and Guilt*. Amsterdam: Benjamins.
Wunderlich, D. 1979: Was ist das für ein Sprechakt? In G. Grewendorf (ed.), *Sprechakttheorie und Semantik*.

2 Intervention in psychotherapy:

A qualitative analysis of persuasive therapy*

Peter Nowak

Theoretical background

This analysis is based (as was my main investigation, Nowak 1984), in many respects on Wodak's papers published on conversational behaviour in a therapy group. A central point is the application of a 'three-level model' when describing the complexity of the meaning of a given therapeutic communication situation. The three levels do not represent different languages which are used simultaneously but different approaches to the complex meaning of a text (Wodak 1981).

In accordance with this 'multi-level model' I have developed four different groups of categories in order to do justice to the special situation of persuasive one-person therapy. Persuasive therapy works first and foremost with the latent meaning of interventions, which cannot be grasped on the level of a 'one-dimensional meaning model'. It is exactly this therapeutically effective type of communication which has been given special attention in this investigation. The analysis aims to show that a qualitative linguistic 'multi-level model' can accurately grasp the appearance of a client's resistance,[1] even though it may not be directly expressed on a manifest linguistic level. Beyond this, the real handling of this common phenomenon in psychotherapy (Langs 1981) with persuasive means, and their latent effects, should be accurately grasped. In this chapter I will describe these analysis steps, which I will then elaborate with the help of two text sections. I will also present the theoretical framework of these analysis steps.

* I would like to thank Professor Becker and Professor Wodak for their help and comments.

The first level is the manifest colloquial level of the interventions by the therapist. In my main investigation (Nowak 1984) — a comparison of psychoanalytic, client-centred and persuasive intervention behaviour — I developed a group of categories in order to grasp the function of intervention in the different forms of therapy, with their manifest differences. The seven categories summarize 'speaker strategies', which are to be understood as superimposed, functional units, which can be expressed not only as single speech acts, but also through other types of texts (for example, short narratives). With these categories as the starting point, the manifest linguistic means of persuasion are represented in this analysis step. I will, at this point, give a brief introduction to these seven categories and give examples from the texts. The transliteration system used is summarized in the appendix to this chapter.

Supportive intervention (Nowak 1984: 19ff.) All speech acts which show the client that he has protection, assistance and support, and all forms of intervention which are made to help raise a client's self-esteem (praise, 'mitigation'[2]: Labov and Fanshel 1977) are contained in this category. Since there is no example in the texts of a purely supportive form of intervention, I have decided to use an example which took place just a few seconds before text 2. It is very typical of the therapist's praise.

T: You dealt flexibly, didn't you. You arranged it well —
and you'll go on doing it that way yes, actually
C: oh yes
T: I'm pleased about that, are you satisfied with yourself?

Understanding intervention (Nowak 1984: 23ff.) The therapist remarks that he understands the client. Of course, every good therapeutic intervention is an expression of the therapist's ability to understand. But in this case we find a special group of intervention forms, which only fulfil this function, and which are often characteristic of client-centred therapy.

C: and this I understand, but you know when the
T: yes but when you are in the
C: going gets rough
T: situation it's still difficult to act like that.

The therapist can either (as shown here) complete what the client has started to say, or paraphrase his remarks, or simply use an understanding listener's signal.

Advisory intervention The predominance of this group of speaker strategies is characteristic for this type of persuasive therapy (Nowak 1984: 25ff.). In particular, it consists of advising, explaining, giving the reason for things, and giving instructions for a client's action. All of these are applied in a persuasive manner:

T: he is — you know why — you've changed so — you have new ideas new goals new methods — you won't let yourself get up tight anymore
C: yes, yes, oh, yes — well, I don't know
T: you will maintain your calm manner — which also makes your work very precise — so you are more or less free from outside disturbance — which is very advantageous — it proved itself in the first week and it will continue to do so in the weeks to come until finally you have a new feeling about your job — that's our goal — that your job becomes something for you where you say — today is another work-day — and I'll show them what I can do.

Clarifying intervention This group consists of all questions and clarifications — that is to say, attempts made by the therapist to ensure that he has correctly understood the client.

T: We have already uhm, uhm, reduced your consumption, right?

Interpretative intervention The interpretation, which is especially important in psychoanalysis represents a contextual hypothesis in which different remarks made by the client are newly related. Since interpretative forms of intervention are very rare in this persuasive therapy, I have decided not to give any examples.

Confrontational intervention The therapist proceeds to refer to clarified material in such a manner that contradictions or unnoticed aspects can no longer be ignored by the client. In this manner the client is provoked into reacting. There is no example of this during the therapy session, since confrontation does not usually play a part in persuasive therapy (Nowak 1984).

Rejective intervention Openly rejective intervention, as given in the following example, is rare. It is more common to find a rejective attitude which is expressed only at an implicit level:

T: but soon we won't need it any more but I
C: well, I don't know
T: know.

In summary, it should be emphasized that the therapist is not totally aware of his use of these linguistic means of persuasion (as I will discuss), but is led by several basic rules to intervene intuitively (Nowak 1984: 103ff.). Several of the linguistic characteristics of the texts and their latent meanings, were not apparent to the therapist until he listened to the playback.

The second analysis step is the latent level of intentions, which the therapist pursues by using the linguistic means described above. Persuasive therapy is built upon the fact that the real intentions of the therapist are not known to the client. The client's rational ego should be avoided so that the therapy is not hindered by its limited imagination and habits (Becker in press; Rossi *et al.* 1978). This latent level of intentions was analysed together with the therapist, using the playback methods as applied by Labov and Fanshel (1977) in their qualitative analysis. I would like to give an example here:

T: still keep on 'snacking' on Umbrium — if you so desire.

Before this intervention, the therapist and the client were talking about the fact that the client takes medicine which gives the client short-term relief from his sufferings without much effort. In the playback, the therapist explains that the client should slowly start reducing his dependence on the drug. On the manifest level the therapist seems to be permitting the use of the drug, but suggests through several words with implicit meaning that the client should put an end to it soon. *Snacking* implies that one likes to do it, but it is frowned upon or does not occur often; *still* implies that there will soon be an end to the snacking; and *desire* also has the connotation of being sinful, and thus of some habit which should be brought to an end. The latent intention, which is expressed here through subtle linguistic means, is really: 'Stop taking those pills!'

The next analysis step illustrates the interactive dimension on the manifest level. The reactions of the client are categorized and subjected to detailed analysis. I have taken the categories in their entirety, with two modified points, from Wodak 1981: 182ff. The modifications (new aspects, agreement) result from the change in the communication situation (persuasive one-person therapy) in comparison with Wodak's investigation. The modifications were established individually in the descriptions of the categories. The classification is based on Wunderlich's (1976: 179ff.) division of speech acts, and on Labov and Fanshel's (1977: 59ff.) taxonomy of 'actions' in the therapeutic situation, which are realized by 'speech acts' (Wodak 1981: 243). The seven categories I use are briefly defined and demonstrated below, with examples from the text.

Rejection The client explicitly rejects advice or support without further comment:

C: Well, Dr Becker, I'm not really up to it at the moment, uhm, I need the Umbrium, you know.

Counter-question The client does not respond to the content of the intervention, but withdraws to the metacommunicative level (Wodak 1981: 183). There is no example of this type of reaction in the text, which is due in particular to the differences in setting (Nowak 1984: 60).

Repetition The client repeats his problem, as if no intervention had preceded it. This reaction is due to resistance to the therapy:

C: Yes, Dr Becker, but you know-well fear most often stems from irregular brain waves.

New aspects Wodak (1981: 183) sees this reaction only from the point of view of a breakdown in resistance and progress in the therapy. But it must first be determined on a latent level of meaning if, in a given case, one can speak of resistance or progress.

C: Because, Dr Becker, I think that my brain lacks some chemical . . .

Conflict 'The patient rejects the intervention and begins a conflict with the intervening person' (Wodak 1981: 183). This also seems to be a very rare reaction in persuasive therapy, since one of this therapy's goals is to avoid direct conflict (Rossi *et al.* 1978). There is no obvious example in the text, so I will not give one here.

Insight 'The patient accepts the interpretation and begins to work with it. The next step is usually explicit acceptance' (Wodak 1981: 183).

T: the will is there but the body is weak that's what the
C: yes yes,
T: Bible says
C: exactly, exactly (*laughs*) — exactly — so I am not the first.

Agreement I developed this category in order to distinguish between real insight and agreement, which is often formally given in my material and then followed immediately by an expression of resistance (Langs 1981). To what extent agreement is an expression of resistance or real consensus can, once again, only be determined by studying the latent level of meaning.

C: Well, because I think, as you say, you know that I tell him you'll get what you're waiting for — as soon as I've finished, that's it and until I've realized that, all that, and
T: yes, yes
C: this I understand, but you know . . .

In the last analysis step the latent level of meaning of the client's remarks are illustrated. In the playback method with the therapist, the latent effects of the intervention on the client were analysed in particular. Special attention was given to the points where the degree of resistance and emotional expression could be registered.

The text analysis

Form of therapy, setting and session context

Motivated by the works of Erickson (Haley 1967; Rossi *et al.* 1978), Becker (in press) developed his own type of persuasive therapy. Erickson tries, within the framework of his 'hypno-therapy', in particular to block out the client's conscious rational ego in order to have direct contact with the client's unconscious. This type of treatment is based on the theoretical assumption that the client's conscious ego limits his great unconscious possibilities through fixed ideas and habits, inhibitions, anxiety and many other things. The client's difficulties stem from these limitations. When the client's conscious ego is blocked out, the therapist should be able to guide the client's unconscious in such a manner that these difficulties disappear. I have discussed the problems of such treatment in detail in my main investigation (Nowak 1984) and they will be briefly mentioned here after the analysis.

Becker's persuasive therapy does not work with a deeper hypnotic state, instead he switches back and forth between light persuasive exercises (similar to autogenic training) and persuasive conversation sequences which have a setting similar to a normal psychotherapy session (the therapist and the client sit facing each other). The goal of the therapy is the short-term relief of symptoms ('medicine without side-effects' Becker) and not modification of the entire personality.

The two text sections I have chosen are from the penultimate therapy session[3] with a man aged about fifty, who suffered from severe anxiety as soon as he had to walk longer distances by himself. Because of this anxiety he was forced to stay home from work on sick leave. The declared goal was to have the client ready (within an eight-week period) to make a new, successful attempt at working because he would otherwise have to retire prematurely, and would no longer be able to provide for his children. After the first few hours, the symptom was really reduced so much that he was able to work for a week.

The session itself is dominated by the client's resistance and the therapist's persevering efforts to deal with this resistance. The main point of the resistance are the psychotropic drugs which the client is taking, in addition to undergoing psychotherapy. The therapist tries to convince him to reduce his pill consumption and to have more faith in his own abilities to deal with the situation. The resistance, as we will see, not only stem from the client's own problems, but also from a real conversation the client had with another doctor who made negative statements about psychotherapy (text 3). Text 1 took place just after the session began. After the client has talked about many things which he has experienced in his first week at work, the subject of psychotropic drugs comes up for the first time in this session. The conflict between the therapist and the client comes to the fore at this point.

Text 2 is taken from about three-quarters of the way through the session, at a point where the resistance is (at least briefly) replaced by some agreement.

Finally, in text 3 we find the story told by the client about his experience with the other doctor, which really makes the persistent resistance in this session comprehensible. The immediate reason of the resistance becomes apparent only a few minutes before the session is over.

Text 1

C: ah I think when somebody works a little bit slower we'll
see how things work out with him (*bang of a door, a woman's voice*)
how things work out with him you know — I don't know either he's
a nice person to work with or not but I think he is
T: a nice person to work with — you know why — you have become a new
person — you have new ideas new goals new methods — you won't
let yourself get up tight anywhere
C: well yes OK — you know that
T: you will maintain your calm manner — which also makes you
work more precisely — that makes you independent from outside
disturbances — that's very advantageous — it proved itself in the
first week and it will continue to do so in the following weeks —
more and more — until you have a new feeling about your job — that's
our goal — that your job becomes something
for you — where you say — OK today is another work-day —

and I'll show them what I can do
C: you know I was there because of
the medicine I take they dry me out so I went to the throat
specialist and he said I should take something for my nose and
T: yes
C: gargle little you know he told me to ask the other
T: yes yes yes
C: doctor if there isn't something else I could take but I'm not
going to take anything else because they make me feel better
T: yes
yes but we've already reduced your consumption you know
C: well you
know
Doctor Becker I'm not really up to it at the moment I need the
Umbrium you know
T: is well then let's just leave the situation with the
Umbrium at this point but you but you have little ah with ah those
C: in the morning I take a double dose
T: Saroten — with Tryptizol we reduced your con-
C: well the Tryptizol you know well I think
T: sumption
C: I still need it in the morning and at noon but when I go home I
don't really need it anymore yes yes yes well
T: that's we decided on — that's good
C: but you know the Umbrium I would like to increase the dose in
T: look if you
C: the morning and at noon
T: if you need the Umbrium — — just go on
snacking on it — yes — but soon we won't need it anymore
C: well I
don't know hm
T: but I know — go on snacking on the Umbrium — if you
desire so — yes — — — yes
C: because you know it takes effect so fast
with this Umbrium and I get (clears his throat) the feeling that
T: yes yes I know yes
C: I never was sick — and if someone asks what is fear
T: I know I know what is fear
— it's no problem for me — but listen we want to get the same
feeling without Umbrium — without crutches — without artificial
limbs for the soul — yes — because that's what they are you know
C: yes
but
Becker most of the fear stems from irregular brain waves
T: yes I know
C: and when I see I'm not going to be able to finish a job
and he's already waiting then before I know it I'm panicking
T: that
could be but doesn't have to be — will become more and more rare
and our goal is — life without Umbrium

64 C: well you know OK I agree
65 with you — I just tell him look you'll get that soon enough when
66 I've finished it OK I can see all that but you know
67 T: yes yes yes yes but
68 when you are in the situation it's still difficult to act like
69 C: when the going gets rough
70 C: well I just tell myself you can't be so fast as the others too well
71 T: that nó can't and I don't want to
72 and I surrender we won't bother
73 C: my ambition plays a role here too
74 T: with that we'll put them in a bottle and throw them out to sea
75 C: (*laughs*) no Dr Becker
76 you know it's so much easier said than done but …

The interventions of the therapist

The first intervention of the therapist (5–16) has already been given as an example of advising intervention. This is a case of typical 'recitation', as Becker calls it. Special notice should be given to the rhythmic setting of pauses which are usually underlined by a slight up-and-down movement of the right hand and synchronic nods. This rhythmic quality is intensified by suitable rhythmic emphasis through which one particularly gets the impression that it is a recitation. Repeated use of subordinate clauses and complicated sentence structure are also important in persuasive therapy.

Similar parts of sentences which are linked are a typical characteristic of these 'recitations' ('new ideas, new goals, new methods' (6)) which, as here, often consist of three parts. The same holds true for the sentence structure in 11–13, which also exemplifies the use of a description of a better future and in which similar parts of the sentence produce the impression that things will improve (more and more, 13). An interesting characteristic of indirect persuasion can be found in the use of the future tense (6, 9, 12). It remains unclear whether the therapist is using it as an imperative, or whether it is purely a description of a future situation. It is only clear that things will be as the therapist has predicted.

We should not forget the beginning of this intervention, in which the therapist repeats the positive remarks made by the client ('a nice person to work with' (5)). This repetition of the client's words is often used in persuasive therapy.

Even though rhythmic emphasis is only based in 'recitation', emphasis in itself can be used to stress important words (9, 46, 71).

The meaning of the personal pronouns in the plural (14) and short lapses of 'code-switching' in Viennese colloquial speech ('today is another . . .' (15)) only becomes really clear when the latent intentions have been considered.

The therapist's two clarifying questions as to the medicine (25–6, 33–5) are more like statements because of the final 'you know' and the weak rising intonation in the second question. Also, the two 'buts' (26,31) stress the pressing quality of these two interventions. That is why the therapist's sudden submission ('that's what we decided on — that's good' (38)) comes more or less as a surprise.

The unsuccessful attempt at making a statement (40) clearly shows that the client does not really want to listen to the therapist. The intervention which helps the therapist to take over the speaker's role (42–3), is once again an interesting form of persuasion, in two different ways. First, as mentioned above, this point in the text is important because of the implicit meaning in the choice of words. Secondly, it is also typical that the therapist interrupts the client when the client starts to comment on a subject about which the therapist does not want to speak.

The clearly rejective intervention (46) immediately after the client objects comes as a surprise. The therapist makes his statement with a greater emphasis, as a contrast to the client's point of view, and afterwards repeats the preceding intervention. Through the use of the expression 'desire' here, the therapist chooses yet another word with negative connotations.

The repetition of the remark 'I know' (50, 52) hardly seems to make an impression on the client, who continues to speak about the medicine. The therapist's subsequent intervention begins with the client's own words ('what is fear' (52)). Further examples of characteristics of persuasion already mentioned can then be observed: the speaker's perspective 'we'; similar sentence parts repeated three times ('without Umbrium — without crutches — without artificial limbs for the soul' (54–5)). The final 'you know' belongs to a type of structure which helps persuade the client to agree with the therapist.

The intervention (61–3) after the remark made by the client shows a sequential structure in which the present is transformed into a better future ('that could be but doesn't have to be — will become more and more seldom' (61–2)). Owing to the additional use of the 'we' mentioned above, and the slogan-like formulation 'life without Umbrium', this intervention appears to be a well thought-out suggestion.

In the lines 67–8 the therapist completes the client's remarks, thus showing his understanding of the client's situation. The subsequent rejection (71) comes as a surprise, just as in line 46. As the intervention develops, we find a characteristic peculiar to indirect persuasion. At this point the therapist switches to the speaker's perspective of the client ('I'). In the closing advisory intervention in this text (74), the therapist makes use of the client's preceding remarks to make a joke.

The latent level of intentions

The rhythmic quality of the different 'recitations', which is produced by means of emphasis, pauses, gestures and repetitive structures, corresponds very closely to the therapist's mode of speech during hypnotic and persuasive exercises. By changing to the mode of speech in persuasive exercises, the client's readiness to take on persuasive formulas should be taken advantage of. This readiness is also maintained by a flowing transition between the exercises and other conversation sequences, whereby the client should remain in a light state of hypnosis.

According to Becker, a second effect of the rhythmic quality is that it makes the texts more impressive, like a classical epic, a religious recitation or a magic formula. In this moment the authority and dignity of such texts can be transferred to the words of the therapist, the more so as this client characterized himself as being religious. Becker himself called this way of speaking a 'preaching style', which is a good description of the impression it makes.

The effect of the complex sentence structure lies in the confusion it creates in the client. Here the therapist follows a way of acting created by Erickson (Rossi *et al.* 1978), using the confusion of the client's rational ego to break through his confining ideas and habits. So the client becomes ready to accept the formula of persuasion flowing directly to his unconscious self without rational criticism.

The effect of the confusion is also produced by the two surprising rejections (46, 71) in this text. The surprise should make the client more receptive to further persuasive efforts.

Becker himself also called these two passages 'authoritarian', for here he uses all his authority to corroborate his point of view. But, in spite of this pressure, the client's resistance cannot be broken at any point.

The use of the future tense can be interpreted as an imperative or merely as a description of future happenings. Although it is not a definite imperative (which would surely increase the client's resistance), the implicit imperative has an effect on the client. The description of an agreeable future in this context gives the client the feeling (without his explicitly noticing it) that everything will work out for the best. Here again, the basic idea is that the negative attitude of the client's rational ego towards the future is eliminated, and the client (unknowingly) takes on a positive image of his future.

Using the client's words, as it is done at the beginning of the first long 'recitation', is also one of the basic rules of indirect persuasion. The client is supposed to get the feeling that he is understood and that he himself developed the content of the suggestions. Furthermore, the therapist stresses those points which correspond to his therapeutic intentions (5). The special emphasis the therapist uses (9) serve the same purpose.

The use of the plural speaker's perspective 'we', and the short shift to Viennese colloquial language at the end of the first intervention (15), should give the client a feeling of solidarity with the therapist, in order to keep the client's resistance at the lowest possible level.

The whole action of intervention is at this point determined by a tenacious confrontation with the client's resistance. Since the client's only reaction to the well formulated suggestion is to mention the psychotropic drugs he takes, the therapist himself seems to become impatient in both clarifying questions (25–6, 30–5). It is not until the following agreement (38) that he returns to an important strategy of indirect persuasion, which is not to work directly on the client's resistance but rather to avoid it. Becker himself, as concerns the two 'authoritarian' passages (46, 71), calls this approach a continual shift between directing and avoiding.

The special choice of words has already been mentioned above as an example for conveying real intentions by using implications. The use of the future tense, which implicitly contains the imperative form, is also an example of this.

The following interventions contain many persuasive means of language whose latent intentions have already been explained above in other contexts: the use of 'we', to convey solidarity; using the client's formulations ('what is fear' (52)); groups of similar constructions (54). The final 'you know' belongs to a group of constructions which suggest that the client agrees with the therapist. Erickson describes this approach as the establishment of a 'yes-attitude' in the client (Rossi *et al.* 1978). The client's open and uncritical attitude should be maintained with the use of such constructions.

Slogan-like formulations ('life without Umbrium' (63)) are intended to create more impressive effects, as is quite commonly seen in advertising and journalism. The latent meaning of the harsh rejection at the end of this text has already been described. The following shift to the speaker's perspective of 'I' is interesting. By taking up the client's 'inner dialogue', the therapist tries to induce the client to identify more strongly with him. This makes it very difficult for the client to break away from the therapist's point of view, and to formulate an opinion of his own.

The joke that appears at the end of the last intervention should also help loosen the client's resistance, but in this case it did not succeed. When reading through this text one can find a great number of persuasive means, all of which were unsuccessful in neutralizing the client's resistance.

The client's reactions

The client's short objection (8) during the long 'recitation' of the therapist seems to be ambiguous; on the one hand the client agrees ('yes, yes, yes') but on the other hand the 'well you know' is the typical beginning of a negative reaction, of which we can find three more examples in this text (27, 48, 64). (See also the detailed analysis of the beginnings of the client's rejections in Nowak 1984: 107ff.)

The short passage on psychotropic drugs (17–24), which will later become so important for this session, must at first be called a new aspect, and seems to appear independently of the preceding long 'recitation' of the therapist. It is not until the context of the whole session and the latent level of meaning of this reaction are considered that its significance can be fully understood. It is also worth mentioning that, while saying this, the client straightened his back as if he could speak more emphatically that way.

After the first clarifying question of the therapist there is a rejection typical of this client (27–9). The use of the therapist's academic title, which appears directly after the client's rejection 'well, but', is also noteworthy. Also the expression 'you know' is common in the client's rejections (27, 34, 39, 48, 64, 66, 76). Very often this expression directly follows a 'but' (39, 66).

After his answer to the therapist's second question, which on the manifest level could not definitely be interpreted as agreement or rejection, the client repeats his rejection (37–41) of the idea that he should reduce the Umbrium on his own. While he says this, he changes the position he is sitting in and seems to be excited. Also, during the open rejection of the therapist's next intervention (44–5) the client straightens his back. Again we have the typical beginning of a rejection with 'you know'. In the next repetition of his rejection the client adds a new aspect: 'it takes effect so fast'. While saying this, he moves forward as if to make a stronger impression. During the words 'I get the feeling that I was never sick' he leans back again and looks out of the window.

He also reacts to the next intervention by repeating his rejection, and he adds to it by using a rational medical explanation ('most often stems from irregular brain waves' (57)) and a new description of his difficulties at work. It is not until the client reacts to the phrase 'life without Umbrium' (69) that we can observe him becoming more reasonable. The client then says 'well you know, OK I agree with you' (64). But still this remark ends with the familiar 'but you know'. The client then continues to speak of his feelings ('you can't be as fast as the others' (70)) in a new, somewhat excited description (gesturing of the hands). Even the closing joke made by the therapist leads to a repetition of the rejection (75).

The latent meaning of the client's remarks

The unbroken resistance which dominates this text section can only properly be understood in conjunction with the story of the doctor. This story gives the client's doubts a so-called official quality. This is a prime example of the social and institutional influence which is most assuredly of importance in every therapy. A social and political conflict between psychotherapist and some doctors, for whom the psyche still seems to belong to an exotic marginal branch of neurology, can be observed here through the client's resistance.

The client's seemingly inconsistent reaction to the long 'recitation', in which he speaks of the medicine for the first time (20–7), is an interesting point. It can be assumed that the client unconsciously chooses this subject because he sees here, with the experience with the other doctors as a backdrop, the best chance of showing his resistance, which he felt in any case. With this in mind, the final comment of this remark 'but I'm not going to take anything else because they make me feel better' (26–7) becomes especially interesting. The phenomenon which can be observed here is called 'allusion of the transference' (Gill and Hoffman 1982) in psychoanalysis. What is meant here is that comments which superficially have nothing to do with the therapy are made by the client because they unconsciously deal with his relationship to the therapist. In this case, it means that the client says: 'I'm not going to take anything else because they make me feel better!'; put another way: 'I'm not going to give you (the therapist) the chance to get me back on your side.' This is a very harsh way of expressing the client's feelings,and only represents one aspect of these feelings. In contrast, the other aspect is very willing to cooperate with the therapist, even though this aspect may be somewhat in the background at the time.

The many rejections in the text can be attributed to this one great resistance within the client. This resistance is also strongly expressed on the nonverbal level.

Another small hint as to why the client is discontented with the therapy is given by the client in his reaction after the first 'authoritarian' intervention by the therapist (48–9): 'because you know it takes effect so fast'. The same cannot, of course, be said for the therapy. In addition, therapy takes more effort.

The reaction (34–7) which could not be clearly categorized on the manifest level can, with the help of the words 'I think' (34), be seen as an unconscious effort to limit the previously mentioned identification with the therapist and to break away from the therapist's point of view.

The effort to rationalize in 57 ('most often stems from irregular brain waves') is an example of the rationalizing defence mechanism, but we must not forget that it also results from the tension between psychotherapy and traditional medicine, and especially from the experience that the client had with the other doctor (see text 3).

Overall, it can be observed that this text is totally dominated by the client's resistance, which remains unchanged to the end.

Text 2

1	T:	You just have to see it as a picture of the future which we
2	C:	mhm
3	T:	slowly want to make reality — without you having to sacrifice
4		anything — you see and if I do something like this I start out
5	C:	mhm
6	T:	small so that someone doesn't even notice that one is taking less
7	C:	aha
8	T:	véry slowly decreasing dosages véry slowly — and if we notice
9	C:	mh
10	T:	that we need it we take more
11	C:	mh you know it's like this (*clears*
12		*his throat*) like well ah ah —— ah the faith is here — but deep
13	T:	yes
14	C:	down inside something wants to erupt like a volcano

T: the will is
there but the body is weak — — that's what it says — in the bíble
C: exactly exactly — exactly yes exactly
(*laughs*) — — — exactly — — so I'm not the first I'm not the
T: of course not
C: first
T: yes of course you see it happens — happens everywhere all
the time — you know that one starts out with good inten-
C: yes yes
T: tions — but one can't fulfil them — you know it doesn't matter
C: yes
T: because it is only important that one doesn't take it seriously
but that you tell yourself the next time it'll be better the
next time I'll try again
C: because the medicine takes effect so fast.

The interventions of the therapist

The therapist begins with the advisory intervention (1–10) which has the well known characteristics of a suggestion (the 'we' which conveys solidarity; the emphasis put on particular words (8)). The impersonal manner of referring to the client as 'someone' and 'one' (6) is conspicuous.

The next intervention (15–16) is also of an advisory nature, and offers a commonplace expression as an explanation for the client's resistance and fears. The explicit reference to the Bible, which is also given additional emphasis, is noteworthy.

The client's insight is followed by a commonplace expression as a further explanation (21–8) for the client's difficulties. The 'you know' phrases, which are interspersed (22, 24), are important for the latent effect. The impression of a commonplace expression is also made through the use of the impersonal 'one' (22, 24, 26).

The latent level of intentions

The impersonal manner of addressing the client in the first and last interventions of the text section should, on the one hand, emphasize the general validity of the remark and, on the other, deny the client the possibility of resistance on a personal level, since it is not a personal address at the manifestly colloquial level. But it is clear at the *latent* level of intention that it is the client who should be persuaded.

The use of commonplace expressions to underpin suggestions is a technique also found by Erickson (Rossi *et al.* 1978). Commonplace expressions are generally recognized to be acceptable, and thus it is difficult for the client to question them. This suggestive technique is also helpful when trying to establish a 'yes-attitude' in the client, as was mentioned above. The therapist added to his description of the effect of this intervention (15–16) the comment that this commonplace expression, because of the solemn exaggeration, could have a humorous effect, which would also help to break down resistance. The explicit reference to the Bible gives the therapist the unquestionable authority of a priest and the dignity of age-old wisdom ('preaching style').

The 'you know' phrases which are interspersed in the last intervention (22, 24) also belong, as is explained above, to the linguistic means used to establish a 'yes-attitude'. Thus, on the whole, this text section is dominated by interventions which have as a goal the establishment of a 'yes-attitude' in the client. They are also intended to lead the client to accept the suggested goals through impersonal and generally valid expressions which avoid a confrontation with the client's resistance.

The client's reactions

After the understanding listener's signals and the 'aha' (which shows insight) during the first intervention, the client only hesitatingly begins to introduce a new aspect. The typical introduction of a slight rejection (Nowak 1984: 107) 'you know it's like this' (11) is followed by the client clearing his throat, empty pauses and filling pauses, before the client finally begins what he really wants to say. Even later, in this significant description of his inner state, the client still hesitates to say everything he wanted to say.

The agreement with the 'Biblical' statement made by the therapist is very strongly expressed by the 'exactly', which the client repeats several times, and through the client's relieved laugh. The client then goes one step further into the problem ('so I am not the first' (18)), so that this reaction could be considered insight.

The repetition of the problem with the medicine after the last commonplace expression only seems surprising when it is considered on the manifest level. The 'because' used at the beginning of the remark was interpreted in my main investigation as an introduction form used by the client to express a slight contradiction (Nowak 1984: 108).

The latent meaning of the client's remarks

The distinctive cases of hesitation in the first long reaction by the client (11–14) are a sign of how emotionally involved the client is in what is being said. The strong emotions stem from two sources. The first source is the fear he experiences, which is very difficult to keep under control ('wants to erupt like a volcano'), and which makes the client very unsure of himself. The second source is the real situation between the therapist and the client. This comment is also to be understood as an 'allusion of transference', as discussed above. The client, by his impressive picture of a volcano, expresses also his resistance towards the therapy and the therapist. Unconsciously he makes it clear to the therapist that on a superficial level he has faith in him, but that 'deep down inside' he really doesn't want to have anything to do with him.

From this point of view, the subsequent intervention by the therapist becomes interesting because the therapist takes up this resistance but, at the same time, closes the matter with a commonplace expression.

There is obviously a difference here between persuasive therapy and psychoanalysis, because in psychoanalysis (and the forms of psychotherapy derived from it) this hint of the client would have been pursued in some way. On the other hand, the therapist's intervention at this point clearly shows how resistance can be avoided in persuasive therapy.

The reason why the client reacted so strongly to the Biblical words used by the therapist could not even be completely clarified while watching the playback of the session together with the therapist. The client was most likely so relieved 'not to be the first one' because his fears of, and resistance to, the therapy had made him believe he could be crazy and not a 'normal' person. So this commonplace expression showed him that there had been other people before with similar feelings who were considered quite 'normal'.

The effect of the 'you know' used in the therapist's next intervention can be measured by the client's 'yes' which immediately follows. On the other hand, this 'yes-attitude' is not very far reaching; the client's final reaction shows this clearly. After a short period of agreement with the therapist, the resistance breaks out again. Here again, as in the first text, the client points out that the psychotropic drugs take effect immediately; but what he really wants to say is that psychotherapy works too slowly.

Considering the client's reactions in this text in comparison with the first one, a slight withdrawal of the resistance can be noticed; but then it comes back, although not quite as strongly as at the beginning of the session.

Text 3 and final remarks

At this point I would like to quote the part of the session where the client describes his experience with the doctor who gave him the psychotropic drugs; this takes place near the end of the session. The experience completely explains the client's uncompromising resistance, in spite of all the therapist's efforts and the use of many elements common to persuasive therapy as we have seen in this therapeutic session.

Text 3

C: so my boss well my doctor there signs everything which is which is ordered you see there he writes according to the hospital do you know what he told me — because I asked him about psychotherapy well I can tell you — he said well
T: yes yes
C: without medicine it wouldn't work out anyway
T: — — so he said without medicine it wouldn't work out anyway yes yes
C: yes well you know it's it's also I I do believe you more than him you see but I just want to say that a lot of things can be messed up by a doctor you know because . . .
T: yes of course
C: Because (*clears his throat*) now now I think he's a doctor you're a doctor now who is right . . .
T: sure

The tension between clinical medicine and psychotherapy, and thus the conditions under which the therapy has to work and the resulting problems for the client, are clearly shown in this text. Evidently the other doctor's irresponsible comments did not *produce* the client's resistance, but rather backed it up by giving it a so-called official quality. But it is not my intention here to investigate or clarify the complicated institutional and ideological problems suggested here.

Concerning the manner of resistance in persuasive therapy, one main point can be particularly stressed in the detailed linguistic analysis of these texts: persuasive therapy, according to Becker (1984), provides little help for the real work on the client's psychic problems (see especially text 2); but for a limited period of time it can overcome the client's resistance so far that it makes his symptoms disappear — or at least their intensity decrease. As long as this remains the only goal which the therapist strives to attain, as Becker does, this kind of therapy as a 'medicine without side-effects' should be preferred to medical treatment to deal with the symptoms. But it should be made quite clear that this method does not affect the cause of the troubles at all. Thus, as we also see in this case, it cannot be expected to improve the client's psychic condition on a long-term basis. One year later the same client had to be treated again for a new symptom (writer's cramp)! Again, this symptom disappeared soon after the beginning of persuasive therapy.

The problems arising from using persuasive therapy to change a whole personality, as Erickson does (Rossi *et al.* 1978), are treated in detail in my main investigation. There is also a comprehensive summary of the means of speech used in persuasive therapy by Becker (Nowak 1984: 100), so this topic will not be dealt with here. The most important of these means of speech and their latent meanings have been discussed briefly above, in the analysis of the texts.

As far as linguistic methods and theories are concerned, it can be said that a phenomenon as complex as persuasion can only be analysed within the framework of a 'multi-level model', according to Wodak (1981). The many levels of latent intentions, unconscious emotions and manifest colloquial formulations can only be fully comprehended through the use of this model. Quantitative investigations are valuable, and necessary to avoid subjective opinions and distortions and to complete a qualitative analysis of such relatively short texts, but they cannot replace the use of this model. A true-to-life picture of what really happens in therapeutic situations can only be given through the use of a 'comprehensive analysis' (Labov and Fanshel 1977).

Notes to Chapter 2

1 'Resistance: everything in the words or actions of the patient that obstructs his gaining access to his unconscious' (Laplanche and Pontalis 1973).

'Defense mechanism: a reaction pattern, usually unconscious, which serves the purpose of protecting an individual from anxiety, guilt, unacceptable impulses, internal conflicts, or other threats of the ego. Defensive behavior is a common, normal means of coping with problems, but excessive use of any mechanism, such as displacement or repression, is considered pathological' (Goldenson 1984).

2 In their investigation of therapeutic discourse Labov and Fanshel (1977) describe four modes to realize 'mitigation' (playing down): euphemism; diffuse reference; intonation; and narratives (335f.). Although the authors described 'mitigation' in the patient's speech, similar phenomena seem to occur in Becker's supportive interventions (see Becker (in press)).

3 This is also one of the two sessions used in my main investigation (Nowak 1984) for quantitative comparison with the other forms of therapy.

References

Becker, A. M. (in press): *Hypnotherapie und andere suggestive Verfahren insbesondere Autogenes Training*.

Flader, D. and Wodak, R. (eds.) 1979: *Therapeutische Kommunikation*. Königstein/Ts: Scriptor Verlag.

Gill, M. and Hoffman, I. 1982: A method for studying the analysis of aspects of the patient's experience of relationship in psychoanalysis and psychotherapy. *Journal of American Psychoanalysis Association* 30(1), 137–67.

Goldenson, R. M. (ed.) 1984: *Longman Dictionary of Psychology and Psychiatry*. New York: Longman.

Haley, J. (ed.) 1967: *Advanced Techniques of Hypnosis and Therapy: Selected Papers of Milton H. Erickson*. New York and London: Grune & Stratton.

Labov, W. and Fanshel, D. 1977: *Therapeutic Discourse: Psychotherapy as Conversation*. New York: Academic Press.

Langs, R. 1981: *Resistance and Interventions: the Nature of Therapeutic Work*. New York: Aronson.

Laplanche, J. and Pontalis, J. B. 1973: *The Language of Psychoanalysis*. Frankfurt/Main: Suhrkamp.

Nowak, P. 1984: *Die Intervention des Therapeuten — eine vergleichende sprach wissenschaftliche Untersuchung von psychoanalytischer, klienten-zentrierter und suggestiver Therapie*. Unpublished dissertation: University of Vienna.

Rossi, E., Rossi, S. and Erickson, M. H. 1978: *Hypnose. Indikation — Psychotherapeutische Anwendung — Beispiele*. Munich: Pfeifer.

Wodak, R. 1981: *Das Wort in der Gruppe. Linguistische Studie zur therapeutischen Kommunikation*. Vienna: Verlag der Akademie der Wissenschaft. Translated as *Language Behaviour in Groups*. Los Angeles: University of California Press, 1985.

Wunderlich, D. 1976: *Studien zur Sprechakttheorie*. Frankfurt/Main: Suhrkamp.

Appendix 1 Transcription system

The transliteration system includes the following signs:

—, — —, — — —	short pauses of increasing length
( )	paraverbal events (e.g. bang of a door, laughter)
/ ( )/	the text between the diagonal strokes is articulated in a special manner (e.g. laughing)
xx́xx	emphasis on this word
(. . .)	incomprehensible parts

Appendix 2 German texts

Text 1

K: ah i glaub wann aner a bißl langsamer is also jetzt werma
ja segn wie si des einspielt mit erm net (türnkrachen, Frau-
enstimme) wie sis einstellt mit ihm net — i was ja net ent-
weder angenehm oder unangenehm aber i glaub eher angenehm
T: eher angenehn — wissen Sie warum — — Sie sind ein neuer ge-
worden — Sie haben neue Absichten neue Ziele neue Methoden
— Sie werden sich ńicht mehr aus der Ruhe bringen lassen
K: hm
ja ja ja — naja des
T: Sie werden Ihr ruhiges Tempo das außerdem
gen aue Arbeit liefert — durchziehen — dadurch sind Sie — von
äußeren — Störungen — weitgehend — unabhängig — — das ist
der große Vorteil — — — das hat sich schon — in der ersten
Woche bewährt — — und es wird sich in den weiteren Wochen
— immer mehr bewähren — — und schließlich — werden Sie
ein neues Betriebsgefühl haben — wir wollen des erreichen
— — daß für Sie die Tätigkeit dort — zu einer Sache wird wos
hingehen und sagen no heit is wieder Arbeitstag da zeig i
wieder was i kann — —
K: wissens jetzt war i da weil die Sachen
da die Medikamente die was i da nimm die trocknen a bißl aus
jetzt war i beim Hals und Nasenarzt der hat gsagt ers ers i
T: ja
K: soll immer a bißl gurgln net er sagt vielleicht fragens
T: ja jajaja
K: den Arzt vielleicht gibts andere aber i stell mi jetzt nimmer
um weil die Ta die tuan ma guat
T: ja ja wir haben aber schon ah ah
herabgesetzt net?
K: naja oba Herr Oberarzt momentan geht des net
sagma mit dem Umbrium wissen Sie
T: (. . .) is naja mit dem Umbrium laß mas
vielleicht aber mit die anderen mit die mit die die mit
K: in der Früh nimm i des doppelte

T: die ah Saroden mit Tryptizol hamma weniger
K: mit die Tryptizol naja i bin i bin
der Meinung also früh mittag nimm i schon aber wann i zhaus
kumm brauch is eigentlich net jajaja na
T: ja hamma ja ausgmacht — na fein
K: und aber des Umbrium wissen Sie des mecht i schon sagma in
T: ja schauns
K: der Früh verstärken und Mittags verstärken
T: wenn Ses schaun Sie wenn Sie
am Umbrium hängen noch — ja — — — ah naschen Sie ruhig davon
ja — — — aber wir werdens bald nimmer brauchen
K: naja i was net
T: aber í was — naschen Sie noch am Umbrium — wenn Ihnen danach
K: mh ja ja
T: gelüstet — — —
K: weil wissen Sie die die Wirkung tritt nam-
lich sofort bei dem Umbrium ein und kommt (*räuspert sich*) a
T: jaja i was schon
K: Gfühl als wie wann ma nie was ghabt hätt und wann ma zu an
T: ja i was schon i was schon
K: sagt was is Angst —
T: was is Angst? Kein Problem für mich ja
aber passens auf ja wir wollen dasselbe Gefühl bekommen —
K: wissen Sie (*räuspert sich*)
T: ohne — Umbrium — ohne Krücke — ohne Seelenprothese — ja —
weil des san alles Seelenprothesen net ja
K: naja schon Herr Oberarzt
K: aber sagma ah wissen Sie mit der Angst des draht si in erster
Linie um Erregungszustände — und wann i siech sagma i werd
T: i was
K: mit aner Arbeit net fertig und der wart schon ja — na göns da
dann brauchts net lang und i bin wieder im Wirbel drin
T: ehii
des könnte sein muß aber nicht sein wird immer seltener sein
— und wir haben das Ziel — Umbriumfreie Lebensweise
K: weil
schön i bin ja der Meinung wie Sies sagn net daß is erm
sag schau du wirst des scho kriegn bis is ebn fertig hab und
áus net und bis i mir ja an dem des erkenne ich alles und
T: jajaja ja
K: seh ich auch ein aber wissen Sie wanns drauf an-
T: die Durchführung is no schwie-
K: kommt ja sag i ma do na herst i kan ah kannst
T: rig is no schwierig
K: net a so schnell sein wie die anderen —
T: néin — ich kann nicht
und will nicht und verzichte allmählich den
K: naja spielt halt der Ehrgeiz a mit
T: laß ma den ziegn ma auf und tuan ma im Vorzimmer aufhänga
K: (*lacht*)
naa Herr Oberarzt is alls so leicht gredt göns aber ah

Text 2

T: ·also nehmans des nur als a Zukunftsbild — dem wir uns — nähren
K: mhm
T: wollen — ohne daß Sie dabei — irgendwelche Einbußen haben — gö
K: mh
T: ich mache es wenn immer gánz kleinstufig ja abwärts daß jemand net amal merkt daß a weniger nimmt ganz schleichend ausschlei-
K: aso mh
T: chend gánz langsam — wann ma merken ma brauchts ja dann laß man wieda
K: mh wissen Sie es is so sagma (*räuspert sich*) wie ah ah — — ah
der Glaube is hier — aber die Tiefen also des Innere im Körper
T: ja
K: des ah ah will oft raus wie a Vulkan
T: der Wille is da aber das Fleisch ist schwach — –– so heißt es — in der Bibel
K: ja genau genau — genau genau (*lacht*) — — — genau — — so bin i net der erste bin i net der erste
T: freilich net ja
freilich na schaun Sie kommt — kommt überall ständig vor — net
K: ja
T: daß ma gutn Vorsatz hat aber — ma rutscht aus — und ma erfüllt
K: ja
T: ihn net ganz — net aber des macht nix wichtig is daß ma des net
K: ja
T: ernst nimmt sondern des nächste Mal si sagt nächste Mal gehts besser net nächstes Mal mach is wieda
K: weil die Medikamente ebn die die wirken direkt schlágartig

Text 3

K: also mei Chef also mei Arzt dort der unterschreibt direkt alles was was angeordnet wird net er schreibt da laut ah ah Kranken-haus wissens was der mir gsagt hat — wei i hab gsagt ob von der Psychotherapie Ihna kann is ja sagn — der hat gsagt naja ohne
T: ja ja
K: Medikamente gingas eh net
T: — — hat a gmant ohne Medikamente gingas eh net ja ja
K: ja ja na is a i i glaub natürlich mehr ihnan göns aber i wü nur sagn was a Arzt a verpfuschen kann net wei
T: (. . .) ja sicher
K: wei (*räuspert sich*) jetzt jetzt i denk ma Sie san Arzt er is
T: sicher
K: Arzt ja wer hat jetzt recht net . . .

3 Confrontation in psychotherapy:
A Conversational analysis

Susanne Bleiberg Seperson

Introduction

Psychic change and growth is one of the main goals of psychotherapy. Confrontation is an activity which may be used to promote such growth. However, while the therapist provides the encouragement to change, it is the patient who changes himself. This chapter examines the activity of confrontation, which is viewed as a strong encouragement to achieve psychic change from a conversational point of view. However, the term 'successful confrontation' as used here means only that the conversational activity has been completed. We do not know if psychic change has been achieved. I leave this determination to the psychotherapists and patients themselves. While a few therapists have written about the activity, it had not, until my work with Churchill (Bleiberg and Churchill 1975), been analysed in terms of its production in any detailed way. We defined it as an activity where the confronter, in this case the therapist, brings the confronted, the patient, face to face with a fact that the patient cannot be permitted to avoid facing. By doing so, the therapist is disagreeing with the patient's initial assertion.

Confrontation, as an activity, has been accomplished using audiotapes and videotapes as well as verbal exhortations. Here I concentrate on the activity as a speech event. The data is based on transcripts of audiotapes of psychoanalytically orientated psychotherapy sessions.[1] All patients had agreed to be taped, and all identifying information has been changed. The chapter provides a brief literature review before offering an analysis of completed confrontations, confrontation variations and incompleted confrontations. The focus is on features of the activity essential for its accomplishment. The theoretical roots of the analysis come from ethnomethodology and conversational analysis.

Literature review

A number of researchers have discussed the use of confrontation in psychotherapy. For instance, Paredes and Cornelison (1965: 28) have written about confrontation as follows:

> . . . self-confrontation in the presence of and with the assistance of a trained therapist may help patients to better understand the self-deceiving and self-defeating mechanisms they have been using to deny or conceal their conflicts and low self-esteem. Following such understanding they may be motivated to work toward finding ways of handling or solving their conflicts.

Milton Berger (1970: 34) writes:

> I must state unequivocally my belief that confrontation alone is not enough to bring about the kind of characterological change and growth which is the usual goal of psychoanalytically-oriented psychotherapy. Almost any confrontation can be accepted and assimilated to some degree if a patient is prepared for the work of psychotherapy, is in a state of positive transference to his therapist or group and there is enough mutuality, caring, regard, trust and intimacy present.

Evaline Schulman discussed confrontation as an expressive skill of communication in the helping interview: 'The essential purpose of confrontation is to produce suitable circumstances that encourage an individual to look at and hopefully to find ways to change his behaviour' (Schulman 1974: 156). Harry Garner is the only psychiatrist who has discussed confrontation as the accomplishment of an activity. He writes:

> The techniques of therapy applied in confrontation problem-solving psychotherapy include the presentation of a statement and a question . . . An alternative is to express the end results of a continued maladaptive activity in so exaggerated an expression that the person would wish to discontinue such behaviour . . . It is as if the therapist's repetitious question acts as a continuous pressure to force the acceptance of a need to explore and solve a problem (Garner 1970: 14).[2]

However, none of these writers has analysed the activity in a detailed way. In this chapter, I examine the work of Bleiberg and Churchill,

Schulman, and Churchill, who have begun a conversational analysis of confrontation. Bleiberg and Churchill (1975: 276) began such an analysis formulating the following paradigm of confrontation:

TABLE 3.1 *Paradigm of ideal reality-confrontation*

Step	Actor	Behaviour
1	Confronted	Makes a general statement.
2	Confronter	Asks a closed-choice (yes/no) quesion about a particular aspect of the general statement.
3	Confronted	Picks the answer that shows that the particular aspect under question is an exception to the general statement.
4	Confronter	Asks a second closed-choice (yes/no) question about another particular aspect of the general statement.
5	Confronted	Picks the answer that shows that the particular aspect under question is another exception to the general statement.
6	Confronter	Asks rhetorical question that contradicts the confronted's original general statement.

However, as I continued this analysis, it became clear that there are many variations of this paradigm which we, as competent users of the English language, still recognize as confrontations or as confrontation-like activities. Thus, I conclude that the activity does not rest on following the structure presented in the paradigm, but rather rests on its essential features. Thus, Schulman's examples of two-liners and even one example of a one-liner (which are discussed later on) are still recognizable as confrontations. Similarly, Churchill's analysis of 'three-liners' which are denigrations (Churchill 1978: 132) shows them to have confrontation-like features which result in our being able to recognize when we have been 'put down'. Since Churchill's three-line denigration is actually based on an initial asssertion or action (really the first of four lines), I conclude that it is essential to analyse the features or elements of the confrontation activity, rather than the form *per se*. In addition, the fact that no strict form is followed automatically lends credence to Garfinkel's (1967) assertion that we are not norm-followers but rather norm-users.[3] The confrontation model is used creatively, since we are thinking, creative beings, and not robots. Thus, in this chapter I turn to an analysis of (1) completed confrontation, (2) confrontation variations, and finally (3) incomplete confrontations.

Completed confrontations

The development of a six-line paradigm was based in part on the following two examples and numerous variations:

Example 1 Jill

1 Pt: I don't want them [my parents] to have anything to do with my life, except (*pause*) security (?).
2 Dr: You live at home?
3 Pt: Yes.
4 Dr: They pay your bills?
5 Pt: Yeah.
6 Dr: How could they not have anything to do with your life?

Example 2 Jill

1 Pt: I don't—have much—faith—in therapy or anything any more.
2 Dr: You don't have any faith in anything?
3 Pt: No.
4 Dr: You want to live? Or you want to die?
5 Pt: I don't want to die, I'd be dead (*very low voice*).
6 Dr: OK, so there's obviously some evidence that you want to live. Is that right?

They were analysed by Churchill and myself[4] as follows.

The confronter facilitates the activity by his tone of voice and rapid-fire nature of his questions. If we look at the examples, we see that the questions demand yes/no answers, *not* carefully thought-out answers. In reality-confrontation, the question-answer sequence leaves no room for a middle ground, a grey area.

The tacit consent of the confronted to this activity is evident when we look at her responses to the direct yes/no questions. The patient agrees to supply the alternative answer that will support the confronter's later 'punch line'. For instance, she answers *yes* she lives at home, and *yes*, her parents pay her bills, in example 1. Thus she accepts the confronter's 'invitation' to continue their joint production of reality-confrontation. Similarly, in example 2, Jill provides the preferred answers to the doctor's yes/no questions. In addition, the patient does not object to the 'stretches'[5] the doctor has made, and thereby participates in the joint production of the activity.

The confrontation or 'punch line' comes after the 'funnel-like' yes/no question-answer sequences, and refers back to something spoken about in the immediate previous past. (By 'funnel-like' we mean that, so long as the patient answers in the prescribed way, i.e. using the alternatives that support the therapist's position, it will be increasingly difficult for her to avoid facing the logical conclusion of the therapist's punch line.) Her options are progressively closed in this funnel-like process, and then, quickly, she is confronted with the punch line. The conclusion is self-evident and, short of appearing stupid, one cannot find an alternative conclusion.

Thus, in each case the therapist has contradicted the patient's initial statement; in the former, her parents *do* have something to do with her life, and in the latter, she *does* have faith in something, since she doesn't want to die.

Yet Schulman (1974: 150) presented the following examples in her description of confrontation which are only 'two-liners'. In analysing these examples, it became apparent to me that it is the constituent elements of confrontation, which will be discussed later in the chapter, and not the form of confrontation that will lead us to recognize the production of this activity.

Example 3 Tom

1 Tom: If only my wife wouldn't make so many demands on me, I wouldn't drink.
2 Mr O: Ten years you've been drinking, Tom. You've been married for five. How come you drank before you were married?

Example 4 Wilma

1 Wilma: My mother was just like that. I know I'm like her. She and my father would argue about such petty things as how high or how low the window shade should be. Then she would get more and more upset . . . throw up . . . my father would shut up. I'm just like her.
2 Dr N: Are you saying that you can't be different just because of your mother?

Example 5 Ted

1 Ted: You're a jerk. You don't understand anything.
2 Mr R: Aren't you foolish talking to a jerk who doesn't understand?

The problem of form became secondary, since it is possible to re-create these excerpts in the form of the six-liner. They are condensed forms of the activity which illustrate that confrontation is based on disagreement. In each case, line 1 is a statement and line 2 is another statement which disputes the original statement. Similarly, line 6 in the paradigm disputes the contention made in line 1. In each case here, the middle part of the yes/no question-answer sequence is elided. This condensed form has less force than the full version, since the confronted has not participated in his own 'destruction', so to speak. The punch line is based on inconsistency, and is a surprise; the confronted did not know that this activity was going to occur. This supports the disagreeing maxim: disagreement can occur at any time (Bleiberg Seperson 1981). In both Tom's and Wilma's examples, however, the doctor's statement of the punchline presupposes prior knowledge of the patient (e.g. knowledge of when the drinking began, and of how many years Tom had been married; and knowledge of Wilma's relationship as well).

In the following hypothetical re-creations of examples 3 and 4, the premisses on which the conclusion is based are publicly admitted. In Tom's case, the change is minor. The doctor's lines 2 and 4, *How long have you been drinking?* and *How long have you been married?* are, then, rhetorical questions,[6] since the answer is already known to both participants. In Wilma's case, there is an implied disagreement over whether she can be different from her mother: she thinks she can't, the therapist thinks she can. In the hypothetical re-creation below, the confrontation is based on *I'm just like my mother*.

EXAMPLE 6 HYPOTHETICAL RE-CREATION OF 'TOM' EXCERPT

1 Tom: If only my wife wouldn't make so many demands on me, I wouldn't drink.
2 Dr: How long have you been drinking, Tom?
3 Tom: Ten years.
4 Dr: How long have you been married?
5 Tom: Five years.
6 Dr: Then how can you say you're drinking because your wife puts so many demands on you?

EXAMPLE 7 HYPOTHETICAL RE-CREATION OF 'WILMA' EXCERPT

1 Wilma: My mother was just like that. I know I'm like her. She and my father would argue about such petty things as how high or how low the window shade should be.
2 Dr N: Have you ever argued with your [father, husband, etc.] about how high or low the shade should be?
3 Wilma: No.
4 Dr N: Did you ever throw up after an argument?
5 Wilma: No.
6 Dr N: Then how can you say you're just like your mother?

In example 4, the doctor confronted Wilma about whose responsibility it is that she is the way she is, and not about what she specifically said in line 1. In example 7, on the other hand, the doctor confronts Wilma about whether she really is the way her mother is. Thus, if Wilma had hypothetically responded in line 3 (of example 7), *I've never argued about the height of the shade, but I have argued about some other equally ridiculous thing with my husband,* the doctor can still follow up, *But did you throw up after the argument?* If the patient says no, then he can still confront her with his punch line, *Then how can you say you're just like your mother*? Of course, she could reply, *But I cried after the argument.* However, the doctor could say, *OK you cried, maybe it's something that you could learn not to do, but you didn't throw up — so you're not just like your mother.* However, in the example the doctor shifts and says, *Are you saying that you can't be different just because of your mother*? That starts the patient thinking about her responsibility for her behaviour. The shift is a good one therapeutically, and, from the example, one that the patient doesn't disagree with.

Before continuing with the analysis of form, it is important to clarify the *yes, but* and *no, but* issue. *Yes, but* is a qualified agreement which means in essence 'no'. *No, but* is a qualified disagreement, which means in essence 'yes'. These are weak agreements and disagreements, respectively. In addition, the *but* or explanation which follows qualifying the initial *yes* or *no* is a completion of reason invitation (Bleiberg Seperson 1981: 41; Churchill 1978). The speaker who adds the reason or qualifier thus holds the floor for a longer time and is in control of the situation, determining when he shall return the floor to the questioner. This delay in the confrontation sequence has the effect of blunting the contradiction the confronter wishes to make. As Churchill notes in discussing this issue in terms of the 'three-liner' denigration, it can also be used to beat the confronter to the punch line. However, the punch line works 'only if no objections to it remain on the floor' (Churchill 1978). Thus, the *but* strategy can be used during the activity of confrontation to do two different things: to control the floor and to give the punch line. In both cases, however, they serve to derail the confrontation sequence. This, as a strategy, will be discussed in the last section of this chapter.

I turn now to Schulman's third example, a two-liner which varies slightly from her other two examples. Example 5 is compounded by name-calling. In addition, Mr R responds to the name-calling by placing Ted in a double-bind. The problem for Ted is that he either must accept that he is a fool (for talking to a jerk) or that Mr R is not a jerk, in which case Ted must admit that he was wrong. This punch line has particular force in that the inconsistency does not follow from the initial premiss, but from the name-calling. For example, this confrontation could be based on the second half of Ted's statement, *You don't understand anything*. The following hypothetical re-creation then results in an inconsistency in the punch line, following from the initial premiss that Mr R doesn't understand anything.

EXAMPLE 8 HYPOTHETICAL RE-CREATION OF 'TED' EXCERPT

1 Ted: You're a jerk. You don't understand anything.
2 Mr R: Who did you come running to when you had a problem at the school?
3 Ted: You.
4 Mr R: Who had to talk to the judge when you were in trouble?
5 Ted: You.
6 Mr R: Then you couldn't possibly mean it when you said I didn't understand anything and called me a jerk.

Schulman (1974: 157) provides another example of confrontation which is even more condensed — the one-liner:

EXAMPLE 9

2 Counsellor: You say you're perfectly satisfied with your sexual relationships with your present husband. How, then, do you explain what you said after your recent 'fling' with your former husband?

In this example, the disagreement is implicit. The therapist responds to something his client said previously, and then not necessarily directly. In this case, the punch line and implicit disagreement alone result in the accomplishment of the activity of confrontation. But even this extremely condensed version of the activity can be recreated as follows:

EXAMPLE 10 HYPOTHETICAL RE-CREATION OF EXAMPLE 9

1 Client: I'm perfectly satisfied with my sexual relationship with my present husband.
2 Counsellor: Didn't you have a fling with your former husband recently?
3 Client: Yes.
4 Counsellor: Didn't you say that you went to him because he alone satisfied you as no one else can?
5 Client: Yes.
6 Counsellor: Then how can you say you're perfectly satisfied with your present husband?

This very short confrontation again points to the fact that recognition of the activity of confrontation results not on its overall form but on its constituent elements, which we know include an initial disagreement and a punch line.

I now turn to Churchill's 'three-liner' before focusing on the necessary elements of confrontation, and on how the activity is actually accomplished.

Churchill's discussion of the three-line form of denigration follows from our analysis of reality-confrontation. In terms of the six-line paradigm presented earlier, Churchill concentrates on lines 4–6. Churchill notes that line 4 (his line 1) is used 'to disagree with some prior utterance or action by H (the hearer) that he feels is silly or stupid or obtuse' (Churchill 1978: 132). Hence the three lines are an indirect response to a prior first line. Churchill writes that his first line of the potential three-liner rests on loaded questions — either a rhetorical question or an attitude question, although these do not exhaust the possibilities (Churchill 1978: 135). He also discusses the non-required answer as potentially denigrating to H, and the self-denigrating question (Churchill 1978: 136).

I have thus presented some of the forms confrontation may take. Given their variety, even at this point (others are considered in the next section), how is it that we are still able to recognize a confrontation when we hear one? As competent members of the American culture, who understand and speak English as normal persons do, we hear the necessary elements constituting a confrontation, and recognize when one has occurred. I turn now to these features, and to the reasons for the effectiveness of this particular kind of disagreement.

Analysis: Necessary elements for a confrontation

Confrontation is a disagreeing activity; the punch line contradicts the first speaker's first line. It is also a denigration; completing a confrontation results in the first speaker having been subject to a 'put down'. Thus the essential elements are:

1 a general proposition or idea on the floor which can be refuted;
2 a punch line which refutes the above; hence, a disagreement;
3 the unforeseen aspect of the punch line: the twist;
4 a punch line in the form of a rhetorical question.

The fact that the 'checkout' or verifying procedure is carried out through questioning means that the confronter will keep 'getting the floor back' after the confronted answers. It is this feature of asking questions that gives the confronter the immediate next 'slot' in the conversation for his punch line (see Churchill 1973). Also, rhetorical questions have an air of inescapable logic to them which makes it difficult to argue against their implication. The unforeseen aspect of the punch line, and the fact that it takes the form of a rhetorical question, makes the confrontation different from a simple contradiction. Contradiction is a direct response; the punch line in confrontation is arrived at indirectly.

There are four basic reasons for the power and effectiveness of the confrontation activity:

First is the relationship of this activity to logic. The punch line is logically unexpected, and the first speaker/hearer cannot be sure in what direction the second is heading. The punch line is a conclusion arrived at inductively rather than deductively. If it were a deductive conclusion, the premisses and logical steps would be readily apparent, and the confrontation would not be a surprise to the first speaker. Instead, the punch line is arrived at inductively; the conclusion follows from an initial statement and instance, and the first speaker is unaware of the direction in which the second is heading. The former does not know what kind of category packages the latter will construct and use against him, since the package in its totality is not presented; hence, the punch line appears as a surprise and even as a shock.[7]

Secondly, the confrontation activity is a violation of the rules of talk.[8] We speak inexactly, and assume others will understand in essence what we are saying, even if only by waiting for later statements to clarify earlier ones. Thus, springing the punch line removes the basic trust between speakers. This on its own is a surprise, even a shock, to the confronted. That is, the confronted makes a general statement, rather than a particular statement, in line 1. The confronter shows the statement is false by pointing out one or more facts that contradict it. He relies on the principle that general assertions of fact cannot be absolutely true because they overlook exceptional cases that the asserter would exclude if he were talking more carefully.

Thirdly, there are the denigrating aspects of the activity. Here there are five aspects to consider. (1) The confronted has participated in his own 'destruction', so to speak, by providing the preferred answers to the yes/no questions in the checkout process. (2) By co-operating, he shows that he has little 'savvy': because he fails to realize where the confronter was going, 'his own action denigrates himself as stupid or slow-witted' (Churchill 1978: 139). (3) The punch line is used to disagree with the first speaker's statement. The disagreement alone is a denigration, as it puts the first speaker's statement into a category of incorrect remarks; hence, the first speaker is sanctioned for being wrong. (4) By being inconsistent, the first speaker leaves himself open to being sanctioned for his behaviour, as it violates a fundamental assumption in conversation: people are expected to be consistent in their remarks. The inconsistency pointed out in the activity appears to sanction the confronted for violating this assumption. Thus, not only did the confronter disagree with the confronted; his disagreement had added force in that it operates as a sanction for improper behaviour as well. (5) If it is the therapist confronting the patient, the additional authority of his position adds strength to the sanction.

Fourthly, there is the power of the rhetorical question. The question is difficult to refute, since it seems to be correct.[9] As a conclusion or punchline, the confronted must show where the question is faulty. This could be accomplished by noticing any 'stretching' that may have been used, or by showing any faulty logic on the part of the confronter; specifically, where the conclusion might not follow from the premiss, or a faulty initial premiss. In short, the confronted would have to refute the punch line by violating the rules of talk himself. In addition, since the rhetorical question implies that the confronter knows for a fact that the confronted's statement is not true, it makes the confronted appear to have lied, or to be mentally incompetent, i.e. stupid or crazy. In any case, such indirect name-calling is seen as such a personal attack, and demands such a strong response, that it usually receives one. Not responding, either by silence or by an unrelated or inappropriate statement, would support the appropriateness of the denigrating label which the rhetorical question implied. For these reasons, confrontation is persuasive as a disagreeing activity.

Other than refuting the conclusion, once it has been reached, there are only three ways of stopping the confrontation process. It is certainly in the potential confronted's own interest to do this, if he wants to avoid being confronted. He should stop the confrontation process before the conclusion has been reached, rather than refuting the conclusion afterwards, since he would thus not have participated in the joint production, and would show that he knows in which direction the confronter is heading. He could do this by not responding as requested to the yes/no questions if they are asked. That is, the first speaker/hearer could answer (1) *yes, but* or *no, but*, as discussed earlier, or respond with (2) a 'misfire', (a disallowed or botched utterance) which would have to be cleared up before the routine could continue. Such a *maybe* response would effectively sidetrack and stop the confrontation process. Or, (3) the respondent could also refuse to answer the question. This would leave him open to appearing mentally incompetent, unless such a refusal were a response to the loaded question which damns the respondent no matter which way he responds, as in the question, *Are you still beating your wife?* (Churchill 1978: 136).

Thus, confrontation is a rude, impolite activity, not often found in natural conversation. It is a disagreement which is also persuasive. It was used on occasion in these psychotherapy sessions since, as a motivational device, it often works. However, as noted earlier, the term 'successful confrontation' as used here means only that the punch line was reached. No assumption is made as to whether the confronted 'truly accepts' the confronter's point of view or not, of whether, as Allen Wheelis (1969: 59) noted, the conclusion lies 'inert in the patient's mind' for any length of time, or is incorporated into the patient's behaviour or attitude or not. As will be seen shortly, confrontation as an activity is available to any speaker/hearers. I turn now to a discussion of variations in completed confrontation routines.

Confrontation variations

The confrontation variations discussed in this section include only those where the four necessary elements are present, but differ in some respect. These elements are: (1) the general statement under consideration, (2) the disagreement in the form of a punchline, (3) the unforeseen aspect of the punch line, and (4) a punch line in the form of a rhetorical question. As will soon become apparent, the essential elements of a confrontation can be reduced to a *contradiction heard as a rhetorical question*.

Consider the following kinds of variations: In example 11 from Ellen, the *yes/no* question has been replaced with a *why* question. Churchill (1978: 138) has discussed this kind of question briefly, so I mention it here only as a variation. Ellen had been talking in great detail about her relationship with her husband, which caused her to feel great anguish.

EXAMPLE 11 ELLEN

1 Pt: And I don't know. It's all too, it's all too confusing for me. It's all too deep for me. It's all too confusing for me. I don't know. there seem to be so many things going on on at so many different levels, that I don't know if there's ever a way out.

2 Dr: You did something just now. After saying all that you said you know, you then said, 'I don't know'. How come you then said 'I don't know' after you said all that you said?

As Churchill notes, a *why* question is only partly loaded. If the respondent can answer to the questioner's satisfaction, then she will have escaped the potential denigration. However, in this excerpt, the *why* question is also in a sense a rhetorical one. The doctor's question, *How come you then said 'I don't know' after you said all that you said*?, implies that the patient (a) should not have said what she did, and (b) should not have needed to say that kind of thing either. These aspects of the therapist's question are denigrating in themselves. The implication of the confrontation is that the patient should focus on her need to feel that way. This is what he is confronting her about — bringing her need from a subconscious to a conscious level.

The next three examples of confrontation are also undertaken to raise the level of conscious awareness of the patient's behaviour. Example 12 from Jill is about the therapist trying to make the patient more aware that she is not living her life fully:

Example 12 Jill

1 Pt: I want to be alive. But I *can't*. I mean . . .
2 Dr: You want to be alive where? You want to be alive like an animal in a cage?
3 Pt: No.
4 Dr: Who's fed?
5 Pt: No. I mean, I, would, I . . .
6 Dr: You think that'll do you . . .
7 Pt: Of course I'd like to be alive like anybody else, and healthy, and creative and productive and . . .
8 Dr: Yeah, but what?
9 Pt: But I can't do it. I've tried all my life.
10 Dr: Now we're back to 'I can't'. Now look, I won't accept 'I can't'.
11 Pt: So I won't. Well, I've tried.

The variations in example 12 include (1) the compound nature of the general statement in line 1; (2) the confronted beating the confronter to his punch line in line 7; (3) the rhetorical question taking the form of a *why* question line 8; and (4) the possibility of another confrontation routine starting in line 10, but a comparatively direct disagreement being offered instead. These variations are discussed in turn.

(1) Problems arise from the patient's initial statement, *I want to be alive. But I can't*. The problem is: which aspect will be confronted? Two different definitions of reality are involved: *I want to be alive/I don't want to be alive* and *I can/I can't*. At the beginning, the therapist deals with the patient's use of the word *alive*. He offers one definition of *alive* as *alive like an animal in a cage*, which the patient does not accept. The

funnel grows narrower as the therapist refines even further: *Who's fed*? Again the patient chooses not to accept this definition of reality. The general statement being repudiated is that she doesn't want to be alive in the full sense of the word, or she wouldn't be living a life as though she were an animal in a cage.

(2) The patient accepts the therapist's interpretation of reality and recognizes her position by her outcry, *Of course I would like to be alive like anybody else and be healthy and creative and productive*. Since she has beaten him to the punch line (by cutting off his line 6, assuming he was going to make one), we can see that the punch line can be given by the confronted as well as by the confronter.

(3) The therapist then offers his own form of a punch line in line 8, asking a *why* question. The assumption is that there really is a difference of opinion at the subsconscious level, i.e. that the therapist believes that the patient does not really want to be alive in the full sense. This is similar to the issue in the previous example.

(4) At this point the conversation turns to the second part of the patient's initial compound statement. Beginning in line 10, the therapist might have begun another classical reality-confrontation, in the following way:

Example 13 (hypothetical)

9	Pt:	But I can't do it. I've tried all my life.
10	Dr:	Did you ever write a short story?
11	Pt:	Yes.
12	Dr:	Did you ever hold a job?
13	Pt:	Yes.
14	Dr:	Then how can you say you can't do it?

However, the therapist short-circuits this process by expressing his own position directly in line 10 of example 12: *Now we're back to 'I can't'. I won't accept 'I can't'*. That is, rather than posing a rhetorical question, he states his position directly. Nevertheless, example 12 is included here as a successful reality-confrontation on the grounds that it has been completed. There is a contradiction present, heard as a rhetorical question on the basis of lines 1 and 8.

The next example, again from Jill, includes two variations. Line 1, the intitial statement, and line 6, the disagreement statement or punch line, are variations on the model presented earlier. Consider the following:

Example 14 Jill

(1 Pt:)
2 Dr: Your behaviour and your functioning says, 'I'm a little girl. Take care of me. Enter my life, take over, and maintain it. Keep me as a little girl.' And you're bitching, 'I don't want to have anything to do with them. I don't respect them. I want to be independent.' You sound like that's, that's crazy. Would you agree with that's crazy?
3 Pt: (*pause*) Yeah. Well, I know I'm crazy. (*chuckle*)
4 Dr: Or would you rather be, um, intellectual, and we'll say that's ambivalent? How would that be?
5 Pt: No, I don't like that. That's not me (*?*). (*chuckle*)
6 Dr: Hah, isn't that nice? An intellectual? That'll get you, you know where that'll get you? Don't you? I'm telling you that's downright crazy.

Line 1 (the line left blank) of the disagreement is clearly a variation on the classical model of confrontation in which an explicit statement is made in the first line, since here there is no such explicit statement. The therapist, although he begins as if he is confronting the patient's immediately preceding statement, *I am not crazy*, is trying to confront her, not with any specific statement, but rather with a conclusion that he infers from her remarks throughout the conversation: that she really doesn't believe that she's crazy, even though she has shown crazy behaviour in the past. The general statement which is disagreed with, then, need not be made specifically, but can be inferred by the confronter from the confronted's other remarks. Line 6 is also a variation, in that the punch line, *You know where that'll get you, don't you*?, makes it sound as though there is a disagreement between them, even though there is not, since in line 3 the patient has already agreed with the therapist that she is crazy. Nevertheless, this example is included here on the grounds that the therapist is talking to the patient's subconscious level as much as to her conscious level of awareness.

Example 15 is the last of the 'variations' that deals with an appeal to the subconscious as well as the conscious level of awareness. It is quite far from the initial paradigm presented, and from earlier examples. Nonetheless there is a disagreement with a punch line. However, the punch line is not clearly in the form of a rhetorical question. Rather, it is a statement with an implied rhetorical question, *How could you be doing this*?, coming after the doctor's statement in line 14. The disagreement is also about the patient's action which is inferred in line 1, rather than about something that she has said. Finally, in line 21, the patient, in effect, 'steals' the real punch line by supplying the correct answer (she knows the nasal spray is addictive) to the therapist's inferred punch line in line 20. It is also, however, a more direct response as an elision, plus a reason to the therapist's yes/no question of line 20.

Example 15 Ellen

1 Pt: (*sniffs something*)
2 Dr: Can I ask you what were you just sniffing?
3 Pt: Neosynephrine.
4 Dr: Do you know what's in that?
5 Pt: No. I mean . . .
6 Dr: Just something you bought on the counter?
7 Pt: Yes.
8 Dr: Did you ask your doctor if you could use it?
9 Pt: I've always used it. No. Why do you say that?
10 Dr: Well, it's something like in the direction of the adrenalin family, epenephrine.
11 Pt: Is it really?
12 Dr: It affects your circulation.
13 Pt: . . . phenylepenephrine, hydrochloric . . .
14 Dr: And you who are pregnant and are so concerned about taking substances into your body that can affect your biology . . .
15 Pt: I never even thought about this, really.
16 Dr: This is a vaso-constrictive . . .
17 Pt: I never thought of it as a drug. You know, I never . . .
18 Dr: Adrenalin is something that relates to people's periods, and contractions of the smooth muscle . . .
19 Pt: Really?
20 Dr: . . . and little things like that, so I would wonder about your use of that. I would check it with him, would you? I had a vague feeling it was that, neosynephrine. I'd better tell you the second story about neosynephrine. It gives you relief for a while, doesn't it?
21 Pt: I know it's addictive, I know it. I'm so hooked, it's terrible.

In this excerpt, the potential for the punch line comes often and early. However, the doctor does not offer one, possibly because there is no statement 'on the floor' to be disagreed with. Instead, the doctor poses four quick questions to her which require brief answers (one fill-in and three *yes/no* questions in lines 2, 4, 6 and 8). Thus, in line 9 the patient takes control of the conversation, posing her own question, *Why do you say that*? The doctor's questions are in response to the patient's action: she has taken out a nasal spray (possibly) and used it. The punch line finally appears in line 14. The rhetorical question inferred is: *Why are you using neosynephrine if you are concerned with your health since you are pregnant*? The disagreement is also implied: the therapist doesn't think she should be using it; the patient obviously does, since she *is* using it. This is thus a major variation from the elements proposed as necessary for the successful completion of a confrontation; the disagreement is implied, and the rhetorical question aspect of the punch line must be inferred. However, this example is included as a variation of confrontation since, as in the last two examples, the therapist has moved the patient from possibly subliminal awareness to direct awareness. This confrontation is, then, a mild one. That it has been successful is evident, however, since in line 21 the patient 'steals' the punch line — she really does know that the drug she is using is addictive.

This next example from Jill is another variation of the confrontation routine. The essential elements are present in lines 1 and 10. There are two variations: the first is minor. That is, rather than a verifying procedure in the form of *yes/no* question/answer sets to ascertain if the punch line/conclusion is warranted, they speak almost simultaneously. There are three such verifying sequences. In addition, in the process, the doctor stretches each category presented. He shifts *appear strong* to *tough*, and adds *fuck you, tough*. She accepts *tough*, but rejects *fuck you*. The second variation is more important; that is, the punch line appears in line 10 in the form of a statement, *and yet, at the same time, you function on such a dependent level.* The unspoken, rhetorical question following that statement would be, *How come you do that*? This inferred punch line would then be analysed in the class of *why* questions already discussed.

Example 16 Jill

1 Pt: I felt, I have always felt that if I ever showed somebody how much I needed them, that they'd reject me and that the only way I can receive love is by, is by playing the role of not needing it, and of being kind of admired.
2 Dr: mmhm.
3 Pt: And, and ap, appearing strong. You know, this is how I was always
4 Dr: Tough.
5 Pt: brought up
6 Dr: Fuck you, tough.
7 Pt: to act.
8 Dr: Tough.
9 Pt: This is how both my parents wanted me to be. Not fuck you, but tough, and independent. And, uh, anyway I always had to put on this attitude of not needing anything, emotionally from either of them.
10 Dr: And yet, at the same time, you function on such a dependent level.
11 Pt: I know.

The therapist thus points out the inconsistency of her behaviour, which she accepts. This is permissible precisely because this is a therapy situation. For a friend to do so would appear impolite. In terms of the process, he encouraged her to state her position openly and directly and then without her being aware of it, he changes his position (having been previously agreeing with her) and then presents the punch line. While it is possible for her to disagree with his punch line and say, *I do not, I'm very independent. I've travelled all over the world, myself*, she does not. Hypothetically, she could disagree and provide a reason for disagreeing. As stated earlier, however, it is difficult for her to disagree, not only because the punch line is coming out of nowhere, but also because the therapist is the acknowledged expert. By making a professional observation, she would then have to question his expertise, something she is unlikely to do.

The last two examples presented in this chapter are variations in quite different ways. Example 17, taken from the Talmud, is a confrontation within a three-person conversation; and example 19 can be heard as a joke. Example 17 also contains an analogy.[10] It is rewritten in conversational form and presented here for its confrontation features:

Example 17

1 Emperor: (*to Rabban Gamaliel*): Your God is a thief, for did He not cause Adam to fall asleep and then steal one of his ribs?
2 Rabban Gamaliel's Daughter: Call the police!
3 Emperor: What has happened?
4 Daughter: A thief entered my house last night, and took away a silver pitcher; but left a gold one in its place.
5 Emperor: Would that such a thief would come to me every night.
6 Daughter: Why then do you decry our God? Did he not steal a rib from Adam only to enrich him with a wife?

What this example shows us is that confrontation as an emerging event can occur at any point in a conversation. The fact that three people are involved in the conversation is extraneous to the activity. The confrontation essentially occurs between the daughter and the Emperor, who is the confronted. Certainly, the fact that the daughter is the third person enables her to speak line 2, *Call the police*! which does not follow directly from the Emperor's line 1. Had the Rabbi tried that, the Emperor could have asked in line 3, *What are you talking about? We're talking about God; why are you calling the police all of a sudden?* However, the essential elements of the confrontation are present, including a general statement which is presented in line 1 and a punch line presented in line 6. The punch line is 'unexpected', and in the form of a rhetorical question. The form of this confrontation follows the paradigm presented earlier; presentation of a general statement, movement to a specific statement (which turns out to be an analogy), and return then to the general statement in the form of a rheorical question. The disagreement is about what real theft is. The confronted, the Emperor, doesn't know where the 'specific' is going to be connected with a 'general'. Hence he is led down the primrose path and, in a sense, duped. He has participated in his own 'destruction'. The use of the analogy also makes this confrontation example a variation of the form.

The excerpt below is a hypothetical re-creation of this piece of conversation, which lays out the grounds for the disagreement between the confronter and confronted in a two-person conversation:

Example 18 Hypothetical re-creation of example 17

1 Emperor: Your God is a thief, for did He not cause Adam to fall asleep and then steal one of his ribs?
2 Daughter: If a thief takes a silver pitcher, but leaves a gold one, has he stolen anything?
3 Emperor: No.
4 Daughter: If God takes a rib but leaves a woman, has he stolen anything?
5 Emperor: No.
6 Daughter: Then why do you call our God a thief?

Implicit in this discussion is the agreement to the statements that gold is more valuable than silver and that a woman is more valuable than a rib.

Finally I come to the last of the variations in example 19, which has the character of a joke. It was offered by the sociologist Paul Lazarsfeld (1973) by way of a comment on the use of the word 'success' in confrontation. As will be very evident, 'success' refers only to reaching the conclusion, and does not imply that the confronted was convinced, although this also occurs. He points out that 'a clever patient could probably always turn the skit around. I recall the story about the patient who believes he is dead. The doctor asks him whether he knows that dead people cannot bleed; upon agreement, the doctor pricks his finger and the patient bleeds. He reaches the conclusion that, after all, dead people can bleed'. I have rewritten this in conversational form as follows:

Example 19

1 Pt: I'm not alive, I'm dead.
2 Dr: Do you know that dead people can't bleed?
3 Pt: Yes, I know that.
4 Dr: (*pricks patient's finger; patient bleeds*)
5 Pt: So dead people bleed after all.

This example contains the essential elements of a confrontation, including the general statement in line 1 and the punch line in line 4. What makes this a variation is the fact that the punch line takes the form of a demonstration, rather than a spoken rhetorical question, which is here merely implied. The joking character comes from the patient's response to being confronted; he draws a false conclusion from a faulty premiss. In addition, this example varies in that only one *yes/no* question is asked, which suggests the direction from which the punch line will come. Nevertheless, I imagine that actually having his finger pricked and really bleeding would still come as a surprise to the patient.

Summary of confrontation variations

Thus, to conclude the description of variations of confrontation, the necessary elements of a confrontation need to be present in order for the confronted to recognize that the activity has been accomplished. It is the punch line which makes the disagreement overt. However, either the general statement or the punch line, in the form of a rhetorical question, can be implied rather than be stated directly. The examples presented thus far employ finding an exception, shifting, making inferences and using the confronted's own logic against him. The examples suggest that a confrontation can potentially be located after any statement, since a confrontation is a disagreement. The disagreement maxim states that anything we say is subject to being disagreed with.[11] What makes these disagreements different are their persuasive character, encouraging the confronted to change his original position. I turn now to confrontation 'failures'.

Incomplete confrontations

This last section considers those excerpts which might have completed confrontations, but which did not. From the examples below, we will find that most often the punch line is not presented; hence, there is no confrontation and no overt disagreement between the two speaker/hearers. In addition, the punch line on occasion is replaced by an explanation of psychodynamics, i.e. an interpretation is offered. Thus, if the punch line is not offered, the conversation may become a different activity. The therapist instead explains the rules and goals of therapy to the patient.[12] Finally, if the *yes/no* question/answer format is not accepted by the patient (confronted) — for example, if an equivocal *maybe* is given instead — the reality-confrontation is again subverted. Confrontation can be subverted, then, temporarily or permanently if any of the basic elements for its production are absent. I turn now to these kinds of examples.

In the examples presented below, the punch line is not present in the proper form of a rhetorical question, and therefore the activity of confrontation has not been completed.

Example 20 Jill

1 Dr: I can't tell yah [what's schizophrenic about your appearance]. You're not that much different than a lot of the younger people today. OK?
2 Pt: They're all schizophrenic?
3 Dr: But from my point of view, they all look, a lot of them look schizzy to me.
4 Pt: Oh see that's where I feel that I can't relate to you.
5 Dr: You can't relate.
6 Pt: Because it's a whole different world.
7 Dr: A whole different general (?)
8 Pt: And I don't see it as schizophrenic. It's just a different set of esthetics and a different set of values.

This example is interesting because the patient attempts to confront the therapist. She disagrees with his assertion that her appearance is schizophrenic. However, the confrontation is not successful because the patient aborts her own beginning confrontation by not coming back in line 4 either with another closed-choice question or with the punchline. For example, a second closed-choice question might be, *How about Mark Spitz, the swimmer? He's only twenty-two. Is he schizophrenic?* Instead she says, *Oh see that's where I feel that I can't relate to you*. She has introduced a new subject, her ability to relate. And at this point the therapist ceases to co-operate in being the confronted; he becomes nondirective. Or she could have posed a rhetorical question as her punch line, as follows: *How can you say people are schizophrenic just because of the way they dress*? However, later on the therapist admits that they will have a problem. He says, *OK, here's an area where we'll have difficulties, where as a result of my not being on your generational level, I still have a problem*.

The next example, also from Jill, also lacks a punch line and is therefore not completed:

Example 21 Jill

1 Pt: Well, all I can gather is that there were just never any standards set for me.
2 Dr: By whom?
3 Pt: By my parents.
4 Dr: You just grew. They didn't ask anything of you? They were completely permissive.
5 Pt: Completely. I mean, they asked things from me, uh, you see I can't explain it, easily (?)
6 Dr: Don't explain it. Tell me. Do not explain it to me. I'm not a judge. You don't have to justify, just tell me. And I'll try to be of help.
7 Pt: I was brought up with the feeling that I was, well, first of all, basically alone, with nobody to rely on.

While this excerpt had the potential for a confrontation, the therapist does not speak in a confrontational way. This is probably due to the fact that the therapist has spent most of the session trying to motivate her to be co-operative, and just when it appears that she is being co-operative, he would not want possibly to undo the work he has done by such 'harsh' treatment. There is the possibility that the therapist might begin a confrontation sequence in line 4, since he asks two *yes/no* questions, *They didn't ask anything of you? They were completely permissive.* (The second sentence is heard as a question.) The patient, however, does not co-operate; that is, rather than giving a simple *yes/no* answer, she attempts to amplify her statement. It is possible that she has learned from her experience in the prior conversation where such brief answers might lead. She subverts this potential occurrence by amplifying her remark.

It is possible that line 4 might have led to a confrontation; we see this in the following hypothetical re-creation:

Example 22 Jill (hypothetical)

1 Dr: Your parents were completely permissive.
2 Pt: Yes.
3 Dr: You could come and go as you pleased?
4 Pt: Not exactly. I had to be home at certain times.
5 Dr: You could do whatever you wanted?
6 Pt: No.
7 Dr: Then how could you say they were completely permissive?

In addition, in line 6 of example 21, the therapist does not offer a punch line. Instead, he says, *Don't explain it. Tell me. Do not explain to me. I'm not a judge. You don't have to justify, just tell me. And I'll try to be of help.* Thus here he uses this opportunity to teach her the rules of therapy, how she should behave. And so, in line 7, she begins, *I was brought up feeling that I was, well, first of all basically alone, with nobody to really rely on.* This is really a victory for the therapist, as we see here the beginning of her co-operation from which a therapeutic alliance may be developed. In order for him to help her, she must begin by presenting personal material, which she does. This is an indication that she is co-operating and hence wants to get well.

Similarly, if the therapist does not follow the closed-choice questions with a punch line, there cannot be a successful completion of the activity. We see this in Example 23:

Example 23 Jill

1 Pt: Then I got very sick.

2 Dr: While you were away?
3 Pt: Yes.
4 Dr: What'd you get? Hepatitis? Or something?
5 Pt: No. Amoebic dysentery.
6 Dr: From needles or from other things?

The therapist's last line is not a punch line based on the immediate past question/answer sequence. For example, if he had said in line 6, *Why are you lying to me? I know for a fact that you've never had amoebic dysentery either here or away*, we would have had a confrontation sequence based on the *why* question. In fact, the therapist is trying to gain information in this sentence. He does not disagree with the patient's initial statement, and therefore an essential element is missing from the reality-confrontation paradigm.

From line 1 of example 23, we see that virtually any general statement can trigger a reality-confrontation production. It may seem unpromising to start with: *Then I got very sick*. But consider the following hypothetical example:

Example 24 Jill (hypothetical)

1 Pt: Then I got sick.
2 Dr: Were you ever nauseous or achey?
3 Pt: No.
4 Dr: Did you have an elevated temperature?
5 Pt: No.
6 Dr: Then how can you tell me you were sick?

In the next example, 25, instead of having a punch line in line 8, there is an explanation of the dynamics of the patient's past behaviour. That is, the patient starts out in line 1 with a statement of his behaviour. The therapist asks three *yes/no* questions (lines 2, 4, and 6) which are slightly longer than anticipated, and are spoken in a gentle tone of voice. If they are not answered in the *yes/no* format, it becomes harder to come back to the initial statement, since the second speaker would then control the floor. However, here the patient gives the expected brief and correct answers for a potential confrontation. But instead, in line 8 the doctor offers an interpretation where the punch line would come. The therapist uses another rule of therapy, namely, that the doctor can make an interpretation at any time. Of course, the doctor could have offered the punch line and confronted the patient; however, he chose not to and worked toward the same end, helping the patient become more aware, by offering an explanation. The key difference between the interpretation made in line 8 of this example and the hypothetical punch line in line 6 of example 24 is that, in this example, the interpretation is offered without any disagreement or hostility apparent in the preceding question/answer sequence. Therefore, while the form of a confrontation is followed, the disagreement and punch line in the form of a rhetorical question are not there for its accomplishment.

Example 25 Bill

1 Pt: (*coughs*) I guess I get into wanting some, well, like I said, when a paranoia starts, paranoia started, when I felt very isolated after coming out of the hospital and ta-, I wanted to talk to somebody, so here they are talking, talking to me.
2 Dr: Is that how it sounds to you like it began?
3 Pt: Yeah.
4 Dr: Being isolated, so you created a world within which you had a dialogue, huh?
5 Pt: Yeah.
6 Dr: Even though the world was a world giving you a rough time?
7 Pt: Right. Yeah. That's the way it,
8 Dr: That's fascinating, you know, what you're saying (*?*). Like kids who are isolated, live in imagination, and have imaginary playmates. Huh?
9 Pt: Um-mm.
10 Dr: You've heard about that. Did you do that as a kid?
11 Pt: Yeah. We used to make up stories about deers. Y'know. After seeing *Bambi*. Heh. (*laugh*)
12 Dr: What kind of stories?
13 Pt: I think there were a number of deers and, I pretended one time I was one of them. I feel like I kind of made an ass of myself during the whole, because I remember when I was much too old I imitated a deer, —

Finally, the last example of an uncompleted confrontation is based on supplying a non-preferred answer during the *yes/no* question/answer checkout phase of the confrontation routine. If other responses are offered, the continuity of the confrontation sequence may be destroyed, and the activity is at least temporarily foreclosed.

Consider the following example:

Example 26 Jill

1 Pt: I just want to be naturally attractive.
2 Dr: You just want to be naturally attractive. Tell me, were you born naturally attractive? Are you physically so constituted that you're naturally attractive?
3 Pt: Yeah, I have been at times. When I feel good.
4 Dr: What do you do about feeling good and being naturally attractive? Do you take care of yourself?
5 Pt: No.

6 Dr: Well how do people take care of themselves who, whose natural attractiveness shows through?
7 Pt: They, it just happens.
8 Dr: It just happens. You know you used that phrase a couple of times already, 'just'. I 'just want to', the 'just', 'just', you mean like (*click*) from the sky?

Here, the patient aborts a beginning confrontation in line 3 by saying *sometimes*, rather than the *no* which would move toward the classic example. Hence, the therapist has to give up confronting *I just want to be naturally attractive*, and finally confronts the general statement, *Natural attractiveness just happens*, that is implied by the patient's answer in line 3. In addition, instead of a punch line in line 8 as a contradiction to line 1, we have an observation. The therapist comments on Jill's use of the word *just* and its implications.

Summary of incompleted confrontations

Thus, whenever the punch line is not reached because it is omitted, or there is no disagreement between the speakers, or the punch line is replaced by an explanation, or the checkout routine is subverted, we have instances of potential, but uncompleted, confrontations.

Summary and conclusions

Reality-confrontation requires as a minimum: (1) an implicit or explicit disagreement between the two speaker/hearers, (2) a punch line arrived at in a nondirect way, (3) a punch line in the form of a rhetorical question which points out a basic inconsistency. We see this in the following paradigm:

TABLE 3.2 *Paradigm of ideal confrontation (revised)*

Step	Actor	Behaviour
1	Confronted	Makes general statement or one is inferred by the next speaker.
2	Confronter	Asks or implies a rhetorical question which contradicts the first speaker's statement.

This model does not imply that the intermediate steps cannot occur. The greater the number of intermediate steps, the greater the possibility of 'turn-offs' or derailments and of not reaching the punch line.

The activity of confrontation rests on its relationship to logic and reason. Its power is based on its ability to sanction inconsistency — an undesirable trait; its violation of the rules of everyday talk; and its denigrating aspects. The rhetorical nature of the punch line also serves to heighten its effectiveness, since it is difficult to respond to, and implies that the confronter knows for a fact that the confronted's statement is not true. This makes the confronted appear to have been lying, or to be stupid or incompetent. Each case of such indirect name-calling demands a response, since it is seen as a personal attack. Thus, confrontation as an exhortation to change is usually responded to, and the work of therapy begins to be accomplished.

Figure 3.1 gives a diagrammatic presentation of how confrontation may be accomplished.

Confrontation may be accomplished in its classical form by using a funnel process which includes two (but not many more) short *yes/no* or closed-choice questions, or 'invitations' which the respondent must take. The checkout procedure to see if the punchline is warranted does not have to be included, however. What is important is that the confronter gets to his punch line by stretching a category in the confronted's initial statement, shifting from a special case to a general proposition, and then basing his conclusion on this general statement, or, vice versa, presenting a specific instance which negates the general rule. Thus, category formation and negative reinterpreting are essential to developing the punch line.[13] The disagreement in the form of the rhetorical question may be strong or mild and stated or implied. Successful confrontation as used here means only that the punch line is reached, not that the confronted necessarily changed his or her mind. Confrontation failures, then, mean that the punch line has not been reached. If the disagreement is not there, or the punch line is not presented, or the routine is side-tracked or stopped, the routine will be subverted.

Without these two essential elements (the disagreement and the punch lines) we may end up as witness to another activity. There is some probability that it will be an interpretation of psychodynamics or the rules of therapy, moves that are always available to the therapist. Confrontation is based on an appeal to intelligence, and to a commonsense understanding of what is logical and what is real. Even someone behaving in a truly 'crazy' fashion has some relation to reality. Confrontation appeals to that connection, however tenuous, and attempts to build on it. Thus, confrontation is a kind of disagreement which is a denigration and, at the same time, an exhortation to change. Confrontation can be used in psychotherapy sessions to encourage the process of change and growth.

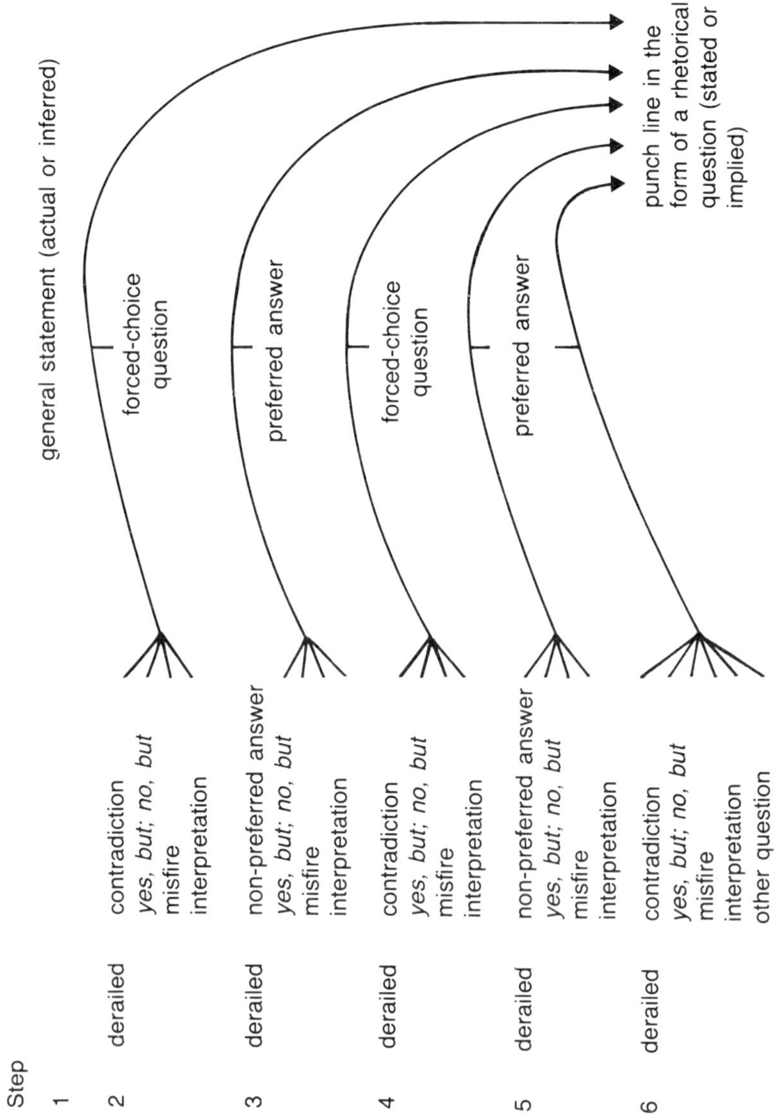

FIGURE 3.1 *Grammatical model of confrontation.*

Confrontation, as a conversational activity, has been analysed in this chapter on the basis of actual conversation, from an ethnomethodological point of view.

Notes to Chapter 3

1 I wish to thank Dr Milton M. Berger for making the data available and thank him and Dr Lindsey Churchill for helpful discussion in formulating this problem.
2 Another work — *Confrontation in Psychotherapy* (Adler and Myerson 1973)˜ came to my attention after my dissertation (Bleiberg Seperson 1981) was completed, and is not, therefore, discussed above. However, all the articles in this volume are psychoanalytically orientated, and have no direct bearing on the analysis presented here. Only 'Confrontation in short-term anxiety-provoking psychotherapy', by Peter E. Sifneos (Adler and Myerson 1973: 371-82) even includes an excerpt from a psychotherapy session as an illustration. My conversational analysis and Sifneos's psychoanalytically based conclusions support each other.
3 See Garfinkel's discussion of the *et cetera* clause in Garfinkel 1967, especially pp. 73–5.
4 Examples 1 and 2 and the analysis are from Bleiberg and Churchill 1975.
5 'Stretches' as the expansion of concepts is discussed in Bleiberg Seperson 1981: 95ff.
6 See Churchill 1978: 135 for further discussion of the rhetorical question.
7 See Clarence Schrag's (1967: 220–53) discussion of induction and deduction.
8 See Garfinkel 1967: 3, 41, 77 for a discussion of how we make ourselves understandable to others, in particular a discussion of the *et cetera* property and the retrospective/prospective properties of talk.
9 See Schopenhauer 1896 for an excellent discussion of argumentation strategies.
10 For discussion of this example as an analogy, see Bleiberg Seperson 1981: 120.
11 Bleiberg Seperson 1981: 79: 'Any statement or specific proposal question offered is subject to being disagreed with.'
12 See Bleiberg Seperson 1981, especially the discussion of rules and goals of psychotherapy in ch. 3.
13 For further discussion of category formation and negative reinterpretation, see Bleiberg Seperson 1981, ch. 5.

References

Adler, G. and Myerson, P. (eds.) 1973: *Confrontation in Psychotherapy*. New York: Science House.
Berger, M. M. 1970: Confrontation through videotape. In M. M. Berger, (ed.), *Videotape Techniques in Psychiatric Training and Treatment*. New York,: Brunner and Mazel.
Bleiberg, Susanne and Churchill, Lindsey 1975: Notes on confrontation in conversation. *Journal of Psycholinguistic Research* 4: 273–8.

Bleiberg Seperson, Susanne 1981: *The Language of Psychotherapy: A Conversational Analysis of Disagreement*. Ph.D. dissertation, City University of New York Graduate Center; Ann Arbor, Michigan: University Microfilms.

Churchill, L. 1973: Answering questions. In H. Ross, ed., *Perspectives on the Social Order*. Revised edn., New York: McGraw-Hill.

Churchill, Lindsey 1978: *Questioning Strategies in Sociolinguistics*. Rowley, MA: Newbury House.

Garfinkel, Harold 1967: *Studies in Ethnomethodology*. Englewood Cliffs, NJ: Prentice-Hall.

Garner, Harry H. 1970: A review of confrontation in psychotherapy from hypnosis to the problem-solving technique. In M. M. Berger (ed.), *Videotape Techniques in Psychiatric Training and Treatment*. New York: Brunner & Mazel.

Lazarsfeld, Paul, 1973: Personal letter to Susanne Bleiberg, 4 April.

Paredes, A. and Cornelison, F. S. 1965: *Development of an audiovisual technique in the rehabilitation of alcoholics*. Unpublished MS, based in part on a paper presented at the 19th clinical meeting of the American Medical Association in Philadelphia, November 1965. Cited in Berger 1970.

Schopenhauer, Arthur 1896: *The Art of Controversy*. New York: Macmillan.

Schrag, Clarence 1967: Elements of theoretical analysis in sociology. In L. Gross, (ed.), *Sociological Theory: Inquiries and Paradigms*. New York: Harper & Row.

Schulman, Evaline D. 1974: *Intervention in Human Services*. St. Louise: C. V. Mosby.

Wheelis, Allen 1969: How people change. *Commentary* (May).

4 A study of the verbal interaction in the initial phase of therapeutic discourse

Agnes Speck and Sabine Stitz

Data and interest of research

In the framework of our DFG-supported project, 'Verbal interaction in short-term therapy after attempted suicides', we have so far systematically analysed the therapy courses of thirty-one patients[1] under two aspects:

1. All session openings, i.e. the first few minutes of the therapy sessions were described with respect to discourse constitution; similarities and differences in speech patterns in such opening sequences were related to one another and to the overall therapeutical concept.
2. The therapy beginnings, i.e. the interactive flow of the respective first hour of a complete sequel, were described with regard to the question, which procedures lead from informal discourse to formal therapeutic communication and are used to guide towards the maxims of therapeutic treatment.

In addition to this, a corpus is being assembled which includes all implicit and explicit allusions and references to the suicide attempt. In a first examination of modes of referring to the suicide attempt (i.e. how utterances refer to this act), directness or indirectness, implicit or explicit reference, as well as the type of presupposition of these utterances, have been taken into consideration. In this context the description of the reciprocal relation of therapeutical interpretation and intervention (modification of the meaning of that which was expressed, reinforcement of the meaning expressed, misunderstanding), and of the process of determining meaning between therapist and patient, became very important (see Speck and Stitz 1984).

The principal concern of this chapter is to answer the question: how do both participants in therapeutic discourse make it clear to each *other* that they find themselves in a specific discourse with one another?

The chapter divides into two parts. First we consider, in fairly general terms, how institutional frameworks and a definition of the situation, which is to be worked out by the participants, can be linked together in discourse. In the second part, characteristics of therapeutic discourse, which formulate the beginning as a recognizable process, will be described.

Institutional constraint and definition of the therapeutic situation

The framework of a situation is determined by the institution within which it is embedded, to the extent that the activities engaged in by the participants are institutionally predetermined. If we assume that 'therapeutic discourse' must be established as the framework for a certain situation (because it initially appears to be just another category of 'conversation'), it becomes interesting to inspect the modalities of this transformation more closely.

For the most part, it is true of public institutions that they premodel the concerns of their potential clients in a sort of self-definition — the revenue and social welfare offices provide examples for this. For the agents of the particular institution, this creates conditions for taking action which imply restrictions on the relevances that may be attended. The external requirements for the analysed therapeutic talks are, among others, the following:

They take place in a clinic and not in a physician's office or at home; there are specific prerequisites for their realization:

1 The suicide attempt of the patient.
2 The hospitalization of the patient, the in-patient treatment which involved the first contact with the therapist; information and encouragement towards accepting the offer of therapeutic care in the clinic by this doctor. This means that the therapy discourse is to large extent institutionally bound: on the one hand by the external commitment to the clinic, on the other by the specific

stipulations which underlie therapeutic discourse. (See Klann 1977, 1978.)

These stipulations are decisively codetermined through expectations, intentions, conscious and unconscious purposes, emotions, wishes, etc., i.e. concealed aspects of mental states). A few remarks about the institutional stipulations should suffice to convey an impression of the experience which a patient has already had when he takes himself for the first time to a therapy session:

1 The procuring authority for the therapeutic relationship is the hospital.
2 The relation between physician and patient was brought about by the institution.
3 Over and above this it is settled that the case doctor (in his function as the first contact person after the suicide attempt) will be replaced more and more by the therapist; the institutional bind however is further ensured by a similar role relationship and the unchanged locality.
4 These therapies are — independently of the clinical stipulations, which must be met at the Münchener Klinik — a social organization, insofar as they 'serve a social purpose with the goal of treating the mentally ill, to free them from their disturbances as much as possible' (Flader *et al.* 1982: 20).

Characteristics of short-term therapy

Another important aspect of these therapeutic conversations is the fact that they take place on a short-term basis, i.e. the time available is extremely limited (twelve hours as a rule). The restricted number of hours, however, affords more than just disadvantages. The time restriction is seen as an important, constructive function in the therapeutic process. One expects that awareness of the time limit will produce greater activity and stronger interest in analysis on the part of the patient (cf. Mann 1978; Balint *et al.* 1973).

The goals of short-term therapy are primary prevention, prophylaxis and alleviation of suffering. The motivation of the patient and his co-operation, the directed interpretation (a repetitive intervention emerging from the attempted interpretations in the first session) as well as non-interpretative interventions (which serve to strengthen a sense of self-value and awareness of reality): all of these are important elements in the therapeutic proceedings.

Presentation of therapy concepts

In this section we shall present a brief characterization of the different therapeutic concepts employed by the doctors in our study.

Client-centred therapy (CT)

In 1942 Rogers, the founder of nondirective client-centred therapy, which was later called 'client-centred therapy' or simply 'Gesprächstherapie', postulated the following psychotherapist's variables as necessary and sufficient for constructive changes in clients in psychotherapeutic discourse:

1. Positive evaluation of as well as emotional warmth of the therapist towards the patient.
2. Empathy towards the patient's internal points of reference and the effort to convey that understanding to the patient.
3. Congruence (authenticity and integrity) in the attitude of the therapist towards the patient. (Tausch 1973: 75).

According to Rogers, client-centred therapy considers the essence of the therapeutic process to be the establishment of an understanding, benevolent relationship which should enable the client to learn to understand himself better. The therapist should restrict himself to simply being interested in the patient's feelings, and to reflecting the patient's utterances in a concentrated manner. This method should not function by intervention (i.e. it is nondirective) but puts great value on the patient finding his own way without being influenced by others.

Jankowski *et al.* (1976) note parallels to Gestalt therapy in the following common maxims:

- emphasis on the here and now (the past should not be explored)
- the 'be yourself' premiss (the patient can find solutions himself, and accordingly the therapist should not be considered an expert)

In the last few years other trends have become important in client-centred therapy; demands for other techniques, such as confrontation, were voiced, and began increasingly to alter the shape of the therapeutic process.

Depth psychology-orientated therapy (DPT)

In contrast to client-centred therapy, depth psychology-orientated models of therapy address to a much greater extent the patient's emotions, and aim to reveal the individual client's idiosyncratic share of perceptions, impressions and feelings.

Here, the therapist's comparatively more active role in the discourse has a greater impact on the delineation of the patient's problem. The therapist's contributions are not only participatory, but also intervening, biased and confrontational. In client-centred therapy, the therapist's effect is more retroactive, and is mediated through the techniques of reflection and the expectation of self-exploration. The early placement of a *focus* (in depth psychology-orientated therapy) is related to the active steering of the conversation on the part of the therapist.

Balint and Malan, who are acknowledged as the founders of so-called 'focal therapy', emphasize the importance of the collaboration of therapist and patient, so that the focus is not chosen, but gradually negotiated between therapist and patient (Balint *et al.* 1973: 197).

The 'crystallization of the focus' (Malan 1975: 210) is laid out in the initial hours of therapy, and further progress of the therapy is based on it; that is, the main theme of each session and the majority of the interpretations can be traced back to the focus. For the ideal case of focus finding (from the patient's point of view), Malan (1976: 256) formulated the following requirements:

(a) the patient has shown a good capacity to think of his problems in emotional terms;
(b) he apparently has the strength to face disturbing material;
(c) interpretations based on the focus have been given during the assessment period, and there has been a reasonably good response to them;
(d) he appears to have the motivation to face the stresses of therapy.

For therapeutic activity, this means a concentration on discovering the focus and its consequent treatment by interpretations and selective attention; the latter does not exclude acknowledging other problems.

Behavioural therapy (BT)

Behavioural therapy procedures are based on results of experiments in educational psychology. They proceed on the assumption that disturbances and modes of behaviour are learned, and that they can be influenced by new learning processes.

The basic principle of the methods of behaviour therapy is to acquire 'adequate' modes of behaviour, and to unlearn 'inadequate' ones. Whether it is sensible to adhere to a certain form of behaviour or not depends predominantly on the positive or negative consequences for the acting person. There is a greater probability that actions which lead to positive reactions or results will be chosen again, whereas the recurrence of modes of behaviour with negative consequences is comparatively less frequent.

In other words, modes of behaviour which are approved of by our environment will be 'reinforced'. Examples of such reinforcements are praise, recognition, love, affection or, in a more material sense, sweets, money, etc. Negative reinforcements, a reversal of the positive ones, are therefore disapprobation, ignoring, denial of sweets, blows, etc.

Behaviour therapy (BT) has long been regarded as an extremely controversial form of therapy; it has been accused of conditioning people, without considering their feelings, drilling them into 'correct' and 'false' modes of behaviour — like a Pavlovian dog. This situation has however changed in the last few years. Indeed, the criticism that behavioural therapy has no interest in the interior life of the patient, in his feelings and discernments, was taken up, and an attempt was made to incorporate thought and emotion into the therapeutic concepts (cf. the concept of 'cognitive behavioural therapy').

This new perspective of cognitive learning is primarily directed towards three therapeutical goals:

- improvement of perception
- improvement of motor or behavioural abilities
- improvement of associative abilities[2]

In psychiatry, behavioural therapy is being given more and more credence. This psychotherapeutic method is considered action-orientated; and 'in the process of therapy, realization ensues in any case after perception' (Dörner and Plog 1980: 398).

Characteristics of therapeutic discourse

In this section, after a discussion of some basic features of therapeutic discourse, we shall present an analysis of the conversational openings of seven client-centred and six depth-psychology-orientated therapies which is inspired by the ethnomethodological approach. In addition to this, twenty-eight sessions of six patients, who were treated by a physician orientated towards behaviour therapy, were examined in the light of two questions:

1 What is the shape of the discourse opening, i.e. the therapist's utterance which introduces the session and the reaction of the patient to it?
2 How does the beginning of the session develop?

The striking fact that the suspension and modification of conventional forms of communication plays a central role in therapeutic discourse has been described repeatedly (by Körfer and Neumann (1982), Lakoff (1980), among others. Familiar forms of (communicative) daily intercourse are replaced by 'new rules' which should be recognized and accepted. In this context, the question arises whether such phenomena can be observed already in the opening phase of the interaction.

We were especially interested in the question whether training in interactive forms of psychotherapeutic discourse takes place through explicit statements or by 'learning-in-interaction' (Körfer and Neumann 1982: 103).

The problem of 'beginning'

In his study of formal characteristics of therapeutic discourse Turner (1976) asks 'which characteristics of therapeutic discourse and of the social event "therapy" are responsible for the fact that the therapist can formulate "commencement" as a visible process (Turner 1976: 143).

Participants in interaction ordinarily know 'when' something begins because they possess methods of interpretation which include 'normal form expectations' and provide for the comprehension and accountability of everyday verbal interaction (Cicourel 1975: 89–94).

To what extent do these methods solve the problems which Turner suspects exist in regard to the beginning in group therapy — namely the transition from the informal to the formal part of discourse (who begins and how, as the first, to talk about himself and how is their activity made plausible in taking over from the preceding one?) These questions are analogously relevant to individual therapy, and should in the following part concern us in the analysis of the materials.

The main problems

Questions which arouse our interest, among others, are:

- how the participants organize a co-ordinated entry into the discourse;
- in what manner they bring forth and develop the peculiarity and typicality of the conversational situation;

- through which interactive procedures do they make their willingness to participate in the discourse accountable.

> The initial problem of availability: "that is, a person who seeks to engage in an activity that requires the collaborative work of two parties must first establish, via some interactional procedure, that another party is available to collaborate. It is clear that a treatment of a member's solution to the problem of availability might, at the time, stand as a description of how coordinated entry into an interactive course of action is accomplished." (Schegloff 1972: 372–3).

In the following sections, selected examples from the beginnings of client-centred therapy and depth psychology-orientated therapy are presented and compared. The final sections of this chapter are concerned with the beginning of behavioural therapy sessions.

Clarification of 'beginning' on the basis of client-centred therapy openings

Example 1

1 T: ya, even as a private person one hardly (.) ah: has the possibility of getting to the bottom of the situation
2 P: [yes exactly]
3 T: Ya, I'd (.) I'd say ah: (2) Let's perhaps *switch* over to what interests us more and where we have the possibility (.) to *do* something and (..) lend a hand where we're not so helplessly at mercy (...h) ah: (h...) (.) and why you also (.) *came* here now (1). For the most part I'll leave the initiative — about what you want to talk about and I'll try also (.h.h) to ask you as few questions as possible ↑ (.) but (.) actually try to make it clear together with you what's happening inside you (.) reflect to you what I (.) have understood ↑ .

Not all of the conversations are recorded right from the beginning of the interaction.[3] Utterance 3 indicates by the interaction-organizing introduction — *ya, I'd (.) say ah: (2) let's perhaps switch over to what interests us more*—that the discourse which had already taken place did not contain the instances of *what interests us more and where we have the possibility (.) to do something*. The therapist makes his activity accountable by 'formulating' it.

Garfinkel and Sacks (1976) regard 'formulating' as a constitutive characteristic of a conversation to the extent that it designates a conventional procedure of participants in interaction: 'saying-in-so-many-words-what-they-are-doing'. The therapist signals that he is aiming at an alteration in conversational activity and a change in the definition of the situation by indicating a 'shift'[4] at the beginning of and throughout his turn.

For the client, the formulation has an orientating function in multiple respects:

1 If the perspective of action of the speakers is made plausible in ongoing turns (3);
2 then it is made clear to him that the previous discourse is obviously lacking in some characteristics (because otherwise one would not have to switch over to something else), which the now-envisaged continuation of the discourse will now contain; and
3 it is signalled that the change of discourse implies a different quality.

With this beginning of the utterance, which is clearly a structuring start for the continued conversation, the therapist initiates a new phase of interaction which seems to be more therapy-specific, and more structurally appropriate than the previous phase: Between the announcement in 3, which alludes to that *(about) why you also came here now*, and utterance 1, a contrast is accented. In therapy there is the possibility of making things clearer; the security is that a professional guarantees the chance of 'lending a hand': the experience of the specialist reverses the layman's being 'helplessly at mercy' into a constructive 'doing'.

In (3) the therapist has visibly made himself available as a participant in the conversation, but not only that: in his reference to the reason for the meeting and his transformation of the (prior) mutual availability within a *we* into a differential distribution of interactive duties, a categorization of the participants takes place in a way which alludes to 'the social positions, which the acting persons have in their "heads"' (Cicourel 1973: 150).

Regardless of the client's 'level of knowledge' about the therapy setting, and the preconditions of therapeutic discourse, the therapist is presented in his function and social position as a professional, of whom it can be demanded that he makes the situation plausible (either in the form of questions which are posed or of expectations which are described). It can therefore be expected that the therapist will, in one way or another, provide an entry into the therapeutic situation at the beginning of the conversation.

Such a transition is necessary for example, when, after greetings, the weather is spoken about: a change of topic must be initiated by one of the participants, be it in the form of 'shifts', as in example 1, or in the form of the patient's initiative, as in the following example 2:

Example 2

1	P:	what should I tell you? Now I'm standing here
2	T:	[hehehe]
3	P:	now we have my problem (..) I mean
4	T:	ya (.) I would I would think (.) you ah should just say whatever is most important at the moment- at the moment (.) what (.hh) (hh.) -what you think is important (..)
5	P:	[Now I have]
6	T:	tell me what-what now is (.h) taking place inside you.

For the description of the sequential organization of the discourse beginning, the term 'slot' should serve to designate the expectancy of specific activities which can only appear in certain positions of a sequence (cf. Sacks 1972: 341).

> For example, a third strike can only be thrown by a pitcher after he has two strikes on a batter. Observations such as these lead to a distinction between a 'slot' and the 'items', which fill it, and to proposing that certain activities are accomplished by a combination of some item and some slot. (Sacks 1972: 341)

The perception of 'slots' and 'items', and the accountable occurrence or non-occurrence of the appropriate activities, is conveyed by rules of relevance; for example a greeting is to be expected as a response to a greeting. As Schegloff and Sacks (1973: 312) have elaborated with respect to the 'opening-up closing' procedures which participants employ to indicate that they intend to end a telephone call,

> . . .there are slots in conversation 'ripe' for the initiation of closing, such that utterances inserted there may be inspected for their closing relevance.

For our purposes, for the analysis of therapeutic conversational openings, we assume that 'slots' are used at the beginning of the session to signal the opening of the therapeutic discourse.

In example 2, the transitions from the informal to the formal part of the conversation is initiated by the patient's statement; her question provides the slot in 3 and elicits, therefore, a directive from the therapist.

A feature common to the discourse openings in examples 1 and 2 is that it is brought to the attention of one of the participants that the current conversation is not yet the 'right' one. Indications are the explicit comment in example 1 on the setting:

3 T: . . .and why you also (.) came here now

and the implicit reference in example 2 and the expectations connected to it:

3 P: now we have my problem,

which should be brought into conformity with the communicative situation.

A second common denominator of the two examples is to be found in the therapeutic directives which (to some extent) instruct the patient in respect to his conversational behaviour.

Clarification of 'beginning' on the basis of depth psychology-orientated openings

Both the previous extracts came from openings in client-centred therapy. By comparison, we would now like to present two depth psychology-orientated therapy openings.

EXAMPLE 3

1 T: if it bothers you [the tape recorder] just say so (*pushing a chair*)
2 T: need a light?
3 P: thanks
4 T: ya (.h) (.) how have you been doing after the (.) hospital?
5 P: ya, first of all I was really unhappy ↑ (.)
6 T: [(ya)]
7 P: that I
was at home and didn't for example never told
my mom (..) because she would've gotten awfully
8 T: [mhm]
9 P: worried and (.) would've gotten scared and
10 T: [mhm]
11 P: things never go very well for her ↑ (.) well she has
12 T: [mhm]
13 P: enough worries and ah I didn't want to (...) do that to her ↑

There is no doubt that the first turns 1, 2, and 3 are conducive to the establishment of the situation as a whole. The therapist's question in turn 4 seems to have a signal effect; the patient begins to report, and the ongoing conversation gives no indication that any lack of clarity exists between the two participants, whether they are already in the 'right' conversation or not.

Example 4

1 T: when exactly released I can't remember anymore
2 P: ah (.) week ago today
3 T: week ago today=
4 P: =ya
5 T: how've you been since then?
(1)
6 P: ya (.) well ah (.) not so hot (1) it had se/seemed
7 T: [mhm]
8 P: when I got home like everything was OK I was first at home on Thursday (.h) started cleanin' and tinkering right away on Friday morning ↑ (.) my friend was at work then . . .

A similar discourse opening in a slightly modified form can be found in this example; utterances 4 from example 3 and 5 from example 4 are semantically equivalent.

Constitutive element of the opening: 'Therapeutic directives'

Anticipating a result from our analysis, we can already make the following comments: there is one constitutive element of discourse openings common to client-centred therapy and depth psychological therapy: in the former the therapist always formulates a sort of directive for the patient at the beginning (with one exception) and in the latter the question *how's it going* is asked in a slightly marked form. The questions introduce a thematic working-out of the stages after release from hospital up to the present state of personal affairs. This observation led us to the assumption that these 'elements' have a therapeutically relevant function. One could then conjecture that, over and above their communicative characteristic, they have an instructive function, through which the beginning of the session is elucidated. In our data, it is obvious that the respective 'opening formula' is connected to the therapy concept: without exception the question is formulated by therapist B and the directive by therapist A.

Before we focus more closely on the patients' reactions, we would like to consider in more detail the problem of 'therapeutic directives'.

Therapeutic work demands from its participants certain orientations to their joint activity (cf. Flader *et al.* 1982; Haubl 1982, among others), which deviate from those customary in daily discourse. These orientations (which, for instance, in psychoanalysis are defined by the fundamental rule) can be designated as the speaker's and listener's maxims; they characteristically differ for the positions of therapist and client.

Instruction: function and meaning (client-centred therapy)

In client-centred therapy the orientations are made explicit by an 'instruction'. In the previously presented example 1, the therapist formulates in a concise instruction the premiss of conversational therapy — 'self-exploration' — for the patient, and indicates that 'reflection' and 'nondirective guidance' are the basic principles for the way the conversation will be conducted.

An obligation is established with the instruction, which makes a specific patient reaction expectable. This aspect of conditional relevance for the successive utterances will be presented in a later example.

Example 1

3 T: . . . For the most part I'll leave the initiative to you about what you want to talk about and want to try (.hhh) to ask you as few questions as possible (.) but (.) actually to try and make clear exactly what's happening to you and (.) to reflect to you what I've (.) *understood* ↑ from it.

This instruction addresses the following partial goals, to be realized in the course of the discourse:

(a) the interest in the inner condition/experience of the patient;
(b) concern that the patient should speak about what seems important to him;
(c) indication that the therapist asks no questions;
(d) indication that the therapist wants to explicate his understanding of the situation described in a parallel reflection.

In the evidence at our disposal, instructions are formulated in a varying complexity of forms in six out of seven client-centred therapeutic proceedings. the partial goal (a), interest in the patient's inner condition/experience, is invariable.

In the client-centred therapy opening which contains no instruction, the patient speaks of her fears on her own initiative. An instruction seems to be superfluous, as partial goal (a), to speak about oneself, is realized.

The observation is not trivial. Because a clear change of frame is in hand (indicated by the instruction) and the invariable element of the instruction contains the invitation 'to speak about his emotions', one can demonstrate on the basis of the data that the therapy situation only 'begins' then, when this invitation is formulated and taken up.

These instructions have a sequence-initiating function, and are conditionally relevant for the addressees, inasmuch as an implicit summons to action goes along with the directive which makes ensuing activity expectable.

One can react in three ways to the 'slot' which one participant assigns to the other. The addressee (in our case the client) can accept the offer (directive); then he behaves in a conditionally relevant manner, but he can also reject the offer or behave neutrally towards it (see Flader 1979: 30). In a reversal of Schegloff's observation that the initiator of the conversation (in his case the caller) has the 'first topic slot', and that there are no restrictions attached to this slot as there are no prior turns to refer to previous turns, the patient is free to choose a topic at his discretion after the therapist's initiative; this, however, with the restriction that he behaves in a conditionally relevant manner in light of partial goal (a).

Let's look at the previous example 2, focusing now on the patient's reaction.

Example 2

1 P: what should I tell you? Now I'm stand here
2 T: [hehehe]
3 P: now we have my problem (..) I mean
4 T: ya (.) I would- I would think (.) you ah should just say
whatever is most important at the moment- at the
moment (.) what (.hh) (hh.) -what you think is important (..)
5 P: [now I have]
6 T: tell me what- what now is (.h) taking place inside you
7 P: for example I have- it was like this ↓ -today it is Wednesday I was just
released=
8 T: =ya=
9 P: =(.hh) and then we go downhill and that's where our friends built the
house (.) . . .

In this example the instruction to the patient is, tentatively at first (5), and then successfully (7) ratified by the patient's performance of the relevant activity. In the organization of the turn assigned to her, she demonstrates that she has understood and accepted the instruction. From the sphere referred to by *whatever is most important at the moment-at the moment (.) what (.hh) (hh.) what you think is important (..)*, she selects an episode for the successive account; she makes this process visible by a structural signal at the beginning of the utterance (7): *For example I have*; thereupon follows the preface *it was like this*, to which she then links the narrative in 9.

The entrance into the conversation is not always free of complications. In the following conversational opening the patient's reaction is disapproving:

Example 5

1 (.hh) I (harumph) actually leave it quite open to you ↑ (.) ah- (..) what you- (.) *about what* you'd like to speak- *what* you'd like to say (1) what's bothering you so much right now (.) (harumph)
2 P: ya ask me something
3 T: mhm (.) I didn't want to actually
4 P: [you more or less know my situation]
5 T: [ya I didn't really want to ask actually- (.) interrogate you but- ah- (.) it's important to me (.hh) that you address *what's* at the moment (.) (.hh) (harumph) *currently* ↑ (1) important to you-(..) eh: on your own initiative=
6 P: =let's say you know the present situation is purely a question of finance.

The therapist's invitation 'to begin recounting' is not accepted, the conditional relevance is not fulfilled. The patient returns the floor to the therapist, in turn 2, in the form of a 'pass-back', and demands a specification of the therapist's instruction. He explains in 5 the part of the instruction in which are described the interactants' duties which are relevant to the client and patient in client-centred therapy. In turn 6, the patient demonstrates willingness to co-operate through her ratification; the information she could supply by (as the therapist asks her to) talking *about what's bothering you so much right now* is presumed to be 'known' by the therapist.

The opening question: function and meaning (depth psychology-orientated therapy)

It remains to be clarified how the therapist's opening moves — question rather than instruction — work in depth psychology therapy. Is it conceivable that this 'question' has a similar function for the opening and for the actual beginning of therapy as the 'instruction'? The conversational openings are introduced with the sequence-initiating questions 'how did it go?' or 'how have you been since release from hospital?'. Although these questions may not seem too fraught with meaning, they are relevant as a connection between that which was, the stay in hospital, and the 'here and now', the first encounter of therapist and client after release from hospital. Freud speaks of a 'Monday crust' (Freud 1967: 187) which forms after such a short pause from treatment such as the weekend, and which must be broken up.[5]

Example 4

1 T: when exactly released can't remember any more?
2 P: ah (.) week ago today
3 T: a week ago today=
4 P: =ya
5 T: how've you been since then?

As a rule the patient's problem range is worked out thematically from 'outside' to 'inside' in the course of the conversation following the therapist's introductory question, and is thereby reduced; i.e. the patient's portrayal of problems, elicited and guided by the therapist, begins with the hospital stay and is then successively narrowed down to personal conflicts.

This 'development-orientated' interest leads to a specific working out of information/questions, which can all be traced back to the openings. When the patient renders a complete account, as in example 4, which ends in a general portrayal of problems, then she is nevertheless requested to terminate the orientation:

Example 4 (continued)

26 P: . . . I would never have had to take that from my husband — none of your goddam business and we never dealt with each other like that. We never spoke like that
27 T: [mhm]
y'know? (.hh) so I can't say it's been goin' good I wish ah
28 T: [how is it ah that we got a bit of a general view how it was up to today (.) how it'll go on]

Thus, at a sequentially propitious position, the patient had placed the prestructuring phrase *ya (.) therefore ah (.) not so good* ahead of her story in reply to the question in 5.

The information/questions have a double function: in that they connect to the last conversation/last meeting they confirm and sustain the interpersonal relation and, at the same time, they serve to achieve a common knowledge-base.[6]

The conversational openings, which are all without exception started[7] with the 'opening question', are ratified by the performance of an appropriate activity; the patient's replies are detailed and centre quickly on problems. Here also it becomes evident that if the patient does not on his own initiative, start speaking about his personal feelings, a problem area is addressed by the therapist.

By formulating 'real' questions, however, the conversational steering is more pointed.

Example 6

5 T: =when did you come back? from the cure?
11 T: you were there (.) at your sister's if I remember correctly? no?
14 T: so you had (.) a real vacation there?
16 T: ya (.) and now you are (.) since when are you back?
19 T: mhm (..) and how are you doing now?

The 'opening question' is formulated in everyday terms; no therapeutical gesture adheres to it. The answer to the question, which usually serves phatic purposes, is hard to withhold since it (1) aims at a convention of politeness between speaker and (2) stresses the 'constitution of normality' in the framework of the therapeutic setting. The 'opening question' signals a stronger symmetry between the two interactants than the 'instruction'.

Moreover, the adressee of the 'opening question' has more alternatives for action at his disposal than in the case of the instruction; he is freer in choosing his 'first topic', and does not have to meet any other restrictions. Evidently a discourse opening organized in this manner is felt by the participants to be 'appropriate'. There are no comparable conversational pecularities as in client-centred therapy openings, whether in respect to a change of frame, as in examples 1 and 2, or a patient's negative reaction, as in example 5.

The comparison of data of openings bound by different therapy concepts confirms this thesis.

Comparison of the therapists' initiatives

To return to the question posed in the earlier sections 'The problem of "beginning"' and 'The main problems', the presentation of different openings should have shown that the explicitness of the setting conveyed by the 'instruction' arouses irritation in the addressee. Obviously the attitude 'what happens here is nothing special' is invalidated by the instruction (cf. Emerson 1974, who characterizes this attitude as a background rule which exercises a normality-constituting function in the context of social interaction) in contrast to the 'opening question' which ensures precisely this attitude.

Concurring features which can be found in both conversational therapy and depth psychology-orientated openings are the following: The therapist-initiated sequence is the rule (two exceptions can be found in the conversational therapy data). The instruction in client-centred therapy fulfils the same function as the question does in depth psychology therapy. Both elements can be characterized as directives which initiate the beginning of therapy. They are located in the same sequential position, and therefore use the same slot. For the participants, the organization of the beginning of discourse is more fixed thematically by the 'instruction' than by the 'question'.

Behavioural therapy: conversational openings

In our exploration of therapy session beginnings, we focused on the point that these beginnings are shaped in a special form, helping the participants to constitute a therapeutic conversation. In the following section, we want to show the composition of this form. As an illustration, we will examine the conversational openings of the behavioural therapy sessions.

At the beginning of each conversation, we observed a specific regularity in organizing the first communicative activities by the participants, which we will call 'normal form' pattern. Methodologically, our analysis is based on the assumption that these conversational openings are constituted by criteria of coherence, formal structure and pragmatic principles. We analysed the function of these utterances, and showed how features of the interactional organization (characteristics of structure, type and place of utterance) are related to the realized form of 'action chains'.

Every therapy session is started by the therapist with the question: 'How's it going? (How are you?)' which the patient learns to answer in slightly changing ways as he accumulates therapeutic experience. In the first session the patient replies:

Example 7

1 T: ya (.) (How's it going?)
2 P: good now actually

The question is therefore answered with the commonly corresponding reply. However, the patient also offers another topic with the time clause *now*: the information that it's going *good now actually* could induce the therapist to ask the question: when weren't you feeling well and why?

The therapist steers towards a different kind of understanding of his question, in that he simply allows the reply to pass (and does not respond to the implicit offer of a new topic):

Example 7 (continued)

1 T: ya (.) (how's it going?)
2 P: good now actually
3 T: ya
4 P: could say so
(2)
5 P: (I) rested at the weekend
6 T: mhm
7 P: got a bit clearer to me (a)bout how it is with my friend (.) moved out of the flat . . .

The patient has confirmed (4) the first reply (2); the theme *how's it going*? is completed after the exchange (3 and 4). She leaves the next move, which initiates a new topic, to the therapist. He, however, leaves the conversational move vacant; the change of topic which is not forthcoming implies an invitation to further discourse. After a two-second pause, the patient changes plans with her answer (5): She translates the therapist's question (1) into the past: 'how were you?' — which she answers with an extensive report.

In the eighth hour's session with the same patient, the beginning of the session looks like this:

Example 8

1 T: how's it going
2 P: very well. I had a nice week (.) Test was pretty good y'know it (.) wasn't (.) at all so bad as he (.) he had said before.

(A detailed description of the test in general follows, in which an account of the patient's special condition is inserted.)

The expectation of courtesy of the 'how's it going? question is minimally fulfilled, and serves as a transition to the report about the most important events of the last week. The question has become the request: 'report on the recent period, that which was important to you.'

In a fashion similar to everyday use of language, therefore, specific (and, occasionally, rather idiosyncratic) interactive routines and conventions are developed over time, and they depend on experience and repetition. These are not general regulations, but the result of establishing certain modes of behaviour as mutually expectable in specific situations. Such an establishment can be achieved not only implicitly (as in these examples) but also explicitly.

The therapist's implicit request to report on the recent past has a further function. The patient is prevailed upon to organize 'her' therapy situation. She does this by bringing the past into the present situation of discourse, and thereby initiating a situation of perception for the therapist and herself which thus becomes a 'show and tell' situation. The complexly organized temporal and personal deictic structure is conspicuous. Referring to Bühler 1934 and Ehlich 1979, Flader *et al.* 1982 suggest three zones of reference which a speaker opens to the listener by means of deictic expressions (in the broadest sense): the (for speaker and listener mutually accessible) 'Sprechzeit- und Wahrnehmungsraum', the 'Rederaum', which is opened when something is shown inside the temporal or local organization of a 'Rede-' or 'Textentwicklung'; finally the 'Vorstellungsraum' (Bühler's 'Phantasma').

Example 7 (continued)

5 P: (I) rested at the weekend
6 T: mhm
7 P: got a bit clearer to me (a)bout how it is with my friend (.) moved out of the flat . . .

The referents of words and phrases which achieve the 'embedding' of the talk within the situation are directly available within the temporal and perceptual space of the situation.

In this example the function is explicitly fulfilled by *now* (2): *now* the patient is *good actually*, and everything else is described by reference to it, either the reasons for this 'going good now' (the 'now' of the situation is always based on past events, actions and emotions) or the previous 'going bad'.

If the 'Vorstellungsraum' in each case is set forth, the speaker specifies the temporal-spatial reference system to orientate the hearer (at the weekend (6)) to the actions and events (7) which he wants to refer to with deictic expressions. If a 'Sprechzeit- und Wahrnehmungsraum' is initiated and marked as a 'Vorstellungsraum' in which the patient and therapist put themselves, then the way is paved towards one of the main goals of behavioural therapy. The behavioural therapist proceeds, not on the premiss that something which happened in the past can no longer be changed, but that from this, something can be learned for the future; and the therapist guides the patient towards realization of this change in therapy.

Behavioural therapy commencement of discourse

The observation of the first five minutes of therapy discourse beginnings has led to the assumption that therapy sessions are opened by 'normal form' patterns of conversational openings.

Structure of phases of discourse openings

1 therapist's question ('How's it going?);
2 patient's reply in the form of a story or report (interrupted by hearer signals, therapist's understanding checks);
3 (reflecting) focusing of the therapist;
4 patient's reaction: comprehension question completion/emphasis on a detail of the description which remained unclear in the reply section;
5 solution by the therapist negotiation or confirmation of the patient's (offered) comprehension (optional link);
6 change of topic/attention.

In this analysis we have given the reply (2) and the focusing—reaction—solution (3, 4, and 5) special attention.

In all cases the *reply* dealt with a report or an account (in the context of the therapist's initiating question); the internal structure of both conversational activities, in light of the connection between the process of presentation and the process of the actions/events portrayed, as well as the *embedding* within the context, have been analysed. A difficult temporal structure can be seen in each one of these discourse beginnings. Surprisingly, discrepancies often appear between the temporal course of that which is portrayed and the temporal structuring of the portrayal, especially in the central part of the patient's discourse. Within the beginning of the conversation, high-grade sensitivity or obstinate insistence (in order to clarify temporal inferences) is exacted from the therapist during the patient's portrayal.

Focusing-reaction-solution stand in a systematic correlation to *reply*. On the basis of our characterization of the individual activities taken by client and therapist respectively, we pointed out that three routinely executed conversational activities are connected as a 'chain of action', bound together by conditional relevancies. Connected to this was the question of facultative versus obligatory members of this chain, and of the reference points of the relevancies.

Information is gleaned from the systematic interrelation of verb tenses and other temporal expressions, and from the reconstruction of the scheme of reference of the utterance in question. That is, the repetition by remembering has two effects; it provides the therapist access to the patient's experience. In the patient it gives rise to the (re)creation of (his) world, to a re-actionalization of experiences in a changed form — even when one supposes that the simple expression in words is such a form. It is important for the therapist to obtain the most exact information about the biographical context of the utterance as well as the actual situation of the patient, if he does not want to be utterly susceptible to his personal interpretations.

At the end of the patient's report a (reflective) focusing by the therapist usually ensues. He selects, either from that which has just been heard, or from what he knows about the patient and his circumstances, an element to which the attention of the discourse should be dedicated. Through focusing, the therapist reduces the margin of comprehension which had been opened for both participants by the patient's portrayal; the therapist refers to/takes a position on a feeling or attitude of the patient which the latter (possibly) had during the portrayal, i.e. in the here and now of the therapy session. If the therapist resorts (for the first time) to therapeutical discourse guidance (focusing), he therefore intervenes in the structure of the patient's experimental world as it is expressed in his words (within which he, the therapist, has installed himself through strategies of perception and interpretation).

Closing remarks

At the beginning of our article we had inquired how the participants in the therapeutical interaction clarified the beginning of therapy. The opening of the behavioural (as shown above), client-centred, and depth-psychology-orientated therapy sessions are realized in a normal form pattern. The specific function of this pattern is to increase the participants' confidence in the situation by using a pattern which has become predictable through repetition. It was easily demonstrated that, in client-centred therapy, a 'pivot' is made visible which, due to its characteristics, announces the beginning of therapy. But what about the comparatively 'inconspicuous' questions of the other two therapists: 'how's it going??

This question is neither more articulate as a therapeutic activity nor more closely linked to the therapy concept. Nevertheless, the question is understood by patients as a signal for the start of therapeutic discourse. Proof of this is to be found in the replies.

We assume that the relevance of an utterance cannot be clarified without taking into account the social context as well as the conclusions, which can be read from the actions connected to them. Means of categorization (used by participants in observers of a certain situation) are applied on the basis of certain rules which facilitate the perception and comprehension of the interactive situation. This 'identification of actors' is designated by Sacks (1972) as a 'membership categorization device'; it results from a categorization of a population or group with some related characteristics, such as sex or age.

For our data we suspect that the operation of the membership categorization device comes from the client's side, and connects with his definition of the situation. He assigns the therapist to a category 'professional/helper', and this category (in this case) is bound up with the execution of certain verbal activities. When the question 'how did it go?' is asked of him at the beginning, he makes use of a specific listener's maxim, induced by the categorization device. Thereby he knows that a different verbal activity is expected of him from that required in an everyday communicative situation.

We have thus ascertained that the therapeutic situation functions by setting up a framework, and also that the comprehension of the particularities of that situation are worked out by the participants and are made reciprocally available. An astounding conclusion lies in the observation that — other than in client-centred therapy — the lack of an orientation to a specific activity is not felt to be a loss but, instead, has a symmetry-creating function.

Notes to Chapter 4

1 An overview of all data can be found in the Appendix to this chapter.
The project on therapeutic discourse, sponsored by the German Research Foundation (Deutsche Forschungsgemeinschaft) was initiated in 1983 by the present authors at the Fachbereich Germanistik of the Free University Berlin under the direction of Norbert Dittmar. We are indebted to the DFG and the FU for their offer of facilities and administrative support. The data of the project come from the Psychiatrische Poliklinik rechts der Isar München, where psychological research on therapies after suicide attempts is done under the

supervision of H. J. Möller. We are grateful for the collaboration of the clinic in Munich. In particular, we are indebted to A. Torhorst for important comments with respect to methodological aspects of short therapies. More detailed information about the project in Munich can be found in *Archiv für Psychiatrie und Nervenkrankheiten* 1982: 232; 1983: 233, and in *Psychiatrische Praxis* 1982: Heft 1 and 4. An outline of the linguistic part of the project carried out in Berlin is available.

2 Cf. the special edition of *Psychologie Heute* 1980.

3 We have used the following transcript notation:

1 ? . = punctuation is used to mark grammatical units
2 (.) (..) (...) = (untimed) intervals between utterances
3 (1) (2) (3) . . . = pause between utterances, timed in seconds
4 = = when there is no interval between adjacent utterances, the utterances are linked together with = signs
5 [ ] the point at which an ongoing utterance is joined by another is marked with a single square bracket; the point where overlapping utterances stop overlapping is marked with a square bracket at the end of the utterance
6 spoken emphasis is indicated by italics
7 (.h) = audible aspiration
8 eh:: = a colon indicates an extension of the sound or syllable it follows
9 [$_{\text{hehehe}}$] = overlapped laughing
10 (harumph) = brackets indicate a nonlinguistic vocal activity
11 ↑ ↓ = marked rising and falling shifts in intonation
12 (a)bout = transcriptionist doubt is indicated by single parentheses which encloses the items in doubt

The transcript notation used here follows the one developed by Gail Jefferson (cf. Atkinson and Heritage 1984).

4 Ervin-Tripp (1972) designated these allusions as 'shifts' (1972: 213).

5 '. . . infrequent work brings with it the danger that one cannot keep up with the patient's real experience, that the "cure" loses control with the present and is forced into byways' (Freud 1967: 187).

6 'In order to communicate about things which are socially recognized and regarded as self-evident, the acting persons in daily life must make certain prerequisites about that which the neighbour knows, and how they know the "same" fact (Cicourel 1970: 304).

7 The 'question' is not always recorded. In two cases it is lacking, but can be reconstructed on the basis of the patient's reply.

References

Atkinson, J. M. and Heritage, J. (eds.) 1984: *Structures of Social Action: Studies in Conversational Analysis*. Cambridge: Cambridge University Press.

Balint, E. (ed.) 1975: *5 Minuten pro Patient. Eine Studie über die Interaktionen in der ärztlichen Allgemeinpraxis*. Frankfurt/Main: Suhrkamp.

Balint, M., Balint, E. and Ornstein, H. 1973: *Fokaltherapie. Ein Beispiel angewandter Psychoanalyse*. Frankfurt/Main: Suhrkamp.

Bühler, K. 1934: *Sprachtheorie. Die Darstellungsfunktion der Sprache*. Jena: Fischer.

Cicourel, A. V. 1973: Basisregeln und normative Regeln im Prozess des Aushandelns von Status und Rolle. In Arbeitsgruppe Bielefelder Soziologen (ed.), *Alltagswissen, Interaktion und gesellschaftliche Wirklichkeit*, vol. 1. Hamburg: Rowohlt.

— 1975: *Sprache in der sozialen Interaktion*. Munich: List.

Dörner, K. and Plog, U. 1978: *Irren ist menschlich oder: Lehrbuch der Psychiatrie und Psychologie*. Wunstorf: Psychiatrischer Verlag.

Ehlich, K. 1979: *Verwendung der Deixis beim sprachlichen Handeln*. Frankfurt/Main, Bern, Las Vegas: Peter Lang Verlag.

Emerson, J. P. 1974: Was hier geschieht ist wirklich nichts Besonderes. *Gruppendynamik* 2.

Flader, D. 1979: Techniken der Verstehenssteuerung im psychoanalytischen Diskurs. In D. Flader and R. Wodak Leodolter (eds.), *Therapeutische Kommunikation*. Königstein/Ts: Scriptor.

Flader, D., Grodzicki, W. and Schröter, K. (eds.) 1982: *Psychoanalyse als Gespräch. Interaktionsanalytische Untersuchungen über Therapie und Supervision*. Frankfurt/Main: Suhrkamp.

Freud, S. 1967: *Studienausgabe. Schriften zur Behandlungstechnik*, vol. II. Frankfurt/Main: Fischer.

Garfinkel, H. and Sacks, H. 1976: Uber formale Strukturen praktischer Handlungen. In E. Weingarten, F. Sacks and J. Schenkein (eds.), *Ethnomethodologie. Beiträge zu einer Soziologie des Alltagshandelns*. Frankfurt/Main: Suhrkamp.

Haubl, R. 1982: *Gesprächsverfahrensanalyse*. Frankfurt/Main and Bern: Peter Lang Verlag.

Jankowski, P., Tscheulin, H., Fietkau, H. J. and Mann, F. (eds.) 1976: *Klientenzentrierte Psychotherapie heute*. Göttingen, Toronto and Zürich: Verlag für Psychologie Dr. C. J. Hogrefe.

Klann, G. 1977: Psychoanalyse und Sprachwissenschaft. In F. Hager *et al.* (eds.), *Die Sache der Sprache*. Stuttgart: Metzler.

— 1978: Sprache in der Psychoanalyse. *Studium Linguistik* 5.

Körfer, A. and Neumann, C. 1982: Alltagsdiskurs und psychoanalytischer Diskurs. Aspekte der Sozialisierung des Patienten in einen 'ungewohnten' Diskurstyp. In D. Flader, *et al.* (eds), *Psychoanalyse als, Gespräch. Interaktions- analytische Untersuchungen über Therapie und Supervision*.

Lakoff, R. T. 1980: *Psychoanalytic Discourse and Ordinary Conversation*. Berkeley, Mimeo.

Malan, D. H. 1975: *A Study of Brief Psychotherapy*. New York: Plenum Rosetta.

— 1976: *The Frontier of Brief Psychotherapy: An Example of the Convergence of Research and Clinical Practice*. New York: Plenum.

Mann, J. 1978: *Psychotherapie in 12 Stunden. Zeitbegrenzung als therapeutisches Instrument*. Olten and Freiburg/Br.: Walter Verlag.

Psychologie Heute, Sonderband 1980: *Neue Formen der Psychotherapie*.

Rogers, C. 1942: *Counselling and Psychotherapie*. Cambridge, Mass.: The Riverside Press.

Sacks, H. 1972: On the analyzibility of stories by children. In J. J. Gumperz and D. Hymes (eds), *Directions in Sociolinguistics: The Ethnography of Communication*.

Schegloff, E. A. 1972: Sequencing in conversational openings. In J. J. Gumperz

and D. Hymes *Directions in Sociolinguistics: The Ethnography of Communication*.
Schegloff, E. A. and Sacks, H. 1973: Opening up closings. *Semiotica* 8.
Speck, A. and Stitz, S. 1984: Entweder Du liebst mich oder ich bring mich um. In H. Krenn, J. Niemeyer and U. Eberhardt, (eds.), *Sprache und Gesellschaft. Akten des 18. Linguistischen Kolloquiums Linz 1983*. Tübingen: Niemeyer.
Tausch, R. (ed.) 1973: *Gesprächspsychotherapie*. Göttingen: Hogrefe.
Turner, R. 1976: Einige H. formale Eigenschaften des therapeutischen Gesprächs. In H. Auwärter, (ed.), *Seminar: Kommunikation. Interaktion und Identität*. Frankfurt/Main: Suhrkamp.

Appendix

Tables

Age Group

Number of patients	Age in years
5	10–20
12	20–30
10	30–40
3	40–50
—	50–60
1	60–70

Number of Therapy Hours

Number of patients	Number of sessions
2	1
5	1-2
1	1-3
5	1-4
2	1-5
4	1-6
—	1-7
3	1-8
2	1-9
1	1-10
1	1-11
2	1-12
4	12 and more

Profession

Number of patients	Profession
2	businessmen
17	employees
1	worker
4	Civil servants in social professions
2	housewife
3	pupils
2	unemployed

Distribution of patients to therapists/therapy concepts (Client-centered therapy: CT; Behavioural therapy: BT; analytically orientated therapy: PA1; analytically orientated therapy: PA2.)

Number of patients	Therapists/ therapy concepts
13	PA1
5	PA2
7	CT
6	BT

Transcripts

EXAMPLE *1*

1 T: ja man hat wohl auch als Privatmann kaum(.) äh die
Möglichkeit die Situation zu durchschauen
2 P: [ja ganz gewiß]
3 T: (.h) ja aber ich würd (.) ich würd sagen äh (2) *gehn*
wir zu dem über was uns beiden vielleicht mal näher liegt
und wo mer die Möglichkeit ham etwas zu *tun* und(.hh)
selber Hand anzulegen wo mer net ganz so hilflos ausge-
liefert auch ist (.hhh) äh(hhh.) (.) und wozu Sie jetzt
auch hierher(.) *gekommen* sind.(1) Ich überlass im wesent-
lichen Ihnen so die Initiative wovon Sie sprechen möchten
und will auch versuchen (.hhh) Ihnen möglichst wenig
Fragen zu stellen ↑ (.) sondern (.h) eigentlich versuchen
mit Ihnen gemeinsam zu verdeutlichen was so bei Ihnen
vor sich geht und(.) Ihnen des widerspiegeln was ich
davon *verstanden* hab ↑

EXAMPLE *2*

1 P: was soll ich Ihnen jetzt erzählen? Jetzt stehe ich da
2 T: [hehehehe]
3 P: jetzt habn wer mein Problem (..) ich mein
4 T: ja(.) ich würd ich würd meinen(.) Sie äh sagen ganz ein-
fach des was Ihnen im Moment im Moment einfach am nächsten
liegt(.) was (.hh) (hh.) was Sie für(.) wichtig halten (..)
5 P: [ich
hab jetzt]
6 T: mir zu sagen was jetzt in Ihnen so (.hh) vor(.) geht=
P: =ich hab zum Beispiel es war so ↓ wir sind doch am am Mitt-
woch bin ich entlassen worden=
7 T: =ja ↑ =
8 P: =(.hh) u:nd da fahrn wir übern Berg runter und da haben un
sere Freunde das Haus geba:ut(.) und da fahrn wir also
vorbei ( ) also ich fahr immer vorbei (.hh) und da sagt
9 T: [mhm]
10 P: mein Mann sagt er "also(.) du kannst dich jetzt entscheiden
entweder X so heissen die mit Nachnamen oder ich"(..)
11 T: [mhm]
12 P: da hab ich gesagt"also du stellst mich ja wieder vor eine(.)
äh äh des ist ja direkt Erpressung" ↑ sag ich (..) ich bin
13 T: [mhm]
14 P: noch net amal zuhause (.hh) und da kommt des scho"(1) ne? (.) . . .
15 T: [mhm]

Example 3

1 T: wenn es Sie stört((das Gerät)) sagen Sie's (Stühlerücken)
2 T: Haben Sie Feuer?
3 P: Danke
4 T: ja (.h) (.) wie ist es Ihnen jetzt gegangen nach dem(.)
Krankenhaus?
5 P: ja erstenmal war ich wirklich froh ↑ (.) daß ich zuhause
6 T: [ja]
7 P: war und hab's aber zum Beispiel meiner Mutter hab ich's
nie gesagt (..) weil die hätt sich jetzt dann wahnsinnig
8 T: [mhm]
9 P: Sorgen gemacht und(.) hätt irgendwie Angst gehabt und ihr
10 T: [mhm]
11 P: geht's selber net so gut ↑ (.) also die hat selber genug
12 T: [mhm]
13 P: Sorgen und äh wollt ich ihr des also (..) auch nicht antun ↑

Example 4

1 T: wann entlassen worden das hab ich nicht mehr genau im Kopf?
2 P: äh(.) heut vor einer Woche
3 T: heut vor einer Woche=
4 P: =ja
5 T: wie ist es Ihnen seitdem gegangen?
6 P: ja(.) also äh(.) net sehr gut(1) es hat den Einschein/
7 T: [mhm]
8 P: Anschein ghabt wie ich heimgekommen bin daß alles in
Ordnung ist ↑ ich war erst am Donnerstag dann zuhause(.h)
hab gleich's des Putzen und des Werkeln angefangen und
am Freitag vormittag ↑ (.) mein Freund war dann in der Arbeit (.hh)
und am Freitag vormittag bin also mit einem Elan
9 T: [mhm]
10 P: an meine Arbeit gegangen (.hh) u:nd hab gearbeitet bis(.)
zehn halb elf sowas hab mir allerhand vorgenommen ghabt
und so um circa um die Zeit um halb elf äh bin i naus zum
Haus und da spricht mich so a ältere Frau da(.h) die ist
scho fast an die neunzig das muß ich also jetzt dazu sagen(.)
11 T: [mhm]
und die kam naus und sagt "na wie geht's Ihnen" . . . . .
28 T: wie ist des äh daß wir da so'n bißchen Überblick bekommen
bis heute gegangen(.) weitergegangen

Example 5

1 T: (.hh) ich(Räuspern) stell's Ihnen eigentlich ganz frei ↑ (.)
äh (..) was Sie(.) *worüber* Sie sprechen möchten *was*
Sie sagen möchten (1) was Sie gegenwärtig so bewegt(.)
(Räuspern)
2 P: ja fragen Sie mich mal

3 T: mhm(.) ich möcht Sie eigentlich

4 P: [Sie kennen an und für sich meine Situation]

5 T: [ja ich möcht Sie eigentlich gar net so gern äh über irgendetwas(.) jetzt ausfragen sondern äh(.) ist mir sehr wichtig (.hh) daß Sie von sich aus (..) äh des ansprechen *was* im Moment (.) (.hh) (Räuspern) *gegenwärtig* ↑ (1) für Sie wichtig ist=

6 P: =sagn' wer die gegenwärtige Situation die kennen Sie die is ne reine Finanzfrage ↓

Example 6

1 P: [mir geht's gut ↑ (...) also vom *gesund*heitlichen Stand-

2 T: [mhm]

3 P: punkt her muß i sagen(.) *da* geht's mir gut=

4 T: [ja]

5 T: =wann sind Sie wieder zurückgekommen? aus der Kur?

6 P: ähm(.) aus der Kur bin i gekommen am dreiundzwanzigsten (.) September und am fünfundzwanzigsten bin ich

7 T: [mhm]

8 P: wieder weggefahren (..) und bin gekommen am vierten

9 T: [ja]

10 P: Oktober zurück

11 T: [Sie warn da bei ner Schwester wenn ich des richtig in Erinnerung habe oder?

12 P: na ich war in (.) bei Verwandten am Wolfgangsee in Österreich und dann war ich noch in Südtirol bei/in nem Hotel (..) bei Bekannten

13 T: [mhm]

14 T: (da haben Sie also (.) vollen Urlaub gemacht? ((leise))

15 P: ja

(1)

16 T: ja(.) und Sie sind jetzt(.) seit wann sind Sie jetzt zurück?

17 P: ähm(.) äh arbeiten tue ich seit vierten äh seit fünften Oktober arbeite ich wieder (..) also des ist die zweite

18 T: [mhm]

19 P: Woche jetzt (.)

20 T: [mhm(..) und wie geht's Ihnen jetzt so? ((leise))

Example 7

1 T: ja(.) (wie geht s Ihnen)

2 P: eignlich gut jetz

3 T: ja

4 P: kann mer scho sagn

(2)

5 P: ich hab mich erholt am Wochenende

6 T: mhm
7 P: bin mir au(ch) e bißchen klarer (da)drüber geworden wie
des is mit meim Freund(.)bin ausgezogen von der Wohnung . . .

Example 8

1 T: wie geht s
2 P: sehr gut(.)ich hab ne schöne Woche gehabt(.h)Prüfung war
ganz gut also des(.)war(.)bei weitem net so schlimm wie
d: der(.) der gsagt hat zuvor . . .

5 Therapy talk: ‘start’, ‘beginning’ and ‘outset’

Karin Kichler and Johanna Lalouschek

Introduction

In this study we shall deal with depth-analytically orientated group therapy sessions. Some of these sessions took place in the Allgemeine Krankenhaus Wien, Institut für Tiefenpsychologie and some in the Kriseninterventionszentrum der Stadt Wien. In the first case, the groups concerned were ‘closed groups’, in the second they were ‘open groups’, i.e. groups in which the number of participants may vary from session to session, because no pressure is applied on the individual patient to take part, and therefore participants may discontinue at will and new ones may join. We obtained transcripts of taperecordings of the sessions.

In the course of processing the material, our interest focused more and more on the analysis of the initial sequences of each session, since we came to attribute to them an important key position similar to the mostly ritualized opening sequences in everyday life situations (greeting, small talk, etc.). Of particular interest were the remarkable initial sequences of those sessions, in which new patients were to be integrated into an already established group.

For the analysis we used the methods of discourse analysis, as elaborated for instance by Stubbs (1983). Kallmeyer and Schütze (1975), and the representatives of symbolic interactionism — especially Erving Goffman. We chose these methods because they are not only descriptive but also interpretative.

Therapeutic communication versus everyday communication

First of all it will be necessary to draw a line between therapeutic communication (TC) and other forms of talk. In everyday life we take part in various interactive situations which arise through various causes and motivations. The manifold variety of these situations reaches from strictly rule-governed, very formal interactions, such as conferences, public speeches, interviews, discussions, via spontaneous, less official ones like so called 'small talk', up to very intimate dialogues between two persons in a familiar relationship (these may, in extreme cases, border upon the therapeutic sphere). Everyday communication (EC) takes place everywhere: in the family, at the place of work, in the street. The length of such interactions varies from short greetings to complex discussions lasting for hours. The number of participants and the kind of person taking part in such discourses vary with the situation and the task of the interaction. The therapeutic setting, on the contrary, is a strongly restrictive, closed form of talk:

> The room is always the same, the time for the meetings is fixed in advance for years, the duration of the interaction is determined from the very beginning. (Wodak 1981: 51; translation by the authors)

The group remains constant apart from a slight fluctuation of the participants. The most characteristic difference to EC is, in our opinion, the presence of at least one therapist:

> The therapist represents the professional authority, nevertheless he is not a member of the group. . . He holds a special position: although he is present in the group and the individual towards whom transfers are directed by other group members, he is always in a marked-off position. (Wodak 1981: 52; translation by the authors)

This study is based mainly on the distinction between EC and 'institutional communication', according to Schlieben-Lange (1979). She limits EC to 'natural' conversations in face-to-face interactions, and contrasts it with 'institutional conversation', by which she means communication at school, in court and in psychotherapeutical settings. Therefore we treat TC as a part of 'institutional conversation'; and in the following pages we shall describe the main differences between these two forms of communication.

Different authors (e.g. Flader and Grodzicki 1978; Wodak 1981) have worked out explicit rules for linguistic behaviour during therapy, and in the following study we want to contrast these rules with those of EC (see Goffman 1963; 1971b; Kallmeyer and Schütze 1975).

We are of the opinion that, especially during the beginning of therapeutic sessions, phenomena will occur which are similar to EC. Our

TC	EC
You can and should say everything which comes to your mind (basic rule)	The structure of turns relative to topic, completeness of detail, adequacy, etc. is highly determined by situational factors
You may talk about yourself as much as you like	You have to consider the interests of the other participants, and therefore talking about yourself should be limited
All topics are permitted	To avoid embarrassment, disagreement or even quarrels (which could disturb the communication) it is necessary to choose topics suited to the exterior situation and to the other participants
Rituals of politeness may be dropped	Rituals of politeness are a basic factor in the constitution and maintenance of social relations
You may cry, laugh, shout, etc.	The exhibition of emotions provokes incidents during communication, because it not only embarrasses the other participants in the interaction, but also constitutes an offence against the presentation of an acceptable image
You don't have to keep up a certain image	To keep the communication free of needless strain one must provide such facts only that are unambiguous and easy to interpret (the socially acceptable image must be maintained)
You may air conflicts and let aggressions take their course	Conflicts should be avoided

assumption is based on Goffman 1971a, according to which the progress of an interaction is largely determined by the events occurring at its beginning.

> We can appreciate the crucial importance of the information that the individual *initially* possesses or acquires concerning his fellow participants, for it is on the basis of this initial information that the individual starts to define the situation and starts to build up lines of responsive action. (Goffman 1971a: 22)

Therefore it is of essential importance for each participant in an interaction to obtain, or to provide, as much information about the situation and the social relations as soon as possible. These critical opening situations occur in social contact all the time, and need to be got over with quickly, unambiguously and economically. This can be achieved by using ritualized patterns of behaviour ('access-rituals', Goffman 1974: 97–137) and through the 'presentation of self' in the form of 'images', by which Holly (1979) means typicalized self-estimations, which represent a certain social value. This minimizes the processing capacity of the participants at the beginning of an interaction, and keeps them at that level throughout the progress of the conversation, because an image, once established, must be maintained and therefore the predictability of the following sequences is high.

> It would seem that an individual can more easily make a choice as to what line of treatment to demand from and extend to the others present at the beginning of an encounter than he can alter the line of treatment that is being pursued once the interaction is underway. (Goffman 1971a: 22)

In TC, 'images' are of secondary importance only, because the opening situation is determined by previously fixed roles (for therapist and patient) and there is no need for rituals to define the relationship. If rituals of greeting or acknowledgement do occur in the opening sequence of a session, the speaker does not behave according to the rules of TC as yet. If we find he uses techniques establishing an image or sequences of small talk, we can assume that he still acts within the rule system of EC.

Since efficient participation in therapy requires that the patient relearns to switch from EC rules to the rules of TC, we expect 'overlaps' of these two systems of rules of speech to occur, especially at the beginning of a therapy, at the commencement of a session, and whenever new patients have to be integrated into a (more or less) established group. We suppose that the occurrence or absence, respectively, of phenomena similar to EC are important and useful to help with ascertaining the stage of integration of a new participant, or of the resistance against the therapeutic process, and to define the boundary between the 'opening' and the 'main part' of a session.

The opening sequence

We shall now deal with the structuring of the opening sequence more precisely. Turner (1972) distinguishes three stages in the course of a group therapy session:

Pre-therapy talk The participants arrive one by one, talk to each other (small talk) and wait for the participants still missing and for the therapist.

Therapy talk All participants are assembled and the therapist gets the session going, that is, he uses explicit verbal orders for the group to begin with the session (e.g. *Well, we might as well start*).

> From the moment the session 'begins', patient's utterances are to be treated as 'data' . . . (Turner 1972: 396)

Post-therapy talk Patients and therapist break up the session: they leave the room.

The first discrepancy arose when we tried to apply Turner's classification to our material, because we needed a different definition for the 'beginning' of a session: our sessions — and accordingly the tape-recordings — began with the entrance of the therapist. Therefore we did not have the opportunity either of finding Turner's 'pre-therapy talk' nor of incorporating it into the analysis. Actually it was pointless to accept Turner's definition of 'therapy talk' since in our data (owing to the different definition of the opening) there was in fact no explicit verbal order of the therapist to begin the session. To assess the boundary of 'therapy talk' it would therefore be necessary to perform a detailed analysis of the opening sequence.

Let us take a look at an example from our data. (The original transcripts, in Viennese colloquial speech, can be found in the Appendix).

Session 1

T:	male therapist
MS:	male, 25 years
FB:	female, 50 years
MM:	male, 27 years
FP:	female, 35 years
FF:	female, —
MR:	male, —

(*noises of chairs scraping, embarrassed giggling*)
T: Don't let this irritate you, you will see you will forget it immediately
(*whispering*)
T: Mr S, you think already
MS: Pardon
T: You think already
MS: Well, hidden camera
(*laughter*)
FB: Nobody dares to speak these one and a half hours
(*whispering, interval, laughter, interval*)

12 T: May I perhaps ask at the beginning: does the
13 microphone irritate you or is this the usual silence
14 that occurs at the beginning of a group meeting until warming up
15 MM: I must say, it irritates
16 T: Why?
17 MM: It disturbs
18 T: What irritates
19 MM: Pardon
20 T: What irritates
21 MM: Yes I think, because, the reason is that nobody wants to
22 say anything, because he doesn't want to be on it
23 MS: No, I don't believe that
24 FP: It wouldn't worry me either
25 (*noise of chairs moving*)
26 FF: How are you today, better, aren't you?
27 MR: Yes, a little
28 FF: In which way
29 MR: Due to the medicine Dr X prescribed, it often makes me
30 sleep for 12–15 hours
31 (*silence*)
32 FF: Did you dream again (to MS)
33 MS: Yes
34 Women simultaneously: Did you write down the dreams?
35 MS: This week I didn't dream anything special, just so, only
36 so, only I dreamt — nothing but crazy things did I dream.

Analysis:

2– 4: Problematization of the situation at the start, because this is the first session to be taperecorded.

5–11: The unpleasant situation is eased by witty comments — a strategy which is a significant characteristic of EC (Goffman 1971b: 106ff.).

12–14: Further problematization and explicit verbal hint of the therapist that the session is still in the opening stage.

15–15: Although the group accepts this, it does so in a neutral way and very cautiously. Here, too, a hint this time made by a patient that therapy has not started yet (21–2).

26–30: Using the form of a question whose strategy corresponds to an EC ritual, FF changes the subject and causes MR to describe his problem.

31–32: A detailed presentation of the problem does succeed; so FF repeats her strategy towards another participant who is known as a less inhibited story-teller (cf. Wodak 1981: 114f.).

33– : Now FF's strategy has reached her aim — a very frank narration about dreams begins, and involves the entire group.

It is obvious that the beginning of the 'presentation of a problem' (PP) which means the 'essential therapeutic discourse' is not identical with the beginning of the session, as the session itself begins with the therapist entering the room. There are several 'beginning strategies' (see Wodak 1981: 116ff.), such as talking about the unusual situation of the meeting being recorded (2, 3), or a provocation made by the therapist (5–7), or silence (31) and also a ritualized question-and-answer game (26–30) of the kind which occurs in EC, to tide over a silent spell, in this case also used to change the subject. A repetition of this last strategy by another participant finally leads to PP, i.e. to a therapeutic discourse in the strict meaning of this word.

Therefore we define the beginning of the session (in our data: entrance of the therapist and beginning of the recording) as START. The moment when a real PP begins, which is dealt with, and only interrupted or relieved by other PPs and their processing, we define as BEGINNING, i.e. the beginning of the 'therapeutic discourse proper' (in the sense of Turner's 'therapy talk'). Therefore the beginning of the problem-orientated therapeutic discourse is not necessarily connected with the beginning of the session (which we call START) at all, but can be pushed far into the session. Neither does it depend on an explicit instruction by the therapist. The period between START and BEGINNING we call the OUTSET, where several phenomena of Turner's 'pre-therapy talk' may occur. These considerations lead us towards another, quite different analysis of the example given above:

START: sitting down
1st strategy: T emphasizes the unusual situation of the session because of the taperecording (2–3)
Reaction: blockage (4)
2nd strategy: provocation by T (5–7)
Reaction: counter-strategy of 'warming up' (8–11)
3rd strategy:(a) provocation by T (12–13)
(b) renewed focusing on the opening situation
Reaction: extension of 3rd strategy: the group accepts the preceding strategy and reacts, without entering into the spirit of the PP; the real reason for the session, i.e. presentation of a problem, remains unresolved.
4th strategy: on the one hand a ritualized question-and-answer game to bridge the silence (in this particular case also to change the subject); on the other hand a firm adherence to one person's problem (26)
Reaction: blockage (27)

5th strategy: repetition of 4th strategy but addressed to a different member of the group (32)

Reaction: extension of preceding strategy which leads to a PP — and therefore represents the BEGINNING

As shown in this analysis, the opening sequence consists of a number of strategies of various kinds and diverse reactions to these. But we can see that there are some strategies more likely than others to lead to a PP. We therefore distinguish between 'warming-up strategies' and 'beginning strategies'. Under 'warming-up strategies' we include joking and small talk, which have the superficial function of delaying the real BEGINNING of therapy talk. 'Beginning strategies' are all those strategies which could lead to a PP and therefore to a real BEGINNING. The very beginning strategy which initiates a PP is called BEGINNING (therefore BEGINNING does not only define the moment the problem-orientated communication starts, but also the strategy that leads to it).

Besides strategies we also find reactions to these:

Extension: the strategy preceding immediately is accepted and carried forward

Blockage: the group does not accept the strategy

Correction: a participant accepts the strategy, but only by, for example, negating the narrated facts.

On the basis of the material at our disposal we suggest the following pattern of the initial sequence of a session:

Turner		Kichler/Lalouschek
	participants arrive	
		pre-therapy talk
pre-therapy talk	therapist arrives	START
	therapist gives verbal order to start	(does not occur)
	beginning strategies	
therapy talk	warming-up strategies	initial sequence
	reactions	(OUTSET)
	beginning strategy that leads to a PP	BEGINNING
		real problem-orientated talk
post-therapy talk	participants and therapist leave	post-therapy talk

The new participant

As mentioned above, phenomena similar to EC may occur very clearly whenever a new patient is to be integrated into an established group — one which has been meeting for some time. We may conclude that a lack of experience with therapeutic groups and with the rule-system of TC are one reason for this behaviour; on the other hand, we may assume it to be the general effect of resistance. We will illustrate this with a further example.

Session 2

T: male therapist
MB: male, 50 years
MA: male, 28 years
MN: male, 50 years (the new participant)
FS: female, 30 years
MZ: male, age unknown

MB: Thanks, yes I have come to terms today — now I hope
that it is the right thing. One can never tell in the
beginning, but it looks pretty good. In fact, it's better
than I have hoped for, isn't it. After I had from . . .
bad luck, I am glad now that finally I — that was im-
possible anyway, I didn't have anything to do the whole
day, that ruined my nerves.
MA: It's unpleasant having nothing to do, hanging around
all day.
MN: I mean that would be the merriest life in the world if
one had no work to do. After all, that's what mankind is
always dreaming about, throughout its lifetime.
FS: I think, it looks differently in reality. One begins
to become depressive, seeing one is useless and super-
fluous
MN: Do you think that work is useful?
FS: Certainly.
MN: I find one thing funny — uh — uh — in the very beginning
mankind worked to one hundred per cent for the production of food,
just to be fed. Today — the Americans have reached an extreme
value of four per cent. Four per cent of the American population are
able to feed the other ninety-six. The other ninety-six are employed
mainly in the so called 'toy industry', that means they produce
machines, where buttons can be pressed, switches turned
and so on; cars, TVs, radios, washing machines, things one
doesn't really need in everyday life.

FS: But you do need washing machines
MN: Once it was said there is a child in every man, in the

30 woman the child can be released through being born.
31 The man is incapable of that, so he remains a child all
32 his lifetime and loves to play and again and again to
33 invent new appliances to play with.
34 MZ: Well, but woman likes to play with such gadgets too,
35 e.g. washing-machine and so
36 (*joking*)

Analysis

In this sequence the new patient tries to avoid the rising problems by turning to a kind of small talk level. This strategy is quite usual in everyday life, but if it occurs in therapy, it should be a starting-point for further treatment.

The example begins in line 1 with the START, but we must suppose that at least one preceding utterance is missing. Therefore our corpus starts with a PP by MB (1–7), which is rather general at the beginning (*one can never tell*), but develops into a very personal presentation, full of emotions (*ruined my nerves*). The syntactically incorrect constructions in the middle part of the utterance (incomplete and broken sentences) indicate that this sequence is produced spontaneously. MA reacts emphatically, but remains very impersonal (*it is — no subject*), which causes a stagnation of MB's beginning strategy; that means a further BEGINNING is possible, but it does not take place.

MN enters the conversation, continuing it on the level of EC; he brings the potential BEGINNING to naught (10–12): he applies the stereotype 'work is a curse' and enhances the impersonal construction in (10) to the universal expression *mankind* (11). Using this strategy, he destroys the justification of the problem presented by MB and MA. We connect this behaviour to considerable resistance against the therapeutic process, which is shown in defence against the problems through rationalization and intellectualization. FS corrects MN and resumes MB's theme, but in a way which is too impersonal and too general to turn the conversation back upon the level of TC. MN enters into the conversation only by picking up *useless* (15) as pivot for *useful* in his question (16). This strategy warrants the cohesion on the surface, but not the coherence, as MN neglects the actual content of FS's utterance (13–15). MN manages to get back to the theme of his turn in 10–12, and also manages to turn the conversation back to the EC-level. With his question *Do you think that work is useful*? he strives for a negative reply, which is not provided by FS (*Certainly*) and he, presumably, interrupts her because of that 'wrong' reply and wants to correct her. He presents a very professional summary of the development of the economic system from the beginning of mankind up to the Americans in the 1980s. He juggles with numbers and percentages; and with the humorously pejorative labelling *toy industry* (23), he tries to establish his own image as that of an 'expert'. The whole utterance (18–27) shows no breaks, and is not only syntactically but also semantically correct. Therefore the whole turn sounds very stereotypical almost like an anecdote, and is certainly not planned and produced spontaneously (compare MB's turn in 1–7).

FS reacts with a candid contradiction (28), applying the *pars pro toto* principle; she frankly shows her resistance to such small talk, but does not verbalize it explicitly, possibly not being able to do so. Through the collocations *child* (29), *toy industry* (23) and *appliances to play with* (32), *buttons to press, switches to turn* (24), MN completely ignores FS's objection and continues his interrupted turn disregarding her comment. Only MZ is able to stop MN's 'presentation of self', without however leaving the EC level. Later in the session MN also uses *the old Greeks, war, capital and interest*, as well as a lot of other catchwords, to maintain his image as a jovial expert and the EC conversation in general. Although the group maintains a critical attitude (e.g. MZ: *I think that the pondering and philosophizing you allude to somehow cannot be a fulfilment of life* and MP: *That leads to nothing, such playing with thoughts*, this behaviour again and again enters into his utterances, and therefore a BEGINNING is prevented. By the use of these strategies the new patient avoids the BEGINNING of a problem-orientated talk for a long time; in the course of the session, however, his behaviour changes and little by little, approaches towards presenting his problems are made. Therefore we may assume not only that his resistance diminishes, but also that he is eventually going to learn TC.

Conclusion

We have set out to show that TC and EC represent different rule systems, both of which have to be acquired. This chapter demonstrates that, in the case of TC, the process of acquisition can be clearly seen during certain stages of group therapy. If phenomena similar to EC do occur during therapeutic discourse, this may allow us to reach conclusions about the progress or stagnation of the therapeutic process, and about the resistance of particular patients to the use of TC, which means a resistance to therapy.

Bibliography

De Beaugrande, Robert-Alain and Dressler, Wolfgang U. 1981: *Einführung in die Textlinguistik*. Tübingen: Niemeyer.

Becker, Alois M. 1975: Psychoanalyse. In H. Strotzka (ed.), *Psychotherapie: Grundlagen. Verfahren, Indikationen*. Vienna: Urban & Schwarzenberg.

Caruso, Igor 1972: *Soziale Aspekte der Psychoanalyse*. Reinbeck: Rowohlt.

Coulmas, Florian 1981: *Routine im Gespräch. Zur pragmatischen Fundierung der Idiomatik*. Wiesbaden: Athenaion.

Eibl-Eibesfeldt, Irenäus 1979: Elementare Interaktionsstrategien. In: W. Heindrichs and G. C. Rump (eds.), *Dialoge*. Hildesheim: Gerstenberg.

— 1980: *Grundriß der vergleichenden Verhaltensforschung*. Munich: Piper.

Flader, D. and Grodzicki, W. D. 1978: Hypothesen zur Wirkungs-weise der psychoanalytischen Grundregel. *Psyche* 7/32.

Flader, Dieter and Wodak, Ruth (eds.) 1979: *Therapeutische Kommunikation*. Königstein/Ts.: Scriptor.

Goeppert, Sebastian and Goeppert, Herma (1973): *Sprache und Psychoanalyse*. Reinbeck: Rowohlt.

Goffman, Erving 1963: *Behavior in Public Places*. New York: The Free Press.

— 1971a: *The Presentation of Self in Everyday Life*. Harmondsworth: Penguin.

— 1971b: *Interaktionsrituale*. Frankfurt: Suhrkamp.

— 1974: *Das Individuum im offentlichen Austausch*. Frankfurt: Suhrkamp.

— 1977: *Rahmenanalyse*. Frankfurt: Suhrkamp.

— 1981: *Forms of Talk*. Philadelphia: University of Pennsylvania Press.

Holly, Werner 1979: *Imagearbeit in Gesprächen*. Tübingen: Niemeyer.

Kallmeyer, Werner and Schütze, Fritz 1975: Konversationsmaximen/Interaktionsrituale. *Linguistik und Didaktik* 21.

— 1976: Konversationsanalyse. *Studium Linguistik* 1.

Labov, William and Fanshel, David 1977: *Therapeutic Discourse*. New York: Academic Press.

Müller, Klaus 1984: *Rahmenanalyse des Dialogs*. Tübingen: Narr.

Rattner, Joseph 1979: *Gruppentherapie*. Frankfurt/Main: Fischer.

Schank, Gerd and Schoenthal, Gisela 1976: *Gesprochene Sprache*. Tübingen: Niemeyer.

Schlieben-Lange, Brigitte 1979: *Linguistische Pragmatik*. Stuttgart: Kohlhammer.

Strotzka, Hans (ed.) 1975: *Psychotherapie: Grundlagen. Verfahren, Indikationen*. Vienna: Urban & Schwarzenberg.

Stubbs, Michael 1983: *Discourse Analysis*. Oxford: Blackwell.

Turner, Roy 1972: Some formal properties of therapy talk. In D. Sudnow (ed.). *Studies in Social Interaction*. New York: The Free Press.

Watzlawick, Paul 1976: *Wie wirklich ist die Wirklichkeit*. Munich: Piper.

Watzlawick, Paul, Beavin, J. H. and Jackson, D. D. 1980: *Menschliche Kommunikation*. Bern: Huber.

Werlen, Iwar 1984: Ritual und Sprache. Tübingen: Niemeyer.

Wodak, Ruth 1981: *Das Wort in der Gruppe: Linguistische Studien zu therapeutischen Kommunikation*. Vienna: Verlag der Akademie der Wissenschaft.

Appendix: Original transcripts

Session 1

(*Geräusche von Setzen, verlegenes Gekicher*)
T: Lassen Sie Sich nicht irritieren dadurch, Sie werden sehen,
Sie habens sofort vergessen.
(*Geflüster*)
T: Herr S., Sie denken Sich schon
MS: Bitte?
T: Sie denken Sich schon
MS: Na ja, versteckte Kamera
(Gelächter)
FB: Traut sich keiner reden, die einendhalb Stunden
(Geflüster, Pause, Gelächter, Pause)
T: Darf ich vielleicht zu Beginn fragen: irritiert sie das
Mikrophon oder ist das das übliche Schweigen, wie es zu
Beginn einer Gruppe vorkommt, bis man sich angewärmt hat
MM: Ich muß sagen, es irritiert.
T: Wieso
MM: Es stört
T: Was irritiert
MM: bitte
T: Was irritiert
MM: Ja, ich glaube, die Ursache, der Grund ist der, daß nie-
mand was sagen will, weil er nicht drauf sein will
MS: Na, des glaub i net
FP: Mich würde es auch nicht stören
(Gerücke)
FF: Wie geht es Ihnen heute, besser ja?
MR: Ja, schon
FF: Inwiefern
MR: Durch das Mittel, daß mir Dr . . . verschrieben hat, da schlaf
ich oft 12–15 Stunden
(*Schweigen*)
FF: Haben Sie wieder geträumt (*zu MS*)
MS: Ja
Frauen durcheinander: Haben Sie die Träume aufgeschrieben?
MS: Die Wochen hab ich nix besonderes tramt, nur so, nur i
hab — lauter irre Sachen hab i tramt . . .

Session 2

MB: Danke, ja ich hab heute abgschlossen — jetzt hoffe ich, daß
es das Richtige ist. Das kann man am Anfang nie sagen, aber
es schaut ganz gut aus. Eigentlich besser, wie ich gehofft
hab, net. Nachdem ich von . . . a Pech gehabt hab, bin ich schon
froh, daß ich endlich — das war sowieso unmöglich, ich hab

den ganzen Tag nix zu tun ghabt, das hat mich nervlich fertig gmacht.

MA: Es ist unangenehm, wenn ma ka Arbeit hat, wenn man herumsteht, den ganzen Tag

MN: Ich find, des war das lustigste Leben auf der Welt, wenn ma ka Arbeit hätte. Davon träumt doch die Menschheit immer, Zeit ihres Lebens.

FS: Ich glaub, in der Realität schauts dann doch anders aus. Fängt man an depressiv zu werden, wenn man sieht, daß man unnütz und überflüssig ist

MN: Glauben Sie, daß arbeiten nützlich ist

FS: Sicher

MN: Ich find eins komisch — ah — ah — zum Anbeginn hat die Menschheit zu 100% in der Lebensmittelversorgung gearbeitet, um sich zu ernähren; heute — haben also die Amerikaner an extremen Wert von 4% erreicht. 4% der amerikanischen Bevölkerung sind imstande, die anderen 96 zu ernähren. Die anderen 96 sind zum Großteil in der sogenannten Spielzeugindustrie beschäftigt, d.h. sie bauen Apparate, wo man Knöpfchen drehen kann, Schalter kippen usw., Autos, Fernseher, Radios, Waschmaschinen, Dinge, die man an sich zum täglichen Leben nicht braucht

FS: Waschmaschinen braucht man doch

MN: Es hat einmal geheißen, in jedem Mann steckt ein Kind, — äh — in der Frau kann das Kind durch das Gebären herauskommen. Der Mann ist dazu nicht imstande, also bleibt er sein Leben lang ein Kind und spielt sich gern und erfindet immer wieder neue Geräte zum Spielen.

MZ: Na ja, aber die Frau spielt sich auch ganz gern mit so einem Gerät, angenommen die Waschmaschine und so

(*Scherze*)

6 'When I was still very small, life was much easier': The manifestation of neurotic disorders in a projective sentence Supplement test for children

Helmut Gruber

Introduction

The aim of this paper is to demonstrate the ways in which text planning and text formation differ between normal and neurotically disturbed children. These differences will be shown by means of quantitative and qualitative analyses of sentence-supplement tests.[1]

A system of categories for the recording of content and structural properties of the test answers is derived from theories of class- and sex-specific language behaviour, and also from a theory dealing with the language of neurotic adolescents. The test consists of thirteen items in the form of incomplete sentences, which the child is told to complete according to his own ideas.

Projective test procedures

Projective tests have a long tradition in clinical psychology. A long time before Hermann Rorschach published his *Psychodiagnostics* in 1922 and laid the foundation for an ever-increasing number of publications on and about the procedure named after him, projective tests were used as so-called 'fantasy tests' (Kerner 1857; Dearborn 1897). According to Frank (1939) quoted in Herrmann, 1976, the projective method operates 'by the creation of stimulus situations, in which it is not the tester who determines what a situation means, but the tested person supplies his own individual interpretation'.

Besides the 'classic' projective tests, i.e. the above-mentioned procedure developed by Rorschach and Murray's TAT (see Murray 1951), a great number of other projective tests were developed. One of them is the sentence-supplement test (SST) developed by Dr. E. Hift, to be investigated in this chapter. In spite of the great popularity and the widespread promulgation of these investigative procedures, most of them lack an explicit theoretical foundation and a uniform method of evaluation (meaning that there exist a number of divergent evaluation methods for each test). This, and the fact that the tests do not provide a direct approach to relevant personality traits, although conclusions on personality characteristics are drawn out of nonstandardized verbal utterances, induced many criticisms of these tests (cf. Fischer and Spada 1973). Experimental investigations dealing with the validity and reliability of some projective tests also produced inconsistent results (for a detailed discussion see Berlach 1982; Meili and Rohracher 1972).

The very fact of the subject's verbal utterance being of crucial importance necessitates the classification of the stimulus material according to linguistic criteria in the particular situation of the SST. This allows the determination of the subject's global situative determination by means of 'items' — not feasible in other projective tests — and at the same time not only justifies but even demands the provision of a socio-psycholinguistic evaluation method for the test. Results from Wodak (1981; 1984) have shown that sex and social class, as well as the presence of a neurotic disorder, influence text planning and text formation. Based on these results, categories of replies and evaluation methods are to be developed which take these three variables into consideration.

Theoretical background

Class-specific language socialization

First I will deal with social class as it influences answers in the SST. The class specific differences can relate to material and social conditions which constitute the reality of the different classes. Aronfreed (1968) stresses mainly the different occupational standards, which allow middle-class people to be more independent of external control and at the same time to have the possibility of changing external circumstances by means of symbol-orientated operations, whereas, for the working class, the extent of active control over their surroundings is restricted through the occupational position, and is limited to the handling of concrete tools of their work routine. These different possibilities of control stipulate different techniques of socialization, too. Kohn (1959) emphasizes that middle-class parents reach their educational goals to a great extent through argumentation, appeal to the guilty conscience of the child, and the threat of withdrawal of love, whereas working-class parents lean towards corporal punishment and the demand for conformity with an external authority.

The differing emotional climate established by different forms of sanctions leads to the development of different intrapsychic systems of behaviour control in the child. Various empirical investigations (Hoffmann and Saltzstein 1965; Sears *et al.* 1957; Aronfreed 1961) have shown that middle-class children are rather more independent of their environment in their moral orientation, while working-class children showed a greater orientation towards external factors. This short sketch of class-specific techniques of socialization already shows the differentiating position of language in them. While Bernstein (1970) argued that working-class individuals are socialized in a language system which differs quantitatively from the middle class system, more thorough investigations, which used more linguistically relevant indicators than Bernstein, show that the language behaviour of both classes varies with and depends upon setting. The differences in class-specific language behaviour are shown to be qualitative (Leodolter 1975; Wodak 1981).

When investigating speech styles of middle-class and working-class members of a therapy group, Wodak (1981) found that members of the working class and women presented their problem in a more emotional and spontaneous way than others. In doing so, members of the working class tended to elaborate on one single event. Middle-class members, on the other hand, presented rather detached and less emotional descriptions of their condition. The meaning of these findings for my chapter is as follows: the influence of external circumstances was kept constant when investigating the normal group, since the test was carried out at school. It is to be expected that, at the age of twelve, middle-class and working-class children are familiar enough with this situation through their secondary socialization. Additionally, the group situation favours the experiences of working-class children because of 'peer-group socialization', rather frequent within this class. Although the clinical group tests were carried out individually, which might be of disadvantage to working-class children, it should be pointed out that the whole test situation (the tests were taken in a psychiatric hospital) was familiar neither to middle-class nor to working-class children, and that in any case, the neurotic disorder influences text formation more than other variables.

Taking as a basis the socio-psycholinguistic theory of text formation (SPTT, Wodak 1984), which assumes that different strategies of dealing with reality — acquired by children of different classes in the course of different socializations — influence the content and structure of verbal utterances, one can postulate that working-class children will appear more influenced from the outside in their SST answers, that they will give scenic descriptions of single events, and that they will express emotions more readily than middle-class children.

Sex-specific language socialization

A child's education is influenced not only by social class, but also by sex. Normally, children are educationally directed (consciously and unconsciously) towards a certain sex role by their parents. In the European — North American culture, this role provides active, autonomous behaviour and the development of analytical thinking for males whereas in females emotional, 'soft' and passive behaviour and holistic (Gestalt) thinking is encouraged. Even in a perception test, which measured field dependency of perception, Bieri (1960) was able to show that women depend more on their environment than men. In this connection one should also point to Freud's view of female super-ego development: according to him, women develop a weaker super-ego than men because of their different psychosexual development. This view (justly) earned him much criticism, since he neglected social factors; nevertheless his position points in the same direction as Bieri's results do.

In the above-mentioned investigation, Aronfreed (1961) discovered sex differences as well as class differences: he found that girls were guided by the external world, but that boys were more independent of their external surroundings. The tradition of sex roles starts very early. Spelke *et al.* (1973) could prove that, at the age of one year, children had spoken significantly more often with the parent of the same sex. This stimulates, by means of imitative learning, the acceptance of sex-specific language and behavioural styles. It also explains the often registered verbal superiority of girls by the attitude which parents take in expecting the greater verbal skills from daughters than from sons. In her above-mentioned investigation Wodak (1984) found that, in compositions, adolescent girls rather express emotions, recount stories and assess actions, while boys report upon and describe facts.

Applying the above mentioned SPTT one may expect that responses from the SST of girls will show them to be more dependent on the external world, and that they will express emotions more readily. Further, girls will react by relating, and evaluating events in their answers, thereby differing from boys.

Normal and neurotic development during adolescence

The beginning of puberty confronts the adolescent with a qualitatively new situation in the physiological as well as in the psychological area. While the physical changes (accelerated growth, development of secondary sexual features, etc.) do not concern the scope of this chapter it will be necessary to touch upon the psychological processes which take place during early adolescence.

During this phase, a weakening of object cathexis and a shifting of libido to the self takes place. The ego concentrates on the self, and makes an object out of it (Blos 1978). Additionally, old, apparently outgrown, pre-oedipal conflicts are reawakened during adolescence. These often cause strong regressive wishes for merger and dependence, while the adolescent outwardly shows strong autonomous tendencies. Adolescents often appear moody, helpless and unstable during this phase. Boys often vehemently reject girls and everything female, and develop adoring crushes on other boys in order to defend their regressive, passive wishes to return to their mother. On the other hand, girls often have an increased need for heterosexual friendships, but these also represent the defence of wishes to return to the pre-oedipal mother. Beside these heterosexual needs, girls often show boyish behaviour and act out of their phallic wishes (Blos 1978).

The co-occurrence of all these inconsistent and contradictory forms of behaviour is no reason for serious problems during adolescence; rather it is an expression of the ego's search for stability, and its attempt to establish boundaries. Problems only arise if and when these aims cannot be achieved. The probability of pathological development increases when the development during early childhood has been disturbed. The achievements of the latency period (cf. the development of intelligence and the separation from primary and secondary process) must have been attained, too. If this is not the case, or if there are already mental disorders from early childhood, adolescence — with the increased drive pressure and the flareup of apparently long since overcome conflicts — is the ideal hotbed for the development of neurotic disorders.

So far there are few investigations dealing with the language of normal and neurotic adolescents. Wodak (1984) was able to show that the compositions of normal and neurotic adolescents differed significantly in a quantitative and qualitative manner. Boys from the neurotic group did not choose descriptive text styles but instead argued their relationships and their problems. Girls, on the other hand, wrote significantly more often in a narrative style than in the normal group, where *reflexive descriptions* had predominated. This is interpreted by Wodak as a sign of regression, which manifests itself linguistically in the form of a setback from a more mature form of describing relations to a more childlike one. Additionally, the compositions of the neurotic group were significantly shorter.

The psychological and psycholinguistic facts outlined in this section allow for the following expectations regarding the answers in the SST (and once more referring to SPTT). Within the sample, the answers of the neurotic and the normal group should differ in a quantitative and in a qualitative manner. Boys in the neurotic group should choose answers similar to those of girls in the normal group. They would be expected to express emotions, and to refer to their own identity. The answers of girls and boys should be shorter in this sample than in a normal one.

Furthermore, one might draw the conclusion from the theoretical representation in this section that the differences which were postulated in the previous section would be especially pronounced because of the specific phase of adolescence at which the juveniles were at the time of the tests.

Hypotheses

In the course of this chapter I will deal only with the description and discussion of some results concerning the syntactic-semantic formation of test answers, and with the performance of speaker's perspective by subjects. Out of the above theoretical considerations we can deduce the following hypotheses:

Hypotheses concerning class-specific language use

1 Working-class children present single events concisely because of the specific situation (school and/or clinical test situation).
2 Working-class children include their own person in their answers more frequently.
3 Middle-class children choose longer and more complex forms of presentation for their answers.
4 Middle-class children prefer impersonal forms of reference.

Hypotheses concerning sex-specific language use

5 Girls are more likely to choose answers in which they refer to their own identity.

6 Girls are more likely to choose complex forms of presentation for their answers.
7 Boys will prefer to dissociate from themselves in their answers.
8 Boys will choose shorter forms of presentation.

Hypotheses concerning the difference between the normal and the neurotic group

9 Answers in the neurotic group are less complex than in the normal group.
10 Answers in the group of the mentally disturbed adolescents centre around personal problems, this finds expression in the syntactic-semantic structure of the answers.

Methods

To provide an evaluation method of the highest possible objectivity, it is intended to develop categories which allow us to test the hypotheses sketched in the previous sections by a content analysis with linguistic indicators. Additionally, extralinguistic categories should be made use of to determine membership to class. Here I go along with Oevermann (1972) and use the indicators 'profession of parents' and 'education of parents' to classify subjects either as middle-class or as working-class. Within the clinical group I also used the clinical diagnosis of subjects to explain subtle differences which turned up during qualitative analysis. This procedure ensures that as much information as possible about each subject is under consideration in the course of analysis, and that, at the same time, as much objectivity as possible is upheld.

Test material and categories

Properties of test material[2]

Before looking into the categories provided for evaluation of the SST, I would like to make some fundamental remarks about this test. Even a superficial glance at the individual test items (sentence beginnings) shows that these are not equivalent with regard to content and structural properties of the supplementation they allow for. Therefore it is necessary to classify the test material according to semantic and syntactic criteria to avoid this bias influencing analysis in an uncontrolled way. I therefore postulate two 'scales of openness', whereby a higher degree of openness means that the item allows a greater variety of possible replies.

Scale 1 Syntactic openness In this scale, items shall be classified according to possible syntactic constituents as supplementation. Obviously, every item also permits the adding of coordinate and/or subordinate clauses. The classification shows only the minimum constituent supplementation required to form a grammatically correct German sentence out of the sentence beginning provided. This classification arranges the items according to their valency; verb valency alone cannot be applied because this property is already restricted by other constituents in some of the items, while in other items there is no verb. Using this classification we obtain the following rank order:

(a) items which require either a subordinate clause or a constituent: items 3, 5, 8, 13
- example 1: *The main thing for me is/eating*

or: *The main thing for me is/that I always have enough to eat*[3]

(b) items which require a subordinate clause only: items 1, 6, 7, 9
- example 2: *It bothers me that/we don't have a holiday*[4]

(c) items which require one (or more) constituents: items 2, 4, 10, 11, 12
- example 3: *School is/ boring*[5]

With regard to hypothesis 9 above, one could expect that in items from group (a), children of the neurotic group would tend to complete only the absolutely necessary constituents. Children of the normal group, on the other hand, would complete a subordinate clause in (a), and one could expect additional constituents to appear in (b) and (c).

Scale 2 Semantic openness Unfortunately it is not so simple with this scale to find clearcut viewpoints for establishing a criterion. I choose for classification of this aspect 'type of speech act' on the one hand and, on the other hand, the 'expressed emotional content' of the item, because these have the strongest 'challenging force'. I believe that these two aspects of the item provide the strongest lead to the content of the supplement for the subject. Thus, type of speech act, emotional content and structural possibility of the supplement are those properties of the stimulus material which guide the subjects' projection in the sense mentioned in the previous section on projective test procedures. Ranking the items according to these criteria creates another three-step scale:

(a) neutral items: 2, 6, 9
- example 4: *When I was still very young/ it was beautiful*[6]

(b) wishes, suspicions: 4, 8, 10, 11, 12
- example 5: *If only my parents/ had more time for me*[7]

(c) emotional items: 1, 3, 5, 7, 13
- example 6: *I am very sad/ that I'm so fat.*[8]

Naturally the neutral items are only neutral in respect to the criteria of (b) and (c); and the range of objects for the answers is also limited here. Yet one can deduce the hypothesis from the above scale, that in group (a) items the thematic variance will be highest, and that it will decrease successively in groups (b) and (c) because these items guide the subjects' projection in a certain direction. One may further assume that in groups (a) and (b) no emotions will be expressed explicitly as a rule.

In this special context, or rather in this language game — in the Wittgenstein sense (Wittgenstein 1980) — of SST sentences, it is legitimate to view and to analyse each sentence as a text. According to the principle of projection one may assume that each sentence beginning becomes the subject's point of crystallization for motives and feelings. Thus, the SST sentences are one-sentence texts in Werlich's sense (1975), which acquire textuality through this particular context of utterance. They are not only acceptable, but also 'situation-relevant' in the sense of Beaugrande and Dressler (1981).

After these remarks on the test material I will present the categories for the analysis of the answers.

Categories of answers

Theme This category records the semantic control centre of the supplement. Beaugrande and Dressler (1981) and Beaugrande (1980) believe this concept of a control centre to exist where most semantic relations meet, if the sentence is represented as a semantic network. If the control centre is located within the given sentence beginning (which occurs when the supplement is not only short but lacks any new semantic content), I record that concept in the supplement which is semantically connected in the most relevant way to the theme. The degree of relevance is determined by the rank order of agent categories (see below). The most relevant category is the preceding one within the rank order.

- example 7: *If only I wasn't so fat*[9]
  theme: 'Self' — 'negative feature'

- example 8: *It bothers me that/some people regard children as being too little to discuss problems.*[10]
  theme: 'children'

This category provides the opportunity to investigate which are the preferred themes in connection with certain items, or if (and which) group-specific differencies exist. A cursory view of data showed that the main themes were parents, school, social relations, and disappointment in social relations.

To permit an empirical analysis I drew up a list of the most frequent themes, drawn at random out of 100 tests. A numerical code was assigned to each theme. Highly unusual themes were recorded as 'Varia', although they might have provided useful diagnostic hints in certain cases. This drawback is a part of quantitative analysis, and shows the advantages of qualitative research methods.

In this category it is also decided whether the supplement is a 'trivial answer' (in accordance with the syntactic openness of items — see above) in items of group (a) and (c); if its theme is already present within the given sentence beginning; and if no 'not syntactically motivated' additional semantic—syntactic relation exists in the supplement.

- example 9: *School is/ boring*[11]
  The main thing for me is/ eating[12]
  answers are trivial
- example 10: *School is/ a bore for me*[13]
  The main thing for me is/ that I always have something to eat[14]
  answers are not trivial

A trivial answer in group (b) is scored if the supplement either completes the minimal structurally required constituent, or if the answer is extremely noncommittal.

- example 11: *When I was still very small I wore napkins*[15]
  trivial answer
  When I was still very small everything was better than now[16]
  not trivial answer

The differentiation between 'trivial' and 'normal' answers makes it possible to judge semantic and syntactic complexity simultaneously, and to investigate their distribution through the different groups of subjects.

Identification with self This category notes whether the continuation of the sentence corresponds with the given beginning in regard to speaker's perspective (Werlich 1975). This category is expressed in two ways: Unmarkedness if the speaker's perspective is turned into the contrary of the given sentence beginning. The relevancy of this category is based on the fact that psycholinguistic investigations have shown members of the middle class and men to be more likely to use an indefinite personal speaker's perspective (Wodak 1981; 1983). Furthermore, this shows to what extent subjects are guided by the test material in respect to the formal design of utterances.

Agent structure This category is supposed to record the syntactic—semantic properties of the completed constituents. The selection of classificatory possibilities was made according to the principle of the most economical analysis. This means that a vast number of categories which allow for very precise description, but which demand an enormous amount of coding and computing work (and which are used mostly in the field of artificial intelligence), should be avoided. On the other hand, a highly inexact and schematic classification, as in case grammar (Fillmore 1968) was abandoned in favour of a description which preserves the inherent character of sentences to a high degree. Therefore I decided to use the following categories:

agent: forceful entity, which performs an action and changes a situation
affected entity: entity, which is altered by an event or an action; it is neither agent nor instrument
instrument: an objective entity without own intention, which is used as a means during an event or an action
state: present or characteristic state of an entity
possession: points to a relation where one sensoric entity possesses another entity
cognition: relates sensoric entities to operations of thought, perception and will

- example 12: *It bothers me/ that my brother always hits me with his ruler*[17]
  agent: brother; *affected entity;* self; *instrument*: ruler

The terms and the definitions of categories correspond to Beaugrande 1980 and Beaugrande and Dressler 1981.

These concepts are recorded sequentially and bi-directional analysis is therefore possible: first one can determinate the transition probability with regard to the sequencing of concepts, and then it is possible to analyse the 'filling' entities of each concept (e.g. *agent*: parents). It should be noted here if a category does occur although its content is not clear to the analyser (unclear references, local and temporal deixis). In the course of analysis this will be regarded as an indicator of subject's egocentricity of language (and therefore of thought). Study of the agent structure of a sentence allows the investigation of a subject's experience categories in respect to himself and his environment (e.g. does he/she experience himself/herself rather as an agent or as an affected entity? How does he/she view surrounding persons in relation to himself/herself?)

Quantitative results and discussion

I shall now set out and discuss the first results concerning the hypotheses formulated above. Nonparametric procedures (chi square test) were used because normal distribution could not be assumed.

To begin with, let us discuss the syntactic—semantic complexity of the answers. As we see, the clinical group shows more trivial answers than the normal group, whereas in the normal group this is reversed. This means that answers in the clinical group are not only shorter, but also semantically simpler (significantly so at the 1%– level). Furthermore it is evident that boys and working-class subjects tend to complete the items by trivial answers (Table 6.2 and 6.3; both results significant at the 5%– level). These results support the theory of socio-psycholinguistic text planning, as they show the difference in the formation of answers between

TABLE 6.1 *Group/trivial answer.*

Count Row % Col. % Tot. %	Non-trivial	Trivial	Row total
Clinical	52 45.6 30.8 18.5	62 54.4 55.4 22.1	114 40.6
Normal	117 70.1 69.2 41.6	50 29.9 44.6 17.8	167 59.4
Column total	169 60.1	112 39.9	281 100.0

Corr. chi square = 15.88573 df = 1 $\alpha = 0.0001$

TABLE 6.2 *Sex/trivial answer.*

Count Row % Col. % Tot. %	Non-trivial	Trivial	Row total
Female	94 66.2 55.6 33.5	48 33.8 42.9 17.1	142 50.5
Male	75 54.0 44.4 26.7	64 46.0 57.1 22.8	139 49.5
Column total	169 60.1	112 39.9	281 100.0

Corr. chi square = 3.89450 df = 1 α = 0.0484

TABLE 6.3 *Social class/trivial answer.*

Count Row % Col. % Tot. %	Non-trivial	Trivial	Row total
WC	34 49.3 20.1 12.1	35 50.7 31.3 12.5	69 24.6
LMC	39 65.0 23.1 13.9	21 35.0 18.8 7.5	60 21.4
MC	31 51.7 18.3 11.0	29 48.3 25.9 10.3	60 21.4
UMC	65 70.7 38.5 23.1	27 29.3 24.1 9.6	92 32.7
Column total	169 60.1	112 39.9	281 100.0

chi square = 10.02712 df = 3 α = 0.0183
Abbreviations: WC = working class; LMC = lower middle class; MC = middle class; UMC = upper middle class

boys and girls, (hypotheses 6 and 8 are thus proved). The highly significant result of the comparison between the clinical and the normal group can be interpreted in the following way. The answers of the clinical group are not only shorter (see Wodak's (1984) findings), but also less differentiated in the field of semantics. This can be interpreted as a regression to an earlier state of cognitive development which runs parallel to the psychological disturbance, and with the regression of drives and fixation on earlier states of development. These results correspond to those of Wodak (1984), who obtained similar results when investigating the choice of text type in normal and neurotic adolescents. Class differences in the results relate to the setting of the tests. These results correspond to those of Bernstein 1970.

Looking at the results concerning change of speaker's perspective, class difference is conspicuous. While there is no difference between the normal and the clinical group here (Table 6.4), and girls tend to change speaker's perspective in their answers only occasionally, class difference is very significant. The most interesting fact is that working-class and upper-middle class-children's results are almost identical concerning 'markedness'. This can be interpreted as follows: Markedness is not sensitive towards the direction into which speaker's perspective turns. This means that it does not matter whether a given personal speaker's perspective is changed to an indefinite personal or a given indefinite personal to a personal speaker's perspective — in both cases it is marked.

TABLE 6.4 *Group/identification with self.*

Count Row % Col. % Tot. %	Unmarked	Marked	Row total
Clinical	98 87.5 39.8 35.1	14 12.5 42.4 5.0	112 40.1
Normal	148 88.6 60.2 53.0	19 11.4 57.6 6.8	167 59.9
Column total	246 88.2	33 11.8	279 100.0

Cor. chi square = 0.00913 df = 1 α = 0.9239

TABLE 6.5 *Sex/identification with self.*

Count Row % Col. % Tot. %	Unmarked	Marked	Row total
Female	120 84.5 48.8 43.0	22 15.5 66.7 7.9	142 50.9
Male	126 92.0 51.2 45.2	11 8.0 33.3 3.9	137 49.1
Column total	246 88.2	33 11.8	279 100.0

Corr. chi square = 3.04330 df = 1 α = 0.0811

TABLE 6.6 *Social class/identification with self.*

Count Row % Col. % Tot. %	Unmarked	Marked	Row total
WC	57 82.6 23.2 20.4	12 17.4 36.4 4.3	69 24.7
LMC	51 85.0 20.7 18.3	9 15.0 27.3 3.2	60 21.5
MC	57 98.3 23.2 20.4	1 1.7 3.0 0.4	58 20.8
UMC	81 88.0 32.9 29.0	11 12.0 33.3 3.9	92 33.0
Column total	246 88.2	33 11.8	279 100.0

chi square = 8.30562 df = 3 α = 0.0401

TABLE 6.7 *Group/content of agent.*

Count Row % Col. % Tot. %	Self	Father	Mother	Family	Others	Teachers	Boys	Girls	Animals	Unclear refer-ence	Varia	Row total
Clinical	24	1	11	9	0	0	0	4	0	0	0	39
	61.5	2.6	2.6	23.1	0	0	0	10.4	0	0	0	36.4
	45.3	33.3	100.0	60.0	0	0	0	30.8	0	0	0	
	22.4	0.9	0.9	8.4	0	0	0	3.7	0	0	0	
Normal	29	2	0	6	6	1	11	9	1	2	1	68
	42.6	2.9	0	8.8	8.8	1.5	16.2	13.2	1.5	2.9	1.5	63.6
	54.7	66.7	0	40.0	100.00	100.0	100.0	69.2	100.0	100.0	100.0	
	27.1	1.9	0	5.6	5.6	0.9	10.3	8.4	0.9	1.9	0.9	
Column total	53	3	1	15	6	1	11	13	1	2	1	107
	49.5	2.8	0.9	14.0	5.6	0.9	10.3	12.1	0.9	1.9	0.9	100.0

chi square = 19.93246   df = 10 α = 0.0299

TABLE 6.8 *Group/content of affected entity.*

Count Row % Col. % Tot. %	Self	Father	Mother	Family	Others	Teachers	Boys	Girls	Animals	Unclear reference	Varia	School	Environ-ment	Row total
Clinical	7	1	0	2	5	0	0	0	1	1	0	0	0	17
	41.2	5.9	0	11.8	29.4	0	0	0	5.9	5.9	0	0	0	28.3
	43.8	100.0	0	66.7	50.0	0	0	0	100.0	100.0	0	0	0	
	11.7	1.7	0	3.3	8.3	0	0	0	1.7	1.7	0	0	0	
Normal	9	0	1	1	5	1	3	7	0	0	6	9	1	43
	20.9	0	2.3	2.3	11.5	2.3	7.0	16.3	0	0	14.0	20.9	2.3	71.7
	56.3	0	100.0	33.3	50.0	100.0	100.0	100.0	0	0	100.0	100.0	100.0	
	15.0	0	1.7	1.7	8.3	1.7	5.0	11.7	0	0	10.0	15.0	1.7	
Column total	16	1	1	3	10	1	3	7	1	1	6	9	1	60
	26.7	1.7	1.7	5.0	16.7	1.7	5.0	11.7	1.7	1.7	10.0	15.0	1.7	100.0

chi square = 25.01368 df = 12 α = 0.0148

This might explain the result: members of the working class change given indefine personal speaker's perspectives to personal ones, and members of the upper middle class do the exact opposite (a single-item analysis will provide an exact explanation of this interpretation).

Concerning agent structure, we see that, within the clinical group, the design of content in the categories of agent and affected entity (I have to limit my research to these categories for lack of space) is limited. In both these categories, content centres around the self and the family. 'Others' are experienced only as affected entites. The normal group shows a very much broader spread of content.

The above results concerning the significant increase of trivial answers within the clinical group and the content of the answers show one overall pattern. Neurotically disturbed children not only show simple semantic—syntactic and regressive formation of answers, but their answers are also limited in content. They concern mainly the subjects 'family' and 'self'. These simplifications are in direct connection with their neurotic disorder, and can be interpreted as an overall regression and an impoverishment in the cognitive—emotional field and in the area of experience.

Qualitative analysis of two text samples

Finally, the qualitative analysis of two text samples will reveal phenomena which are typical for the clinical and the normal group respectively, but which would possibly be missed in quantitative analysis because of their rare occurrence. Nevertheless such phenomena might provide useful revelations, as the following texts will show.

Text 1 (normal group)[18]

1 It bothers me, that/ some people consider children too small to talk problems over with.
2 School is/ not as bad as some people think and declare.
3 I'm very sad/ if my parents are angry with me.
4 If only my parents/ would sometimes discuss things with me, which upset me.
5 I hate/ boasting, pride and exaggerated vanity.
6 When I was still very small/ I had a very poor opinion of school and didn't want to have anything to do with it at any price.
7 I'm glad, that/ I am like I am.

8 Perhaps others say about me/ that I'm fat, but I know they are right and don't mind.
9 When I'm at home/ I lie on my bed and switch on the radio.
10 If only I didn't/ get a bad mark.
11 Girls should/ sometimes consider what they say.
12 Boys should/ not yell in class but learn not to hit one another but to argue peacefully.
13 The main thing for me is/ to achieve something at school.

This text of a middle-class boy shows a strong tendency to choose neutral descriptions of state. Thus he tells us about *some people* who think of *children* as being too small to talk problems over with in item 1 In the context of item 4 these *people* might be his own parents. This is another hint on the increase of unclear references at the appearance of conflict themes. Items 2 and 4 show this tendency too (use of *some* and *things*). Regarding surface structuring, the 'argumentative' style is conspicuous in some of the items (e.g. 4, 7, 12). This style is achieved by the use of subordinate clauses and disjunctive or contrajunctive sentence connectors respectively. In spite of this elaborated speech style, the answers are of neutral content: emotions are suppressed even in such items which appeal to them explicitly (the stereotypical answers in items 5 and 7).

Text 2 (clinical group)[19]

1 It bothers me that/ I don't get a good job
2 School is/ over and I would like to go there once again.
3 I'm very sad/ that I don't earn a lot.
4 If only my parents/ were with me.
5 I hate/ Carly.
6 When I was still very small/ was much easier life.
7 I'm glad, that I/ still have a job.
8 Perhaps others say about me/ that they like or don't like me.
9 When I'm at home/ I'm very happy.
10 If only I didn't/ have to get up so quickly in the morning and not so quickly.
11 Girls should/ get along with each other but my sister and I not.
13 The main thing for me is/ that I can remain with my family.

This text was produced by a working-class girl. The supplements are much shorter than those of the normal group. In addition the ungrammatical supplements in 6, 10 and 11 are conspicuous. Obviously *life* in item 6 was added as an after thought to elucidate the utterance. Because *life* (particularly school — the girl has a school problem) is a worry for her, she is so distracted by reminiscences of her happier earlier childhood, that her utterance becomes intelligible to others only by an afterthought, i.e. when cognitive control of text planning reasserts itself. Obviously, in items 10 and 11 too, text planning control was suspended, so that the adverbial *not so quickly*, possibly particularly distressing to her in the real situation, occurs twice. In item 11, the above-mentioned phenomenon even causes the surface sentence to express the very contrary of the girl's intention, i.e. the obvious fact that she and her sister should get along with each other, but do not.

The content of items 1, 3, and 7 is particularly striking, since the theme *job* could not be explained, neither in the girl's case history nor by other signs in the test. Striking is the contradiction between items 1 and 7; also that all three items concern feelings towards self. The girl blocks emotions by these inexplicable answers, much as she does in item 5, where *Carly*, too, remains a mystery. This regression into a kind of private language is a sign of existing problems.

In this investigation, two phenomena were recognizable. When themes are approached which concern the girl's difficulties with and in her environment, text planning control gets out of hand and the girl's answers become ungrammatical, but still intelligible. With intrapsychic problems, though, the girl reverts to a sort of private language, and thereby blocks herself up towards outsiders. In qualitative analysis we could thus discover two text planning strategies typical for neurotic adolescents: disturbance of cognitive text planning, and reversion to a private language. We are thereby put in a position to realize that qualitative analysis provides a more comprehensive overview than quantitative analysis of the text planning of neurotics.

Notes to Chapter 6

1 The texts of the normal group were recorded in the course of a scientific project at the Department of Depth Psychology of the University of Vienna in 1981. Professor Dr H. Strotzka and Dr C. Schmidt were in charge of this project. The texts of the neurotic group were recorded at the University's Neuropsychiatric Clinic for Children and Juveniles, and were kindly made available to me by Dr E. Hift.

2 The test consists of the following thirteen items:
  1 It bothers me, that/
  2 School is/
  3 I'm very sad/

4 If only my parents/
5 I hate/
6 When I was still very small/
7 I'm glad, that I/
8 Perhaps others talk about me/
9 When I'm at home/
10 If only I wouldn't/
11 Girls should/
12 Boys should/ (This item was not used in the neurotic group)
13 The main thing for me is/

3 Original German text (OGT):
Das Wichtigste ist für mich/ Essen *or*
Das Wichtigste ist für mich/ , daß ich immer zu Essen habe
4 OGT: Es stört mich, daß/ wir nicht schulfrei haben.
5 OGT: Die Schule ist/ fad.
6 OGT: Als ich noch ganz klein war/ war es schön.
7 OGT: Wenn nur meine Eltern/ mehr Zeit für mich hätten.
8 OGT: Ich bin sehr traurig/, daß ich so dick bin.
9 OGT: Wenn ich nur nicht/ so dick wäre.
10 OGT: Es stört mich, daß/ manche Leute Kinder für zu klein halten, um Probleme zu besprechen.
11 OGT: Die Schule ist/ fad.
12 OGT: Das Wichtigste ist für mich/Essen.
13 OGT: Die Schule ist/ für mich fad.
14 OGT: Das Wichtigste ist für mich/, daß ich immer zu Essen habe.
15 OGT: Als ich noch ganz klein war/ trug ich noch Windeln.
16 OGT: Als ich noch ganz klein war/ war alles viel besser als heute.
17 OGT: Es stört mich/, daß mich mein Bruder immer mit dem Lineal schlägt.
18 OGT: 1 Es stört mich, daß/ manche Leute Kinder für zu klein halten, um Probleme zu besprechen.
2 Die Schule ist/ nicht so schlimm wie manche glauben und behaupten.
3 Ich bin sehr traurig/ wenn meine Eltern mir böse sind.
4 Wenn nur meine Eltern/ manchmal mit mir mehr über etwas was mich aufregt, diskutieren wollten.
5 Ich hasse/ Prahlerei, Hochmut und übertriebene Eitelkeit.
6 Als ich noch ganz klein war/ hatte ich eine sehr schlechte Meinung von der Schule und wollte um keinen Preis etwas davon wissen.
7 Ich bin froh, daß ich/ so bin wie ich bin.
8 Andere sagen vielleicht von mir/ daß ich dick bin, doch ich sehe ein, daß es stimmt und ärgere mich nicht darüber.
9 Wenn ich zu Hause bin/ lege ich mich aufs Bett und drehe das Radio auf.
10 Wenn ich nur nicht/ einen Fünfer bekomme.
11 Mädchen sollten/ sich manchmal überlegen, was sie reden.
12 Buben sollten/ nicht in der Klasse herumschreien, sondern lernen, sich nicht zu schlagen sondern sich friedlich auseinanderzusetzen.
13 Das Wichtigste ist für mich/ ist, in der Schule etwas zu leisten.
19 OGT: 1 Es stört mich, daß/ ich keine gute Arbeit bekomme.
2 Die Schule ist/ aus und ich möchte am liebsten noch einmal hingehen.
3 Ich bin sehr traurig/ das ich nicht gut verdiene.

4 Wenn nur meine Eltern/ bei mir wären.
5 Ich hasse/ den Carly.
6 Als ich noch ganz klein war/ war viel einfacher das Leben.
7 Ich bin froh, daß ich/ noch eine Arbeit habe.
8 Andere sagen vielleicht von mir/ daß sie mich mögen oder nicht mögen.
9 Wenn ich zu Hause bin/ bin ich sehr glücklich.
10 Wenn ich nur nicht/ so schnell aufstehen müßte in der Früh und nicht so schnell.
11 Mädchen sollten/ miteinander auskommen aber meine Schwester und ich nicht.
13 Das Wichtigste ist für mich/ das ich mit meiner Familie zusammen bleibe.

References

Aronfreed, J. 1961: The nature, variety and social patterning of moral responses to transgression. *Abnormal and Social Psychology* 63.

— 1968: *Conduct and Conscience*. New York: Holt, Rinehart & Winston.

Beaugrande, R. de 1980: *Text, Discourse and Process*. Norwood, NJ: Ablex.

Beaugrande, R. de and Dressler, W. U. 1981: *Einführung in die Textlinguistik*. Tübingen: Niemeyer.

Berlach, G. 1982: *Sequentielle Abhängigkeit der Antworten im Rorschachtest*. Unpublished dissertation, University of Vienna.

Bernstein, B. 1970: *Soziale Struktur, Sozialisation und Sprachverhalten*. Amsterdam: de Munter.

Bieri, J. 1960: Parental identification, acceptance of authority and within-sex differences in cognitive behaviour. *Abnormal and Social Psychology* 60.

Blos, P. 1978: *Die Adoleszenz*. Stuttgart: Klett.

Dearborn, G. V. 1897: Blots of ink in experimental psychology. *Psychological Review* 4.

Fillmore, C. 1968: The case for case. In E. Bach and R. Harms (eds.), *Universals in Linguistic Theory*. New York: Holt, Rinehart & Winston.

Fischer, G. H. and Spada, H. 1973: '*Die psychometrischen Grundlagen des Rorschachtests und der Holtzman Inkblot Technique*. Bern: Huber

Herrmann, M. L. 1976: *Lehrbuch der empirischen Persönlichkeitsforschung*, 3rd edn. Göttingen: Hogrefe.

Hoffmann, M. L. and Saltzstein, H. D. 1965: Parent discipline and the child's moral development. *Personality and Social Psychology* 5.

Kerner, J. 1857: *Kleksographien*. Tübingen; cited in Berlach 1982.

Kohn, M. L. 1959: Social class and parental values. *American Journal of Sociology* LXIV.

Leodolter, R. 1975: *Das Sprachverhalten von Angeklagten bei Gericht*. Kronberg: Scriptor.

Meili, R. and Rohracher, H. 1972: *Lehrbuch der experimentellen Psychologie*. Bern: Huber.

Murray, H. A. 1951: Uses of the Thematic Apperception Test. *American Journal of Psychiatry* 107.

Oevermann, U. 1972: *Sprache und soziale Herkunft*. Frankfurt/Main: Suhrkamp.

Rorschach, H. 1972: *Psychodiagnostik*, 9th edn., Bern: Huber.

Sears, R. R., Maccoby, E. E. and Levin, H. 1957: *Patterns of Child Rearing*. Evanston, Ill: Great Expectations.

Spelke, E., Zelazo, P., Kagan, J. and Kotelchuk, M. 1973: Father interaction and separation protest. *Developmental Psychology* 8.

Strotzka, H., Schmidt, C., Hartmann, C. and Laburda, A. 1983: Das Kind im Spannungsfeld von Eltern — Schule und Gesellschaft. Projektbericht, Vienna.

Werlich, E. 1975: *Typologie der Texte*. Heidelberg: UTB.

Wittgenstein, L. 1980: *Philosophische Untersuchungen*. Frankfurt/Main: Suhrkamp.

Wodak, R. 1981: *Das Wort in der Gruppe*. Vienna: Verlag des österreichischen Akademie der Wissenschaften.

— 1983: Arguments in favour of a socio-psycholinguistic theory of text planning. *Klagenfurter Beitrage zur sprachwissenschaft*, 9.

— 1984: *Hilflose Nähe? — Mütter und Töchter erzählen*. Vienna: Deuticke.

Part 2

Schizophrenic language behaviour

7 'Grammar' and 'language-game' as concepts for the analysis of schizophrenic communication

Hans Rudi Fischer

I am sitting with a philosopher in
the garden; he says again and again
'I know that that's a tree', pointing
to a tree that is near to us. Someone
else arrives and hears this, and I tell him: 'This fellow isn't insane.'
We are only doing philosophy. (Ludwig Wittgenstein, 1969)

Introduction

In this chapter an analysis of the phenomena of schizophrenia is proposed which is orientated to the late philosophy of Wittgenstein. The speech-interactive aspect of deviant behaviour will be stressed, and psychosis interpreted as an expression of a form of family life.

Gaining access to an understanding of schizophrenia must therefore be orientated to the interpersonal context of this phenomenon. Schizophrenic communication styles can only be analysed from this standpoint, as they only make sense in such a framework. First, a methodological reason will be given for the application of Wittgenstein's language-game concept to the analysis of schizophrenic speech; then the constitutive or constructive elements of language as a means of coping with reality and procuring sense will be worked out. Wittgenstein interprets these elements of language as 'grammar'. The main function of grammar in this context is to conceptualize and categorize experience, thus allowing orientation in an intersubjective framework. In pathological cases, this grammar must be seen as disturbed. It leads to the development of atypical perspectives (ways of access) on one's own feelings and experiences, and on the way one perceives others. Normally, the family as a psychosocial organization is the medium of forms of life, such as grammar, and is therefore the location where deviant grammars and the corresponding forms of life are learned by the individual. This reflection concerning madness leads to the positions contained in the family and communication theory in schizophrenia research, and contributes to the theory's philosophical justification.

My intention is not to give a linguistic-grammatical analysis of 'schizophrenic language'. There is no 'schizophrenic language' as such, only resemblances in language and thought structures which are, however, different depending on circumstances. I am aware of the difficulties in defining 'schizophrenia', but in this chapter I shall be using the term uncritically all the same.

In referring to the consequences of Wittgenstein's language-game analysis, I wish to develop a basic perspective on the constructive characteristics of language. This position has validity for 'normal' and 'abnormal' language behaviour, and will be exemplified with two language-games of schizophrenics. At first it may seem surprising to refer to Wittgenstein in relation to insanity, but the strangeness vanishes if we consider the numerous widespread aperçus on the problems of insanity and look at it from Wittgenstein's philosophical viewpoint. In the next section. I shall sketch the main trends of communication theory in schizophrenic research and briefly comment on them.

Patterns of communication and interaction as a focus of the family theory in schizophrenia research

Since F. Fromm-Reichmann's publication (1948) about the schizophrenic mother drew attention to the mother/child dyad, the interest in interpersonal contact within the family has increased. In the following period, family theories were developed which put into focus the family's communication and interaction modes. These theories took this focus as a basis for etiological theses on schizophrenia, or as a new definition of the term 'schizophrenia'. Within the various theoretical positions three major directions can be identified, which, each in different ways, have established basic concepts for analysing and describing the phenomenon of schizophrenia. Bateson, Jackson *et al.* (1956) created a model of schizophrenic communication structure based on anthropological studies with the concept of the 'double-bind'. Lidz (1965, 1973) and Lidz *et al.* (1958) tried to describe disturbed interaction in the family with the help of the concept of 'transmission of irrationality'. Finally, Wynne *et al.* (1958) tried to identify a characteristic deformation in the family relationships of schizophrenics by the notion of 'pseudo-mutuality', and to understand transactional thought disorders in this context. Dell (1981) criticized these positions for mixing individual and interactional views, and confusing systemic epistemology and linear/causal theses.

I do not wish to criticize these theories which, pragmatically speaking, are valuable and fruitful, but to point out the problematic foundation on which the systemic-orientated family theory is based. Bateson (1955) explicitly mentions the theories that he uses as an epistemological basis for his own position: 'Earlier fundamental work of Whitehead, Russell, Wittgenstein, Carnap, Whorf, as well as my own attempt (1951) to use this earlier thinking as an epistemological base for psychiatric theory . . .' (1955: 29). Bateson and Ruesch (1951) place communication in the centre of psychiatric research and refer to the 'theory of types' (Whitehead and Russell), and to Wittgenstein's early theory of language, as well as to Carnap's and Whorf's theories, in order to use and integrate them in his own systemic theory. The crucial point for the entire double-bind theory Bateson had already mentioned in 1951: 'Using an organistic phrasing, one might say that impulses and showers of impulses travelling in the neutral network are an internal reflection or picture of the external events . . . or following mentalistic theories, one may say that ideas and propositions (whether verbal or nonverbal) are the translation or reflection of external events' (169). Referring to Wittgenstein, Bateson formulates his position as analogous to the way language is understood in Wittgenstein's *Tractatus*: 'While is it impossible for a man to have inside himself a tree corresponding to the external tree that he perceives, it is possible to have internal objects or events so related to each other that their relations reflect relationships between parts of the external tree' (170). These passages show the fundamental epistemological model that in Bateson's opinion is valid not only for the neural pictures of our perception, but also for language.

Watzlawick *et al.* (1967) took over the same epistemological premiss and established, with the theory of types and the concept of the double-bind, a 'pragmatics of human communication'. It is hard to understand why the contributors to this influential tradition did not realize that they had taken an incompatible premiss into their concept. When Bateson fell back on early Wittgenstein, Carnap and Russell, they overlooked the fact that these philosophers followed an old epistemological paradigm, which is to be found in a simple form in the philosophy of Democritus: the picture-theory. According to this model, knowledge and language (when describing cognition) is a picture of external reality. The order of reality was presupposed, and the only function of language was to depict this order correctly. (This is incidentally, a completely different position from the relativist proposal by Whorf, also referred to by Bateson.) By using the basis of the picture theory paradigm (which is fundamental to the theories of language in *Principia Mathematica*, the *Tractatus* and *The Logical Syntax of Language*, and connecting it with the clearly constructivist understanding of individual and family reality, Bateson's and Watzlawick's positions become inconsistent. Both Watzlawick and Bateson quote Wittgenstein's *Tractatus* as theoretical support, which has been understood as an attempt to reconstruct from ordinary language an ideal language which is adequate for logical syntax, and which thus renders a theory of types superfluous. Moreover, the radical picture-theory position of the *Tractatus* does not leave room for self-reflexivity (cf. Wittgenstein 1922 (cited in this chapter as *TLP*), 3.332ff.). Furthermore, the theory of types was 'not really a theory but a stop-gap' as Russell stated self-critically later on (cf. Cronen *et al.* 1982: 94).

The original double-bind theory has often been criticized since it was created. Cronen *et al.* (1982) take another approach to modifying the basic assumptions of the double-bind theory, and by this modification to make the original theses suitable for further use in schizophrenic research. (For a further exploration, Cronen *et al.* 1982.) One may also ask why the Palo Alto Group, after having turned more and more towards the pragmatics of human communication, did not take up the late philosophy of Wittgenstein. He is, beside Morris, the father of linguistic pragmatism. By using the methodological construct of the 'language-game', he put into focus not only the context of language use or sign interpretation but also, at the same time, the subject who uses the signs. It is precisely the pattern-orientated epistemology of Bateson that suggests a recourse to Wittgenstein's language-game conception.

The language-game can be understood as an epistemological/reconstructive pattern as well as a technical philosophical one. In the same way, the language-game as a pattern of communication analysis is clearly constructed instrumental-systemically.[1] I do not want to criticize these various theories in detail, but to develop a position based on language-philosophical reflections which allows us to see the various important concepts from one common perspective. It will become evident that the concepts of Bateson (double-bind), of Laing (mystification), of Lidz (transmission of irrationality), of Stierlin (delegation, adaptation to the 'stronger' person's reality) and of Wynne/Singer (pseudo-mutuality transactional thought disorder) can be summarized under the terms of the 'language-game' and the 'grammar' which are central to the late philosophy of Wittgenstein. On the basis of this understanding of language, the positions mentioned are not very far from each other, as they merely stress various aspects of the same phenomenon and organize it differently.

Methodological foundation: Language-games as a focus of observation

The proposal that by way of analysing the language-games of schizophrenics, one can gain a clearer idea of the phenomenon of schizophrenia may seem at first sight to be very limited. For such diseases characterized not only by linguistic deviations but by more complex disturbances which concern the person's thinking, acting, feeling and experience. Orthodox psychiatry, which is physically orientated, has always called whatever insanity produces nonsensical, apart from a few psychoanalytical positions. In this context I want to mention a scientist who has attempted what nobody else had done before, namely to introduce the language-game concept into communication-orientated research on schizophrenia. I am referring to the very interesting and elaborate model by A. Lorenzer (1970a; 1972; 1977). Lorenzer's theory has been directed towards psychoanalytical theory and therapy from the very beginning. In his attempt to explain psychoanalysis metatheoretically, Wittgenstein's idea of the language-game takes up a prominent position. As I have shown in a previous paper (Fischer 1982a), the term 'language-game' is used inadequately here; also, in the light of the analysis of language, the psychoanalytical understanding of the functioning of a neurotically disturbed language appears indistinctly, and metatheoretical substantiation consequently fails. By looking at the patient's specific level of symbols as related to the 'inner reality', psychoanalysis must presuppose a partly privatized language (although unconscious) which functions in the language community.

This comprehension of Wittgenstein's language-game analysis is in radical opposition to the results of Wittgenstein's later philosophy, and is not conceivable as a result of Wittgenstein's descriptions of our language-games. However, the connections between language and forms of life, which are invariably stressed by Wittgenstein, was pointed out by Lorenzer's theory in an extended and appropriate way. As far as my own position is concerned, I have gained, from studying his theory, essential incentives which have become very fruitful for my own understanding.[2] Habermas (1967; 1968) advocates a similar language-analytical position for sociology. The position presented here is mainly in agreement with Habermas. Some aspects, however, such as the transcendental-philosophical interpretation of Wittgenstein, are different. A discussion of Habermas's complex theory is beyond the scope of this chapter. (For a further exploration see Habermas 1967; 1968). In the following pages, I intend to explain the term 'language-game' and to claim that, when analysing schizophrenic communication, the language games in the family have to play a central role in the examination. It has to be mentioned that language or speaking needs to be understood here in a more complex way. 'Language' does not mean only speech, but also paralinguistic phenomena like facial expressions, body carriage and gestures. The 'language-game', as Wittgenstein introduced the term, must be seen as a synthesis of verbal and nonverbal actions. All facts whose existence is a prerequisite for the sense of a sentence must count as belonging to language. At crucial points in the *Philosophical Investigations* (Wittgenstein 1953, cited in this chapter as *PI*), Wittgenstein writes:

> I shall also call the whole, consisting of language and the actions into which it is woven, the 'language-game'. (*PI* 7)
>
> Here the term 'language-game' is meant to bring into prominence the fact that the speaking of language is part of an activity, or of a form of life. (*PI* 23)

The action or cognition aspect that is of great importance in this chapter is often set out by Wittgenstein in the tool analogy. By emphasizing the operational aspects of the application of words in language-games, Wittgenstein overrides the separation between 'pure language' and 'language-independent actions', and understands language itself as a refined action. In order to maintain the usefulness of the term 'language-game', it has to be taken into consideration that Wittgenstein makes no categorical distinction between language and thought. Even in his early notebooks he says that language is irreducible. This statement can be proved above all epistemologically, and this gains decisive significance when examining epistemologies in families. Epistemologically speaking, we have no neutral access to the phenomena of our experiences, no matter whether they are 'inner' or 'outer' experiences. That means the epistemic path to our field of experience is in principle language-dependent or bound to the possibility of verbal description. In the *Philosophical Investigations*, Wittgenstein puts it this way: 'the language is itself the vehicle of thought,' (*PI* 329). According to this position, the mediation of thought structures as far as they are relative to a culture (Whorf 1956; Sapir 1949) must take place through language and its corresponding forms of life. Thus language has a decisive cognitive aspect that becomes especially obvious in the deviant communication styles in the families of schizophrenics (Wynne and Singer 1963). Wittgenstein's understanding of language is also compatible with the premises of family theory above all with regard to the term of interpersonal communication:

> We suggest that the term 'communication disorder' is a more comprehensive and appropriate term. 'Communication' takes into account the transaction in which thinking and language are embedded; it implies a verbal interchange e.g., in patient-interviewer dyads and in family relationships. (Singer and Wynne *et al.* 1978: 504)[3]

In the secondary literature there have been a number of misunderstandings about the term 'language-game', because its ambivalent but nevertheless fruitful structure has not been understood. On this account, I want to characterize the term briefly. Its primary function is to be a line of investigation or a point of view. It focuses on a smaller unit (language-game) that can be easily overlooked, and thus makes it possible to analyse the mechanism of language without battling against the fog of the entire language system. This is the methodological function of the term. It is only the secondary aspect that marks language games as 'complete systems of human communication' (Wittgenstein 1958: 81/121). So within the term 'language-game', line of investigation and object of investigation come together as one. The latter usage is always overshadowed by the former, the methodological approach, so that at an ontological level nothing is prejudiced. Another characteristic of Wittgenstein's understanding of language-games that is methodologically relevant to the analysis of schizophrenic communication is a result of Wittgenstein's philosophy of psychology. The notion 'language-game', with all its implications, turns out to be an instrument of a methodologically behaviouristic psychology of 'inner states'.

As a result of a discussion about the problems of philosophical psychology, these positions are to be found above all in the *PI*, where Wittgenstein takes a stand against the possibility of a private language. He criticizes the model of introspective psychology (in the tradition of William James) which allows access to the mental phenomena of others by drawing an analogy from one's own way of experiencing. The analogy conclusion is due to an attribution which is introspectively justified. In proving that an introspective philosophy of psychology (which is based on self observation) can establish neither criteria of identity for one's own mental events nor a rule-governed usage of such privately constructed mental predicates, Wittgenstein destroys the fundamental position of introspective psychology. But behaviourism, which also justifiably rejects introspection as a legitimate source of knowledge, in principle follows the same misleading paradigm as introspective psychology does. Contrary to introspective psychology, behaviourism is based on the attribution of mental predicates to 'outward' behaviour in order to come to 'objective' statements about mental states. Neither sees the fundamental disparity between the first and the third person singular (present tense) when ascribing mental predicates. Behaviourism collapses the first person with the third by saying that even the first person comes to self-attribution only by observing his own behaviour. In contrast to this, introspective psychology bases the ascription of mental predicates of others on self-observation.

When Wittgenstein stresses the criterial asymmetry between first and third person, he is arguing against the paradigm of the two psychologies. He emphasizes that the first person ascribes the mental predicates to himself without criteria, and, because of this, the self-ascription is in principle incapable of correction. This, however, does not account for the third person (see Fischer 1983b). In spite of Wittgenstein's criticism, he argues in favour of methodological behaviourism when saying that 'an "inner process" stands in need of outward criteria' (*PI* 580). Wittgenstein shows that, when mental predicates are ascribed, ordinary language is grammatically bound to criteria of 'outer' behaviour, and that such 'inner processes' have to be presupposed grammatically if you want to talk about mental events. Therefore, behaviour must be understood as an expression of 'something' that can only be described in language; this 'something', however, is not identical with the behaviour. The denial of such 'inner processes' as practised by radical behaviourism is another inconsistency of the theory.

So we can say that Wittgenstein is an advocate of methodological behaviourism, as far as the language-game concept is concerned; but outward criteria form the basis for the usage of mental predicates with regard to other persons. The position is methodologically behaviouristic; for it does not deny 'inner processes', but shows that our language about mental states presupposes their very existence. In the following, I will take for granted that our ways of thinking and experiencing are determined by language-games and their inherent logic. This is also true, at least in my opinion, of the language-games of schizophrenics. What I have explained up to now has made it obvious that the concentration on schizophrenic language-games does not constitute a reduction of the complex phenomena concerning the problem of language, but is the only possibility of opening a comprehensive path to the experiences of the insane. For indeed, we only have 'outward' criteria (behavioural criteria in a broader sense) to depict the 'inner states' of the insane. One can only speculate about their thinking processes or their subjective experiencing, speculation which from a scientific point of view is worthless. Therefore, all we have is the observable language behaviour in the language-games which are actually played.

That means that a methodological restriction to the observable seems to be appropriate at the beginning. The notion of language-game as a 'system of human communications' has to be seen as a systemic unit, in which the single words and propositions (sentences) acquire their meaning or sense. This is only one facet of the contextual position in Wittgenstein. In analogy to this, I would like to advance the socio-psychological assumption that an individual's behaviour can only be interpreted in the light of the behaviour of the social group of which he is a member (Mead 1934). Wittgenstein usually refers to this by the terms 'forms of life', 'ways of life' or 'culture'. Language-games have to be understood as systems of intersubjectively shared meanings, as well as systems of shared behaviour. Mead developed the theoretical tradition of symbolic interactionism, and he described the way in which interaction and communication systems are of constitutive significance for the disposition of acting. I employ the term 'language-game' as the embodiment of such interaction and communication systems. I take the family as a subgroup of a more complex form of life in which the individual's behaviour has its home.

The concept of grammar and its relation to the form of life

Wittgenstein's usage of the term 'grammar' is indeed unique and not easy to define. The philosophically conclusive usage of the term is developed from the concept of logic in the *Tractatus*(*TLP*). The same usage is relevant when talking about schizophrenic communication, as we are here. The specific logic of each specific language-game takes the place of the logic that in the *Tractatus* constitutes the rationalistic base of language. According to Wittgenstein, the term 'grammar' is almost equivalent to the 'logic' of the language-game.

The following questions can now be put forward. In which way do we need to understand such 'grammatical propositions', and what is their essential function in the present context? In order to understand the term 'grammatical proposition' we need to be aware of the family resemblance to the term 'rule', because Wittgenstein calls such propositions 'grammatical rules' as well. The relationship between grammatical propositions and rules becomes obvious in Wittgenstein's discussion of the foundations of mathematics. With an example from arithmetic, he makes it clear that adopting a 'mathematical proposition' (rule) also means learning a technique. At this point Wittgenstein's term 'grammar' or 'grammatical proposition' becomes important. Learning how to follow a rule — and this is true in principle for all rules — depends on the adoption of the rule and on what is called the 'correct' following, for each rule can be basically ambiguous. This is also reflected in some passages from the *Remarks on the Foundation of Mathematics (RFM)* (Wittgenstein 1980):

> Let us remember that in mathematics we are convinced of grammatical propositions; so the expression, the result, of our being is convinced is that we accept a rule. (*RFM* 162)

Games, languages and rules are institutions and refer to a learned technique or to a custom, as Wittgenstein says, acquired in the process of socialization (cf. *RFM* 334).

> By being educated in a technique, we are also educated to have a way of looking at the matter which is just as firmly rooted as that technique. (*RFM* 243)

On the same page, he describes very impressively the nondescriptive or noncognitive function of such 'grammatical propositions' and their central function in the constitution of language-games. He hints at the fact that the grammatical proposition shows the connections 'that we regard as rigid. But to a certain extent we look away from these connections and at something else. We turn our back upon them, so to speak. Or: we rest, or lean, on them . . .We acknowledge it by turning our back on it.' Such sentences are means of representation but of the things that are being represented (cf. *RFM* 392; *PI* 50). Accordingly these sentences (propositions) also defy empirical examination and verification. Such 'sentences' form an established way of representation and become 'a rule of expression, for speaking about our experiences' (*RFM* 50). On the implicit basis of such 'sentences' (or 'propositions') we describe reality in propositions of experience, which, corresponding to their descriptive nature, can be verified or falsified.

This, however, is not the case with grammatical propositions. When Wittgenstein talks about grammar in this sense, we have to see it as the system of the propositions which circumscribe, or define, the specific game. Such propositions describe the logic of the game, but may not be understood in this game as descriptions. I shall talk about grammar in the same way. It is remarkable that Wittgenstein also wanted the differentiation between grammatical and empirical propositions to be understood as a distinction of logical types: 'All grammar is a theory of logical types; and logical types do not talk about the application of language. Russell failed to see this, (*Lectures, Cambridge 1930–32* (*LI* 12). (In this chapter I cannot go into the Russell criticism which is to be found in the entire early and middle periods of Wittgenstein.)

Some further terms that Wittgenstein employs as synonymous, or at least as having a strong family resemblance, can explain the term 'grammar' in more detail: method of representation, form of representation, system of rules, way of looking at the matter, paradigm, pattern and so on. Grammar taken in this sense forms the co-ordination axis of language, the support on the basis of which we describe and comprehend reality. For that reason, grammar as a form of representation of reality cannot be justified by a recourse to this reality.

> Grammar is not accountable to any reality. It is grammatical rules that determine meaning (constitute it) and so they themselves are not answerable to any meaning and to that extent are arbitrary. (*Philosophical Grammar (PG)*, 184)

Grammatical propositions are thus the verbal formulation of principles of our judgements, and constitute those judgements. To justify those rules on the basis of our experience would therefore be a *petitio principii*. Wittgenstein takes this view, and instead postulates the arbitrariness of grammar. Such propositions as 'there are four primary colours', 'every rod has a length' or 'I know that I am in pain' are various forms of grammatical proposition which have often been taken for propositions of experience; and therefore, as metaphysical pseudo-propositions, they have confused many philosophers.

At this point, I want to put special emphasis on the constitutive character of such propositions or constitutive rules, with regard to the access to reality. This is especially relevant for the area of 'soft reality', which refers to relationships, feelings, dispositions of behaviour and so on; that is the questionable ontological sphere, which Wittgenstein deals with in his philosophy of psychology (cf. Fischer 1983a). It is also of great importance for our social and personal identity. This constructive moment in his conception of grammar becomes all the clearer for being closely related to the 'world picture' or 'Weltanschauung'. In this way the specific access to reality, or 'world', becomes explicit. (For further exploration of this connection see Wittgenstein 1969 *On Certainty (OC)* 141 ff., 162ff.) The propositions that, according to Wittgenstein, describe our world view are those grammatical propositions and rules that underlie our language-games without being noticed. Such propositions have an epistemological and pragmatic function (cf. Fischer 1982a; 1982b), for they constitute the latent basis of our thinking and acting. Wittgenstein's position regarding these constitutive elements of grammar has a definite perspectivisitic element, that shows strong parallels with Nietzsche's perspectivisim. However, unlike Nietzsche, Wittgenstein does not draw any nihilistic conclusions. Language and reality are therefore not considered as two areas that can be ontologically differentiated; but the relationship between language and reality is seen as inseparable and at the same time bound to the grammatical rules of our use of language. At the beginning of Wittgenstein's development towards his late philosophy, which was at the end of the 1920s, this position gains more and more influence and finally dominates in his late works, *Philosophical Investigation* and *On Certainty*. In 1930 he says: 'Grammar lets us do some things with language' and 'We see in a different way according to the system in which we see' (*LI*: 8, 54). This system in which we see or think and speak is termed 'language-game'. Language-games as systems of communication not only govern our speech but also our thinking, as long as there is no categorical difference between the two. Grammatical propositions, taken as a measure of description and as organization of reality, are 'the fixed rails along which all our thinking runs, and so our judgement and action goes according to *Zettel* (*Z* 375). Wittgenstein talks about our 'conceptual world' (*Z* 568, *Remarks on the Philosophy of Psychology* (*RPP*) II, 398) or of 'conceptual glasses' (cf. also Whorf 1956). This also stresses the cultural relativities of grammars or world views. A few days before his death, Wittgenstein beautifully described this component. I would like to quote this passage completely. It starts out with the discussion of whether acting according to the theoretical (grammatical) propositions of physics is acting on 'good ground':

> Supposing we met people who did not regard that as a telling reason. Now, how do we imagine this? Instead of the physicist, they consult an oracle. (And for that we consider them primitive). Is it wrong for them to consult an oracle and be guided by it? — If we call this 'wrong' aren't we using our language game as a base from which to combat theirs? (*OC* 609)

> And are we right or wrong to combat it? Of course there are all sorts of slogans which will be used to support our proceedings. (*OC* 610)
>
> Where two principles really do meet which cannot be reconciled with one another, then each man declares the other a fool and heretic. (*OC* 611)
>
> I said I would 'combat' the other man — but wouldn't I give him reasons? Certainly; but how far do they go? at the end of reasons comes persuasion. (Think what happens when missionaries convert natives.) (*OC* 612)

Wittgenstein also says about these propositions that they 'might be said to be fossilized' (*OC* 657) or that they are 'hard rocks' of our judgements (*OC* 99). If I present grammar as a social consensual process of sedimentation of historical knowledge, the reconstruction of this grammar is comparable to Foucault's 'archeology of knowledge'. The family therapist digs for family communication structures and their underlying myths, attributions and roles. He is also an archeologist, in that he analyses the sedimented structures of a pathological nature. He tries to change the pathological patterns of language and action. It is precisely because of this that he can be called a missionary. The objective, however, is to change not only pathological communication styles but also, of course, the family's ways or forms of life. That leads us to Wittgenstein's other important concept; 'forms of life'. I have said that the term 'grammatical proposition' is used as having a family resemblance with the term 'rule', and that, in being patterns of action, such rules have a highly significant pragmatic function. Wittgenstein compares this function to a path:

> A rule is best described as being like a garden path in which you are trained to walk, and which is convenient. You are taught arithmetic by a process of training, and this becomes one of the paths in which you walk. (*Lectures, Cambridge 1932–5* (*L*II 155)

The image of a road emerges again in a different context and stresses the psychological aspect:

> But our interest does not attach to the fact that such-and-such (or all) human beings have been led this way by this rule (or have gone this way); we take it as a matter of course that people — if they can think 'correctly' — go this way. We have now been given a road, as it were by means of the footsteps of those who have gone this way. (*RFM* 98)

This is Wittgenstein's metaphorical paraphrase of rule and rule-obeying which is very important in socialization. This path leads through a historically formed landscape into which the individual is born. This horizon Wittgenstein calls 'forms of life', 'way of life' and 'culture' (cf. Fischer 1984). He also counts it among the conditions that make language and action possible. Wittgenstein does not want to give a historical/genetic language theory, but to prove that language as a social reality can only become comprehensible if we know the background from which it has grown. It is precisely this aspect that needs to be reclaimed in connection with the language-games of schizophrenics. Again, in the *Remarks on the Foundations of Mathematics*, Wittgenstein makes clear the connection between rules, rule-obeying and forms of life:

> But how then does the teacher interpret the rule for the pupil? (For he is certainly supposed to give it a particular interpretation.) Well, how but by means of words and training? And if the pupil reacts to it in thus and thus, he possesses the rule inwardly. But this is important, namely that this reaction, which is our guarantee of understanding, presupposes as a surrounding particular circumstances, particular forms of life and speech. (*RFM* 414)

We should not think that grammar is determined in a linear-causal way by forms of life, but rather by a systemic unit (open) of grammar (language) and forms of life. A change in the one normally involves a change in the other. Wittgenstein uses another image to show this relationship even more clearly:

> But I did not get my picture of the world by satisfying myself of its correctness; nor do I have it because I am satisfied of its correctness. No: it is the inherited background against which I distinguish between true and false. (*OC* 94)
>
> The propositions describing this world-picture might be part of a kind of mythology. And their role is like that of rules of a game; and the game can be learned purely practically, without learning explicit rules. (*OC* 95)
>
> It might be imagined that some propositions of the form of empirical propositions were hardened, and functioned as channels for such empirical propositions as were not hardened but fluid; and that this relation altered with time, in that fluid propositions hardened, and hard ones became fluid. (*OC* 96)
>
> The mythology may change back into a state of flux, the river-bed of thoughts may shift. But I distinguish between the movement of the waters on the river-bed and the shift of the bed itself; though there is not a sharp division of the one from the other. (*OC* 97)

This gives us another metaphor for grammar: the river-bed. We see that Wittgenstein uses 'world picture', 'grammar' or 'grammatical propositions' (rules), and also mythology, as terms bearing a family resemblance. If we stay with this image we can visualize the landscape within which the river is flowing as the form of life or the river's (language) surroundings.

In comparing this world picture to mythology, Wittgenstein's fideistic position becomes evident. As grammar is arbitrary in the sense that it cannot be justified by means of recourse to experience, it forms an epistemic system which has the quality of a system of belief. Grammar, however, is responsible for the categorizing and conceptualizing of experience, and thus also for what we call our 'rationality'. This makes plausible Wittgenstein's relativizing statement about our rationality being a mythology. In this image, the river-bed consists of empirical propositions which are hardened, and he compares these propositions to rules that, in accordance with a given interpretation, we can understand as grammatical rules. Such rules are supporting elements in our socialization. It should be noted that 'what we believe depends on what we learn' (*OC* 286) and what we learn is taught to us as a foundation of the description of reality. This foundation, however, is the limitation of the game: 'At the foundation of well-founded belief lies belief that is not founded' (*OC* 253). The justification recourse must therefore be stopped at the pragmatic limitations of the game, otherwise it will end in metaphysical no-man's-land.

One epistemological consequence of this fideistic-conventionalistic way of thinking lies in the fact that there does not exist a reality as such ('objective reality') in a nonmetaphysical sense, and accordingly there can be no 'objective knowledge' of this reality. Thus the grammatical/consensual system of description functions as an organizing pattern, and constitutes in this way the linguistic/cognitive foundations of the recognition and description of reality. This grammatical system requires 'a steady way of living (forms of life), regular ways of acting' (*Ursache und Wirkung* (*UW*) 420), which defines this grammar as a frame of action. It is essential to the language-game we play that we utter certain words, and regularly act in accordance with them (cf. *UW* 412). In this manner we maintain recourse to the grammar of the language-game and its corresponding perspective. For this reason I conceive the relation/grammar (language)/form of life as a self-referential system (cf. the river/river-bed metaphor) that is maintained because grammar as a cognitive perspective is related to a specific form of life (patterns of acting). This cognitive reality is sustained in a recursive way by living these forms of life. The relation between grammar and form of life is understood as a homeostatic system which constitutes its own reality and reproduces it accordingly.

The individual who is integrated into this system has a range of experience which is kept in balance because this system determines the cognitive/conceptual experience as well as the concrete experiences of its members. This implies that we construct our reality by means of a specific grammar, and create and maintain it by using it in our forms of life.[4] Such an idea can usefully be applied to the family and made fruitful for schizophrenic communication. Before I explain the logic of language acquisition, I wish to establish a connection between what I have said on this point and communication-orientated research into schizophrenia.

We read in Wittgenstein that within the language there is 'a whole mythology' (*Bemerkungen über Frazer's 'Golden Bough' (BUF)*, 46). Wittgenstein attaches this to the idea of a linguistic world picture as already found in Humboldt's philosophy. He refers to 'normal' and 'undisturbed' speech. The user of the language is not conscious of the inherent world view of our grammar, and this only becomes clear when looking at other cultures or, in the context discussed here, when looking at world pictures of the insane which are different from the myth of our 'rational' languages and actions. It is remarkable that this trait of thought has already found its way into family research. It was Ferreira (1966) who introduced the term 'family myth' into family research, and he understands it in a similar way to that suggested here, that is, as an aspect of deviant family grammar. Such family myths contain many different rules of relationship that find their expression in daily family habits. Ferreira describes these as being integrated into everyday life in such a way that they are inseparable from the experiental context in which the family members live. The opinions formed within the family, which are responsible for the formation, maintenance and justification of many interactional patterns, and which seem to people outside the family an extreme falsification of real events, are accepted by the family members as ultimate truths and remain unquestionable (cf. Watzlawick and Weakland 1979: 87ff.). We can easily see the analogy between this description of family myth and what has been previously called the myth of grammar or language. Such myths are conveyed through language, and this is also true of those obviously deviant grammatical systems which Wittgenstein has postulated for socially valid grammar: '"So you are saying that human agreement decides what is true and what is false?" — It is what human beings say that is true and false; and they agree in the language they use. That is not agreement in opinions but in forms of life.' (*PI* 241) Here it becomes clear how the concept of grammar and forms of life can be integrated into family research. The following sections are devoted to showing how a general perspective can be developed.

On rules and language acquisition and the possibility of systematic misconditioning

Talking about language games, Wittgenstein also refers to situations in which children learn the language through 'primitive forms of language' (language-games). In accentuating the use of language as a social practice, the point that connects language with action is put into focus: language acquisition. In the process of language acquisition, speech and action (behaviour) are connected, and thus actual linguistic activity is constituted. At the early stage of language acquisition, rules are not explicitly taught but shown by example (cf. *z* 295ff.). The rule that is conveyed in the learning situation becomes the path on which walking is learned, as Wittgenstein describes it metaphorically. In this phase of socialization the switches are set that guide verbally dependent thinking and acting, as well as verbal access to our emotions. According to Wittgenstein, the rule-obeying aspect forms the central problem. It precedes the explicit formulation of the rule, and therefore we first need to follow the rule blindly. Because rule following is not governed by a further metarule, the learning situation has the crucial function of conveying socially accepted rule obeying. As, in these early stages, there is not yet any understanding of the explanation of rules, Wittgenstein calls it in this context 'conditioning', 'drill' or 'training'.

Of course, in this learning situation there always remains the possibility that socially deviant rules will be internalized. There are various experimental psychological studies that Wittgenstein's analysis casts light on. I wish to refer to a study by A. Bavelas that is mentioned in a report by Watzlawick (1981). The study belongs to what is called 'non-contingent reward experiment'. In these tests the connection between the subject's behaviour and its assessment by the experimenter is absent. In the study, a long series of number pairs was read to the subjects and they were asked to decide whether the two numbers fitted together. When the subjects asked in which way the numbers were supposed to fit together, the only answer was that the objective of the experiment was to discover the rule behind this connection. Thus the impression developed that it was a 'trial-and-error' study. The subjects were given the answer 'right' or 'wrong' in accordance with the Gauss law of distribution, which takes no account of the answer as such. It is actually a little surprising that, in the course of the experiment, the subjects developed a hypothesis which they held onto even after being told that their answers had been non-contingent.

I shall go on to describe this experiment against the background of

Wittgenstein's discussion concerning the term 'rule'. I shall compare this experiment to a learning situation where the experimenter plays the role of a teacher and the subject the role of the pupil. The pupil starts the learning situation by trying to determine a rule relationship between the number pairs presented — that is, he tries to reconstruct a rule that governs the use of the words 'fit' and 'does not fit' and in this constitutes their sense within the language-game. At first the experimenter is the arbiter, the final authority assessing the rightness of the answer. In the course of the experiment the 'right' answers take shape, with the outline of a rule, its rejection or modification entirely determined by the teacher's judgement. An increasing number of 'right' answers encourages the pupil to establish a seemingly valid rule for the game and also obedience to that rule. In fact we can understand the teacher's answers as positive or negative reinforcement and thus interpret the learning situation as an act of social instrumental learning. We can imagine the language acquisition situation to be similar, with the selective moment, which reinforces what is taken to be 'right' rule-obeying, playing the outstanding role. The pupil gets more and more convinced of the 'rightness' of his outline because of this reinforcement. When, according to the Gauss law of distribution, the frequency of his right judgements decreases, he at first continues to hold onto his belief and defends it against the assessment of the teacher who had just previously confirmed the 'rightness' of this rule. The teacher 'suddenly' wants to convince him of the false nature of the rule which has already pragmatically proved useful.

This experiment explains how a rule is intersubjectively internalized and how, on this ground, a perspective is developed under which reality is seen and organized. An essential element in the formation of a rule is the systematic reinforcement of what is counted as 'right'. If the experiment was set up so that the experimenter would answer 'wrong' and 'right' alternately, the pupil would never be able to establish a rule. He would perhaps determine the reason for the experiment and thus dissolve it. For a rule must be applied repeatedly, and this is not possible in an experiment which has been modified in this way. In this experiment the achievement of the pupil lies in the reconstruction of a grammatical rule. It constitutes the application of the verbs 'fit' and 'does not fit', and hence their sense in the given language-game. The pupil has recourse to this rule when in conflict, for it is the basis of his orientation in the specific experiment situation, and it is to this rule that the pupil will refer when justifying his assessment. The rule is the paradigm which reality and experience is compared to or organized in accordance with. The pupil by himself can no longer justify these grammatical rules theoretically; perhaps he can do so pragmatically, as it is then useful in obtaining the teacher's reward in the form of a 'right' assessment.

At this point the pupil becomes uncertain. In his opinion the rule has visibly proved useful, namely, the rule that he has factually learned through the noncontingent behaviour of the experimenter, which the subject of course is not aware of. The teacher 'suddenly' does not accept the pupil's game any more. The pupil's behaviour is psychologically understandable. In the course of the experiment or learning situation, he has developed a perspective which confirms his behaviour and thus renders it meaningful, at least subjectively. 'Objectively' this assumption seemed to be confirmed by the teacher's assessment. When the teaher factually rejects this rule, an explicit contradiction becomes apparent and the student defends his belief system until the experimenter dissolves the situation (cf. Watzlawick 1981: 13ff.). In the experiment, the adult is able to recognize the contradiction and cope with it intellectually. The contradiction between pupil and teacher in this experiment lies in the fact that the pupil's grammatical rule, that has given him orientation, is suddenly not valid any more, and is now inconsistent with the 'objectively' valid grammatical rule which appears to underlie the experimenter's answers. The experiment shows clearly how uncertainty comes about when the student can no longer act adequately on the grounds of the acquired role.

Another important aspect of such a learning situation is the asymmetrical power structure in the teacher/pupil relationship. It is analogous to the learning situation of the child, in that both experimenter and parents are the final authorities who decide what is 'right' and 'wrong'. The adult in the experiment has the possibility of escape, whereas the child does not have such a chance. This situation is similar to what is called by Laing 'mystification'. With the help of many examples, he shows the ways in which way parents systematically devalue their children's statements and by this disrupt the organization of their perception and feelings, which they have formed on the grounds of their grammatical rules. In this context Laing talks about the parents being arbiters (1964: 43) or representing the orientation axis (1969: 302). Indeed, a functioning grammar is the orientation axis around which our perception revolves. As the grammar, however, is conveyed by the parents, they are the institution that uses grammar as a power factor and as an instrument of control for their own needs.[5]

These elements of unbalanced power relations can be postulated for primary and also partly for secondary socialization. If the children are mystified from early on, then the inequality remains and will become pathological. Besides this asymmetry and its implications, another point in the child's learning situation has to be considered. As a child's ability to express his feelings, intentions or desires is rather limited, it always needs interpretation (cf. Ryan 1974: 199ff.). As the mother must interpret the child's body language, this situation is extremely sensitive for the adoption of a deviant grammar. This will be explained in more detail in the next chapter. The child's early learning situation, which I have characterized as being asymmetrical, is described by Stierlin (1981) as the dialectic between the 'giver of truth' and the 'receiver of truth'. This stands in analogy to the previously presented analysis of the non-contingent-reward experiments. First, Stierlin gives an etymological analysis of the term 'Wahrnehmung' (perception, literally: truth-receiving). Then he draws the conclusion that, at the time of crucial development and separation processes, the members of various generations play the role of both 'giver of truth' and 'receiver of truth'. In this process the reality of the relationship is created and consensually validated (cf. Stierlin 1981: 57). In this article Stierlin does not refer explicitly to the function of speech. For that reason I would like to stress this point, which is of importance for the lingustic consideration of schizophrenia, namely that 'right' and 'wrong' only exist in a conceptualized system of communication. It is clearly shown in the above experiment, where the experimenter plays the role of the 'giver of truth' and by doing so creates that which gives meaning to 'fit' in this language-game. In this process of conveying grammatical rules there also occurs, as stated by Stierlin (1959), an 'adaptation to the "stronger" person's reality'. He also characterizes the early asymmetry of the situation by saying that parents, the administrators of the 'stronger reality', are 'givers of truth' at the beginning and the child is the 'receiver of truth' (Stierlin 1981: 57).

I would like to summarize the main points of my argumentation in this chapter again. Against a background of socioculturally nurtured forms of life, the subject is led to that which Wittgenstein calls 'agreement in action'. It occurs in primary (and even in the secondary) socialization, through rule-governed connection of speech and action. In the process of language acquisition, the individual adopts the grammar presented to it and its corresponding forms of life. In the learning situation, the child is entirely dependent on its teachers (parents) and their standards. Grammar as a way of representing reality becomes an epistemological foundation for the verbal description of the world, and thus governs access to experience and the actions which are pragmatically connected with it.

These grammatical structures constitute linguistic access to reality, and must be understood as operational patterns of reality acquisition and coping with that reality. There is no doubt about the fact that there is great variety in grammatical structures in different cultures. It is also clear that, in spite of major differences, there are also cross-cultural invariances and similarities to be found. This is irrelevant to my study. What is important is that great differences are also possible within one culture. Differences occur not only in grammar but also in the corresponding forms of life. Consider the various subcultures. We can assume that a communication community also has common forms of life. In spite of different grammars and forms of life, understanding is in principle possible. 'Stepping over' into a different system (grammar/forms of life) is only possible to a certain degree. What applies to society as a whole is also true of micro-societies.

The grammar of feelings

In schizophrenia, special importance has to be attached to affective ambivalence, incongruence between emotional and verbal expression, and emotional states with which the individual cannot cope intellectually. Wittgenstein deals with this aspect of the philosophy of psychology by analysing the language-games centring around 'inner states' or 'states of consciousness'. Wittgenstein's insight concerning the connection between mental events and verbal expression leads to the previously mentioned methodological behaviouristic view. He characterizes his position as follows: 'Also what goes on in the inner has meaning only in the stream of life' (*Last Writings on the Philosophy of Psychology* (*LRPP*) 118). The stream of life, Wittgenstein's most important metaphor, refers to the social practice where such mental events have meaning. And this practice is certainly an interpersonal and intersubjective one. In the discussion about deviant communication, the following question is of great interest: in what way can speech be related to the 'inner phenomena' of a third person? This is of paramount importance, because we only have indirect access to these mental events. Given that schizophrenic people do communicate with others in a deviant way, especially in the area of mental events, then the learning situation that impresses such ways of behaviour upon them deserves to be examined.

Wittgenstein has used the paradigm of pain to show how a 'normal' language-game about 'inner states' is built up. A child learns to replace the preverbal expression (e.g. crying) with a verbal one. The language-game 'to be in pain' is based on preverbal modes of behaviour (Mead's 'nonsignificant gestures') and 'is an extension of the more primitive behaviour' (cf. *RPP* 1, 151). The natural expression of pain (crying) has been replaced by the verbal expression. This does not imply, however, that the word *pain* actually means pain, but that the word expression has taken the place of the natural expression and does not describe it. Wittgenstein thinks these words of sensation are primarily expressive and not descriptive, even though there may be language-games where they have a descriptive function. In the learning situation, however, they are picked up as expressive words. Wittgenstein gives the following reason for this assumption. I cannot get between pain and its expression by language (*PI* 245). Ontogenetically speaking, pain precedes natural expression. If there were no natural expression, we would not be able to learn the language of sensation. Thus, natural expression is a prerequisite for our public speech. Wittgenstein talks about this as the 'outward criteria' from which public speech proceeds. In his discussion, pain functions as a paradigm for 'inner states', and we can transfer the result of this use of language to our discussion of other feelings.

This analysis is consistent with various speech acquisition theories in two important ways. (1) Natural behaviour is primarily expressive, that is it has no symbolic function (Mead 1934; Bruner 1974; Ryan 1974). (2) Parents, as teachers of language, are required to 'interpret' this behaviour. The differentiation between the first and third person singular that Wittgenstein has introduced in referring to psychological verbs such as *hope*, *fear*, and *believe* presents an essential addition to our position. When analysing the language-game about 'inner states', Wittgenstein proves that there is an epistemic disparity between the first and third person. He discovered that the usage of verbs directed towards a third person can be verified or falsified by observation, which is not true for the first person. The behaviouristic methodological position corresponds to this differentiation. If I attribute 'anger' to a third person, I need such outward criteria as a red face or a threatening fist. The fact that outward criteria are needed opens up the possibility of wrong attribution. That means that it is possible that the person himself is not in fact in this 'inner state' but is feeling something else. This, however, cannot happen to myself, as I do not need outward criteria to describe my states of consciousness or identify them. There are no 'objective' criteria for myself. So when I say: *I am angry*, the question: how do I 'know' that? is senseless. I attribute my states of consciousness criterion-less. Therefore it does not make sense to talk about 'knowing' when referring to one's own states of consciousness, and it is also senseless to talk about 'not knowing'. (*I don't know that I'm in pain*). This element of consciousness has been fossilized into the bases of language-games about 'states of consciousness'; thus, sentences like *I know that I'm in pain* (cf. *PI* 244), taken as an empirical or cognitive proposition, are senseless, because they do not express genuine knowledge. They are grammatical propositions, and hint at our usage of the verb *to know* in referring to language-games about 'states of consciousness' played by the first person singular. In contrast to this, I attribute feelings to a third person by means of criteria, and thus it is meaningful and also possible to employ the verb *to know*, for this 'knowing' is not necessarily true and can be corrected.

This criteriological asymmetry underlines what has been said above about the early learning situation and the indispensible interpretation of the child's natural expressions. As the infantile *I* is also without criteria and in its egocentric narcissim is not able to take the position of the third person, it is completely in the power of the attribution of others. The child learns at this instant to associate his psychological processes with an 'outward' social situation and form of life, and is not able to correct what is learned in the situation. It is only afterwards that the grammatical difference between the first and third person is built up. On the other hand, in the acquisition of such criterion-less self-attribution lies this instant attribution (like a shortcircuit), the first basis of rudimentary personal identity. Conversely, it remains to be examined whether the origin of later schizophrenia has to be sought in failure of such criterion-less self-attributions. Wittgenstein hints at the possibility of systematic misconditioning in the following passage:

> The behaviour of humans includes of course not only what they do without ever having learned the behaviour, but also what they do (and so, e.g., say) after having received a training. And this behaviour has its importance in relation to the special training. If, e.g., someone has learned to use the words *I am glad* as someone else has learned to use the words *I am frightened*, we shall draw unlike conclusions from like behaviour. (*RPP* I, 131)

In another passage Wittgenstein stresses the aspect of linguistic action and the possibility of an emotional association:

> We say to a child *No, no more sugar* and take it away from him. Thus he learns the meaning of the word *no*. If, while saying the same words, we had given him a piece of sugar he would have learned to understand the word differently. (In this way he has learned to use the word, but also to associate a particular feeling with it, to experience it in a particular way.) (*PG* 64)

In the discussion about the meaning of words, I pointed out that these meanings develop through rule-governed usage. That means that we act in accordance with words; and this leads us back to the interaction context in which words fulfil their function. In the given example, the feeling that is constituted grammatically as 'joy' (that the observer understands as 'fear') would be embedded into the interaction context of 'joy'. So, in the opinion of the outsider, incongruences would occur which the player of such a language-game could probably not see through, because they are part of his grammar.

We can conclude that the normal language-game only functions when the grammatical rules are accepted and used by all participants. This is an essential element of organized behaviour and co-ordinated interaction. It is also true of the single individual, socially organizing his interactions and experiences. Family research has often shown that such deviant grammars can only be maintained in a context that reinforces them (cf. Wynne and Singer 1963: 65). On the other hand, a dissolution of such common grammatical standards seems to lead not only to social disorganization and disintegration but also to a personal one, as seen in the phenomenon of schizophrenia. Wittgenstein's example is surely quite radical. In reality it must be assumed that such systematic of dislocations grammar are more subtle.[6]

I would like to explain the aspect of self-attribution of psychological predicates in more detail. Such attributions as *I am sad* or *I am angry* cannot be corrected and cannot be wrong (the psychoanalytical language-game has to be considered as a special case of a highly questionable nature). Another person cannot in principle 'know' more about my state of consciousness than I myself. It must be resupposed, however, that the basic certainty of the language-game about psychic conditions, which finds its expression in the criterion-less self-attribution of psychological concepts, has already been established. This fundamental certainty is thus included in our language-game, and so I am the 'final authority' of my mental events. The fundamental certainty in this game needs to be conveyed to me earlier, namely that I am the one who has this certainty and, similarly, that I can 'trust' my feelings, that I have them.

Laing has found out that this fundamental certainty is not conveyed in the families of schizophrenics (Laing 1964). We are dealing here with the grammatical aspect that is decisive for what is usually described via the term 'self-awareness'. Grammatically speaking, my expressions concerning my states of awareness constitute the crucial criteria for a third person. That means that the 'privileged access' (not in an epistemic sense) which I have to my states of consciousness enters into the grammar of this language-game in that they are uncorrectable. This also implies that I attribute my states of consciousness beyond 'objective' criteria. Thus, the criterion-less self-attribution of psychological concepts can be looked upon as a grammatical substratum of personal as well as of social identity. My 'subjective' feelings about intersubjective grammar are in the same way 'objectively' determined as the handling of them; we may call it 'the grammar of feelings'.[7] This grammar of feelings, which is acquired in early socialization, enables us to talk about our feelings and the action related to them. If we consider the early learning situation as the location where deviant grammars are inscribed, then this is certainly true of the sphere of emotions, relationships, etc. Unconscious taboos, or even deformed world pictures, underlie this field of soft realities, and force the parents to convey their idiosyncratic, often pathological views to their children. What Wittgenstein suggests as a general possibility is especially true of the language of psychic states.

> I want to say: an education quite different from ours might also be the foundation for quite different concepts. (*Z* 387).
>
> For her life would run on differently. . . . Here different concepts would no longer be unimaginable. In fact, this is the only way in which essentially different concepts are imaginable. (*Z* 388)

'Certainty' is another aspect of the function of language-games that has already been mentioned. Especially in the epistemological discussion of sceptical questions, Wittgenstein takes the position that a doubt without an end is not even a doubt (*OC* 625), and consequently, that certainty is always a prerequisite of doubt. Conversely to this, the learning situation does not begin with doubts but only on the grounds of a basis which has been taught as being 'correct'. This leads us again to the grammatical propositions of language-games. These can be described as pivots functioning as 'fixed propositions', around which the empirical propositions rotate; these grammatical propositions form the epistemologically 'certain' foundations of our language-games, and thus are beyond doubt. It is obligatory that the rule 'can be followed', which means that it contradicts neither itself nor others. The path representing the rule must be apt for walking on, otherwise it is not suitable for orientation and produces uncertainty, as Wittgenstein has correctly stated: 'And a contradictory order, of which it may be said it is not an order at all, could be used to produce uncertainty' (*L* II, 72). But in order to detect a rule as being contradictory, a basis must have been laid. Contradictions can appear in language-games in various ways. In the pathology of schizophrenic language-games, it is the contradiction that has entered the grammar of a single rule and which thus remains concealed from the individual.

Epistemology and schizophrenic language-games

In our consideration of the learning situation, the asymmetrical power structure between pupil (child) and teacher (parents) has become evident. It is clear that, during the entire socialization period of the child, grammatical/social norms are conveyed, and that this transfer does not only occur during the language acquisition period. Therefore, the chance of internalizing deviant grammars is given at various stages of psychological development. As has been shown previously, with regard to linguistic constitution and coping with reality, grammar needs to be understood as an 'orientation axis' which is conveyed by families acting as agents of socialization. If the result of deviant modes of communication can be described as 'ontological uncertainty', as stated by Laing (1960), then in the language being used here it already happens at the grammatical level in so far as the ontology is constituted by the grammar (cf. Fischer 1983b). If the grammar is not clearly outlined as an orientation axis, the basis for the description of experience loses its grounds, and thus orientation in reality is made impossible. Grammar produces 'ontological uncertainty', to the degree that it contains aspects of world pictures, when they are not consistent in themselves and can be transformed on a pragmatic level into actions. Conversely, an adequate grammar produces 'ontological certainty'. The history of scientific revolution has always shown an orientation crisis when the established world picture, the customary grammar, no longer coincides with facts. Wittgenstein proposes the question: 'Should I stay in the saddle however much the facts bucked?' (*OC* 616).

Such occasions present various possibilities. We and the grammar fall off the horse — our grammar loses its supporting function, and we are without orientation until we have found another grammar that allows interpretation of the new facts (Copernican Revolution); or we try to stay in the saddle, as the Catholic Church did when faced with the Copernican Revolution. However, that means living in another world, thus denying or pushing aside many experiences. Such epistemological systems of belief allow change only slowly, and this is true of institutionalized systems of this kind as well as of personal, individual ones. Schizophrenics seem to be in a similar situation. Either they have never had the chance to internalize an adequate grammar, or it is systematically devalued or destroyed. I shall employ two examples from the literature of schizophrenic research to discuss these possibilities. It will thus also become clear that such a grammatical disorientation or grammatical uncertainty is bound to the communication and interaction context of the family.

In a study by Bowen (1977) about the family as a frame of reference in schizophrenic research, he reports on a girl who was living in an extremely symbiotic relationship with her mother. The girl herself was never able to 'know' how she was feeling. In that she was entirely dependent on her mother, who told her how she was feeling. If at times she had a feeling that was different from the one her mother expressed, she devalued her own feeling and felt in the way her mother had told her she should. Against the background of my statements about the grammar of the 'normal' language-game of sensations, I would like to reconstruct the language-game of the girl, who is said to be schizophrenic.

If the girl never 'knows' herself, what she is feeling, or in what state of consciousness she is, the sentence *I know that I am in pain* becomes an empirical proposition. I will substitute the feeling 'to be in pain' by 'anger', because from my viewpoint the specific state of consciousness does not really matter. However, the example of internalized denial of 'being angry' stems from therapeutic practice. The sentence the girl can utter as an empirical sentence comes about as follows. The girl learns from the mother: *You are angry*. Then, in the girl's context, it makes sense to say: *I know that I am angry*. In this language-game, such a statement would be an acceptable empirical proposition. In the 'normal' language-game, we have disqualified such a sentence as being senseless, as this use of 'know' does not express genuine insight.

What does the negation of such a statement look like? In the above example, the girl behaves as follows: If the girl occasionally 'knew' which feeling she had, but this was different from her mother's qualification, then she always devalued her own assessment of the feeling and thus devalued the feeling itself, in order to feel in the way her mother had said. If it still happened that the girl felt: *I am angry* and her mother answered: *No, you are not angry, but you are* (for example) *tired*, then the girl had to negate her first sentence by saying: *I know that I feel no anger, but . . .*, which implies that it is not the 'knowing' of sensation, and thus the consciousness of this sensation, that is negated, but the sensation itself. Therefore, for the girl the verb *know* is not redundant in connection with her states of consciousness, as is the case in normal language-games. The verb expresses a real insight about herself, empirical knowledge that is basically correctable. The grammar of this language-game which has been obeyed unconsciously can be pictured in the following way. (1) The certainty in regard to her feelings does not lie within the child, but is anchored in the mother. (2) In the primitive sense of *to know* that lies in certainty of mental events, she 'knows' nothing about her feelings. She is not able to constitute them grammatically. (3) The mother tells her what she is feeling. (4) Only then has she genuine knowledge about her sensation.

The complex grammar of this language-game shows the way in which the asymmetry that is typical of the early language acquisition process has hardened into a form of life between mother and child. This girl has not been able to develop the indispensable certainty regarding her emotional states that is important for building up her own personal identity. As in an infantile situation, only the mother has at her disposal the standard for the description of her emotional sphere. The mother does not only constitute the criteria for 'right' and 'wrong' of the child's self-attribution, she also provides the defining (grammatical) criteria of the specific feeling. This is an example that demonstrates the way in which the grammar of this language-game has been substantially deformed in accordance with the symbiotic relationship between mother and daughter. As has been shown above, the criterion-less self-attribution of feelings, which is the prerequisite of personal identity, has not been established in this socialization process. The mother is still the final authority for the interpretation (fixation) of the child's feelings. Consequently, individuation cannot happen and the child remains in the power of the mother's attributions. In this sense she is schizophrenic, and has no self-identity.

What does a grammatical proposition of such a language-game look like? From the analysis of the grammar, we know that, for the girl, the uncertainty about her own states of consciousness is normal. The proposition 'I do not know that I am . . .' is a grammatical rule in this language-game. Because of this, it makes sense to talk about 'to know', in this language-game, as the 'not knowing' (e.g. uncertainty) has entered the grammar. It also makes sense to have doubts about the 'knowing', because the 'knowing' about a state of consciousness in this case is not given beforehand and thus criterion-less, but happens through criteria. In the girl's language-game, the doubts as to her own states of consciousness is therefore constitutive. For that reason, each statement about her own consciousness is subject to the 'right/wrong' marking, and is verified or falsified by her mother. What is true of grammatical propositions in normal language-games is also valid here: 'One thinks that one is tracing the outline of the thing's nature over and over again, and one is merely tracing round the frame through which we look at it' (*PI* 114). The grammatical proposition of this other language-game appears as the perspective through which the user of this language-game looks at his own sensations and his reality, and the way in which he organizes it grammatically.

What can be said about the grammatical proposition 'I do not know that I am angry' in view of the normal language-game? For us to have a sensation, or a state of consciousness, necessarily means that we are sure of it. In the grammar of the ordinary language-game, the following is implied: (a) I have the sensation, and consequently (b) I 'know' that I have it. The following contradiction appears when we look at the grammar of the schizophrenic language-game. (a) The girl (G) has the sensation; that has always meant for us that she must know that she has this sensation. Consequently (b) G knows that she has it. In the experience of the girl, however, it actually means that (b) is negative. G does not know that she has this sensation. Therefore, we see a contradiction in the grammar of (b) and non-(b), and it is a paradox, in our opinion. This paradox, however, is only a result of the perspective of the 'normal' language-game, because the girl's language-game is consistent in itself. It functions, and therefore it is not to be considered as 'disturbed'. In regard to our normal grammar and its corresponding form of life, such a game is extremely deviant. It represents the girl's inner splitting on the grammatical level. For the girl herself, the experience in the language-game and the corresponding organization of her emotional sphere is consistent. The experience sustains the mother's and daughter's symbiotic relationship as well as the structure of their communication. This is another proof of the thesis presented here, namely that a grammar has a corresponding form of life. Wittgenstein's following remark is also valid for this language-game:

> Something surprising, a paradox, is a paradox only in a particular, as it were defective, surrounding. One needs to complete this surrounding in such a way that what looked like paradox no longer seems one. (*RFM* 410)

It is the family-theoretical perspective that removes the paradox of such a game and regards it as consistent in this context.

Before giving another example of a disturbed language-game, the idea of certainty will be explained in more detail. As discussed earlier, grammatical sentences, by being a constitutive or defining basis of the language-game, are 'hardened' sentences. At least temporarily, they are beyond doubt like the river-bed metaphor; in fact they *have* to be indubitable in order to be a measure of verbal description and the organization of reality. The sentence *I know what I am feeling* explains this fundamental certainty in regard to the language-game concerning inner states. What we are dealing with here, however, is not only a 'grammatical' certainty, but a certainty that can be seen in our action and interaction patterns, and thus constitutes a certainty of the form of life as well.

> Now I would like to regard this certainty, not as something akin to hastiness or superficiality, but as a form of life . . . (*OC* 358)
>
> But that means I want to conceive it as something that lies beyond being justified or unjustified; as it were, as something animal. (*OC* 359)

In the language-game of the schizophrenic, this fundamental certainty often does not exist. The mystifying parents, as Laing has described them (1964), are not able to convey certainty or even to permit it. They maintain the asymmetry of the valid judgement against the child's needs, and in so doing prevent the development of self-confidence and individuation in the child. Another example given by Wittgenstein is as follows:

> If someone wanted to arouse doubts in me and spoke like this: here your memory is deceiving you, there you have been taken in, there again you have not been thorough enough in satisfying yourself, etc. and I did not allow myself to be shaken but kept to my certainty — then my doing so cannot be wrong, even if only because this is just what defines a game. (*OC* 497)

The structure of this example is similar to Laing's example. He describes how the parents systematically confused their children, as the sceptic does in a philosophical discourse. Here again, an important difference becomes obvious. The adult has the ability to withdraw to his 'certainty', he possesses and lives it ('I kept to my certainty') because otherwise he would have to give up his belief in the grammatical sentences (rules) of the language-game, which however are constitutive to the game. This type of doubt or confusion presupposes a grammatical certainty that has already been estalished. Therefore Wittgenstein characterizes such an act of radical scepticism as an attempt 'to confuse someone with doubts at the bedrock level'.

The following example has been described by Laing (1964; 1969). It deals with a girl whose parents systematically negate her certainty concerning her own psychic states.

> Her parents contradict Maya's memory, feelings, perceptions, motives, intentions . . . and while they spoke and acted as though they knew better than Maya what she remembered, what she did, what she imagined . . . this control was often maintained in a way which was further mystifying (Laing 1964: 42).

As with the asymmetry of the infantile learning situation, the mother was 'arbiter (1) of what Maya recognized, (2) of what Maya "really" wanted, in contrast to what she thought that she wanted, (3) of what was for her own good, (4) of what was a reservation or a change, (5) of what was possible (43). The mother thus does act in the same way as the sceptic in Wittgenstein's example: she just tries to confuse her daughter with doubts at bedrock level'. In the girl's case, she is actually confused, and will remain confused in her life conditions. In contrast to the example by Bowen, the girl has however developed the ability to describe her psychic experiences in a grammatically correct way. However, the statements that describe her needs, wishes and actions are systematically disqualified, so that the girl has to discard them as being uncertain. The certainty concerning her grammar is permanently undermined, the result being disorientation and disintegration. The examples presented attack established norms, in that the certainty regarding the grammatical sentences (the validity) of the language-game are questioned or not accepted. Another contradiction comes about when, in single sentences of the grammatical system, language and behaviour ('objectively' contradictory) are linked 'correctly', which seems to be contradictory from the perspective of the language-game in its socially practised form. Wittgenstein's example — *I am afraid (I am happy)* — and Bowen's example illustrate this. Incongruence also occurs between language and behaviour, and between verbal and nonverbal emotional utterances. At this point, two possibilities for contradiction on the level of grammatical rules can be summarized:

(1) The game has already been defined and the grammatical rules have been conveyed, so that the child is able to use the language adequately. Then the foundation of the game is no longer accepted by the dominating parents, who act as arbiter and set their grammar against the child's, so that the child can only discard his own as being uncertain (just as the subject in the noncontingent experiment and the girl in Laing's example do).

(2) A second possibility is that the contradiction lies within the grammar, so that it becomes invisible from outside and is realized in a specific form of life. Thus, there is no contradiction or conflict between grammatical structures within the family game, as in (1). The contradiction has been taken into the world picture and thus only exists latently.

With these examples of schizophrenic language-games, it has been possible to show the way in which the concepts of grammar and language-game can be valuable for a communication-theory analysis of schizophrenia. It has became apparent that the schizophrenic has internalized a deviant grammar that often allows him idiosyncratic orientation within the corresponding form of life of the family. Either that, or his normal grammar gets into conflict with the grammar of the dominating parents.

This grammar, however, is no longer able to function in regard to normal forms of life; the consequence is disintegration and disorientation. It has also been demonstrated that the various intentions of family-orientated schizophrenia research can be traced back to an understanding of language that is epistemologically and methodologically suited to these positions. The present grammatical analysis of two 'schizophrenic language-games' is an outline of a typology of schizophrenic grammars that needs to be set out in more detail.

Notes to Chapter 7

1 It was not until later that Bateson picked up the language-game term and used it incidentally and in a reduced sense: 'Telegraphist A has written message on his pad and sends this message over wire to B, so that B now gets the same sequence of letters on his message pad. This transaction (or 'language-game in Wittgenstein's phrase) has created a redundant universe for an observer' (Bateson 1972: 102).

2 From my present point of view I would revise some aspects of my criticism.

3 Singer, Wynne *et al.* 1978: 504: 'Having found conceptual and clinical support for the hypothesis that specific links exist between the parent's style of communicating and the severity of diagnosis of their offspring, we evolved a broadened conceptualization of what is usually called thought disorder or language disorder — terms that take thinking and language out of their interpersonal context'.

4 In biological epistemology, Maturana (1982) comes to a thesis that is in remarkable accordance with those by Wittgenstein.

5 Lewis Carroll had already perceived the control function of speech:

> 'I don't know what you mean by "glory"', Alice said. Humpty Dumpty smiled contemptuously. 'Of course you don't — till I tell you. I meant there is a nice knock-down argument for you!', 'But glory doesn't mean a nice knock-down argument', Alice objected. 'When I use a word', Humpty Dumpty said, in rather a scornful tone, 'it means just what I choose it to mean, neither more nor less.' 'The question is', said Alice, 'whether you can make words mean so many different things.' 'The question is', said Humpty Dumpty, 'which is to be master — that's all.' (*Alice's Adventures in Wonderland* and *Through the Looking-Glass* (London 1972), 190).

Compare also Orwell's *1984*, where he also deals with this topic.

6 In this context another element is of great interest, namely 'I-grammar'. The reference of the *I* precedes without criteria and is, in principle, infallible. This is especially interesting for the classic cases of schizophrenia, where the subjects talk about themselves in the third person. The splitting seems to show in the grammar as well, in that individuals also experience themselves in the third person.

7 Cf. Moser 1981. Moser uses the term 'Grammatik der 'Gefühle' ('grammar of feelings') without referring to Wittgenstein. He tries to describe the development of the child's emotional sphere in his psychoanalytical consideration of early childhood. Moser's use of the term 'Gefühle' is similar to its use in this chapter.

References

Bateson, Gregory 1955: A theory of play and fantasy. American Psychiatric Association, Psychiatric Research Reports II. Reprinted in Bateson 1972.
— 1972: *Steps to an Ecology of Mind*. New York: Ballantine.
Bateson, Gregory, Jackson, D. D., Haley, Jay and Weakland, John W. 1956: Towards a theory of schizophrenia. Reprinted in Bateson 1972.
Bateson, Gregory and Ruesch, Jurgen, 1951: *Communication: The Social Matrix of Psychiatry*. New York: Norton.
Bowen, Murray, 1977: Die Familie als Bezugsrahmen für die Schizophrenieforschung. In J. Habermas, D. Henrich and J. Taubes (eds), *Schizophrenie und Familie*. Frankfurt/Main: Suhrkamp.
Bruner, J. S. 1974: From communication to language — a psychological perspective. *Cognition* 3.
Carroll, Lewis, 1972 edn: *Alice's Adventures in Wonderland* and *Through the Looking-Glass*. London: Tavistock.
Cronen, E. E., Johnson, K. E. and Lannamann, J. W. 1982: Double-binds, paradoxes and reflexive loops. *Family Process* 21.
Dell, P. F. 1981: Untersuchung der Familientheorien zur Schizophrenie. Eine Übung in epistemologischer Konfusion. *Familiendynamik* 4.
Ferreira, A. J. 1966: Familienmythen. In P. Watzlawick and J. H. Weakland (eds), *Interaktion*.
Fischer, Hans Rudi, 1982a: Die Psychoanalyse im Lichte der Wittgensteinschen Sprachanalyse. *Zeitschrift für klinische Psychologie und Psychotherapie* 4.
— 1982b: Wahrheit, grammatischer Satz und Lebensform. *Conceptus: Zeitschrift für Philosophie*.
— 1983a: Grammatischer Satz und Lebensform. In G. Frey und J. Zelger, (eds.), *Der Mensch und die Wissenschaft vom Menschen*, vol. 2. Innsbruck: Solaris.
— 1983b: Ontologie and Grammatik. Bemerkungen zum ontologischen bzw. identitätstheoretischen Aspekt der Privatsprachenargumentation. In P. Weingartner and J. Czermak, (eds.), *Epistemology and Philosophy of Science: Proceedings of the 7th International Wittgenstein Symposium*. Vienna: Hoelder-Pichler-Tempsky.
— 1984: 'Die Sprache bezieht sich auf eine Lebensweise' oder wie der Terminus Lebensform bei Wittgenstein zu lesen ist. In R. Haller, (ed.), *Aesthetics: Proceedings of the 8th International Wittgenstein Symposium*. Vienna. Hoelder-Pichler-Tempsky.
Fromm-Reichmann, F. 1948: Notes on the development of treatment of schizophrenics by psychoanalytic psychotherapy. *Psychiatry* 11.
Habermas, Jürgen, 1967: *Die Logik der Sozialwissenschaften*. Frankfurt/Main: Suhrkamp.
— 1968: *Erkenntnis und Interesse*. Frankfurt/Main: Surhkamp.
Laing, Ronald, 1960: *The Divided Self*. London: Tavistock.
— 1964: *Sanity, Madness and the Family*. London: Tavistock.
— 1969: Mystifizierung, Konfusion und Konflikt. In J. Habermas, D. Henrich and J. Taubes (eds), *Schizophrenie und Familie*. Frankfurt/Main: Suhrkamp.
Lidz, Theodor, 1965: *Schizophrenia and the Family*. New York: International University Press.
— 1973: *The Origin and Treatment of Schizophrenic Disorders*. New York: Basic Books.
Lidz, Theodor, Cornelison, A., Terry, D. and Fleck, S. 1958: Intrafamilial

environment of the schizophrenic patient: VI The transmission of irrationality. *Arch. Neurology and Psychiatry* 79.

Lorenzer, Alfred, 1970a: *Sprachzerstörung und Rekonstruktion*. Frankfurt/Main: Suhrkamp.

— 1970b: *Kritik des psychoanalytischen Symbolbegriffs*. Frankfurt/Main: Suhrkamp.

— 1972: *Zur Begründung einer materialistischen Sozialisationstheorie*. Frankfurt/Main: Suhrkamp.

— 1977: *Sprachspiel und Interaktionsform*. Frankfurt/Main: Suhrkamp.

Maturana, Humberto, 1982: *Erkennen: Die Organisation und Verkörperung von Wirklichkeit*. Braunschweig/Wiesbaden: Vieweg.

Mead, George H. 1934: *Mind, Self and Society*. Chicago: University of Chicago Press.

Moser, Tilmann, 1981: *Grammatik der Gefühle*. Frankfurt/Main: Suhrkamp.

Richards, P. M. R. 1974: *The Integration of a Child in a Social World*. London: Tavistock.

Ryan, Joanna, 1974: Early language development: towards a communication analysis. In P. M. R. Richards *The Integration of a Child in a Social World*.

Sapir, Edward, 1949: *Selected Writings*, (ed.) P. G. Mandelbaum. Berkeley: Berkeley University Press.

Singer, M. T., Wynne, L. C. and Tookey, M. L. 1978: Communication disorders and the families of schizophrenics. In L. C. Wynne *et al.* (eds), *The Nature of Schizophrenia*.

Stierlin, Helm, 1959: The adaptation to the 'stronger' person's reality. *Psychiatry* 22.

— 1974: *Separating Parents and Adolescents*. New York: Quadrangle.

— 1978a: *Delegation und Familie*. Frankfurt/Main. Suhrkamp.

— 1978b: The transmission of irrationality. In L. C. Wynne *et al.* (eds), *The Nature of Schizophrenia*.

— 1981: Die 'Beziehungrsrealität' Schizophrener. *Psyche* 1.

Watzlawick, Paul (ed.) 1981: *Die erfundene Wirklichkeit*. Munich: Piper.

Watzlawick, Paul, Beavin, J. H. and Jackson, D. D. 1967: *Pragmatics of Human Communication*. New York: Norton.

Watzlawick, Paul and Weakland, J. H. (eds.) 1979: *Interaktion*. Bern/Stuttgart/Vienna: Huber.

Whorf, B. L. 1956: *Language, Thought and Reality*, (ed.) John B. Caroll. New York: Wiley.

Wittgenstein, Ludwig, 1922: *Tractatus Logico-Philosophicus*. Reprinted in Wittgenstein, *Schriften* vol. 1. Frankfurt/Main: Suhrkamp, 1960.

— 1953: *Philosophical Investigations*. Oxford: Basil Blackwell.

— 1958: *The Blue and Brown Books*. Oxford: Basil Blackwell.

— 1961: *Notebooks*. Oxford: Basil Blackwell.

— 1967a: *Zettel*. Oxford: Basil Blackwell.

— 1967b: Bemerkungen über Frazer's 'Golden Bough'. *Synthèse* 17.

— 1969: *On Certainty*. Oxford: Basil Blackwell.

— 1975: *Philosophical Grammar*. Oxford: Basil Blackwell.

— 1976: Ursache und Wirkung. Intuitives Erfassen. *Philosophia* 6.

— 1978: *Remarks on the Foundations of Mathematics*. Oxford: Basil Blackwell.

— 1980a: *Lectures, Cambridge 1930–1932*. Oxford: Basil Blackwell.

— 1980b: *Lectures, Cambridge 1932–1935*. Oxford: Basil Blackwell.

— 1980c: *Remarks on the Philosophy of Psychology*. 2 vols., Oxford: Basil Blackwell.

— 1982: *Last Writings on the Philosophy of Psychology*, vol. 1. Oxford: Basil Blackwell.

Wynne, L. C., Cromwell, R. L. and Matthysse S. (eds.) 1978: *The Nature of Schizophrenia*. New York: Wiley.

Wynne, L. C., Ryckoff, J. M., Day, J. and Hirsch, S. I. 1958: Pseudo-mutuality in the family relations of schizophrenics. *Psychiatry* 21.

Wynne, L. C. and Singer, M. 1963: Thought disorders and family relations of schizophrenics. *Arch. General Psychiatry* 12.

8 Paradoxical injunctions in everyday language and in the language of science

Stephan von Block

To begin my discussion of paradoxical communication I would like to give you an example which should not be taken too seriously. In the preface to a special edition of *Psychologie Heute* (1980: 5), two types of parents are described. Those belonging to the first group struggle with an immense amount of technical psychological literature, hoping to do everything correctly. The others, misunderstanding the term 'anti-authoritarian', are asked by their children in the relevant situations: 'Müssen wir heute wieder spielen, was wir wollen?' ('Do we have to play what we want to again today?')[1] In the exaggeration of the example its paradoxical nature is clearly expressed. The more 'common' paradoxes of everyday life are more subtle, and only recognizable by the reaction of the receiver of the message. Let us take just one example. If a microphone is examined to see if it functions, the technician is often asked 'just to say something'. As a reaction he normally begins to *count*. Automatisms and stereotypes belong likewise to the typical 'schizophrenic' reactions.

In this context I would like to add some remarks about the term 'anti-authoritarian'. In the public discussion about Neill's concept of 'anti-authoritarian education' (Neill 1970), the terms 'anti-authoritarian' and 'laissez-faire' are consistently confused. In the 'laissez-faire' educational style, parents and teachers behave in a completely passive manner — the interpersonal relation is characterized by indifference (Steltmann 1976: 38f.). The fact that Neill never had this in mind, however, is underlined by the following quotation (Neill 1970: 321).

To the question:

Wie lange dauert es, bis ein Kind, das absolute Freiheit besitzt, die lebenswichtige Rolle der Selbstdisziplin erkennt? Erkennt es sie überhaupt? (*How long does it take until a child who lives in absolute freedom learns to recognize the value of self-discipline? Does such a child ever learn this?*)

Neill answers:

> Absolute Freiheit gibt es nicht. Wer einem Kind immer seinen Willen laßt, befindet sich auf einem gefährlichen Weg. Kein Mensch ist ganz frei; denn er Muß die Rechte anderer achten. Jeder aber sollte persönliche Freiheit genießen. (*There is no absolute freedom. The person who lets a child always have its own way is on a dangerous course. Nobody is completely free, because everybody has to respect the rights of other people. But all people should be allowed to enjoy personal freedom.*)

For further information concerning this question, see also the very instructive contribution of Bettelheim about Summerhill (Bettelheim 1980: 190–206).

My chapter, which will be divided into theoretical and applied sections, deals with paradoxical injunctions in everyday language and in the language of science. First of all, presuppositions of terminology — in particular terms like 'everyday language', 'language of science' and the concept of 'paradoxical injunctions' used by Watzlawick *et al.* are clarified. In the applied section of my chapter, paradoxical injunctions in different social contexts are explored. With regard to the 'language of science', examples of pedagogics are dealt with primarily. In the field of 'everyday language', psychological advice columns will be discussed, as well as the possible connections of paradoxical injunctions with the development of stuttering.

Terminology

I wish now to discuss some presuppositions of linguistic terminology. The terms 'everyday language' and 'language of science' are to be regarded as constructs and abstractions, in so far as a great deal of linguistic, communicative and social facts are grouped together under one general heading. For this reason, only basic communicative strategies are discussed in this chapter. A general definition of these two terms does not seem to be opportune.

'Everyday language' is *generally* connected with the oral/verbal communicational channel (cf. Porzig 1957: 250f.; Söll 1974: 34). Communicative pressures mean that there is not much time in such language for preparation (cf. Söll 1974: 37). Schmidt (1972: 384) mentions the following hypothetical axioms for this kind of interaction: 'Dominanz von Informativität, Intersubjektivität, Pragmatizität, hohe Redundanz im semantischen Bereich.' (*'Domination of the informational, intersubjective and pragmatic aspect, also much semantic redundancy'*). The processes of hearing and understanding therefore take place without too much delay (Schmidt 1972: 397). Between the terms 'everyday language' and 'colloquial language' (*Umgangssprache*) there are intermediate sections. Ungeheuer (1972: 211) points out that the term 'colloquial language' refers to a community of communicative partners, in which the ability to communicate remains intact even if the ideolects of the members of this community belong to different but similar language systems. In contrast, the 'language of science' is often realized in written language, from which it is transferred into verbal language such as lectures or discussions. As distinct from 'everyday language', the long time needed for the preparation of the language of science has to be emphasized. If we disregard discussion, scientific language is realized in indirect or discontinual communication (cf. Kallmeyer *et al.* 1977: 31). Furthermore, the exact terminology of scientific language has to be considered as its most important criterion, alone guaranteeing the communicative success of this kind of language (cf. Seiffert 1974: 30).

But we also have to consider a pragmatic aspect. The 'language of science' deals with the question of how problems can be explained in an appropriate and uncontradictory way, so that the reader or the listener may have an opportunity to familiarize himself with the subject. As I presently hope to point out, paradoxical injunctions are in contradiction to this maxim. They can be understood better if we begin by characterizing the speech act of injunction, which is described in Bühler's 'Organon-Modell' (1978). In this case the language sign is a 'signal', for its function is to *appeal* to the hearer: 'Appell', as Bühler calls it (cf. Bühler 1978: 28). Kainz (1970: 41f.) speaks about the imperative function of language ('imperative Funktion') through which the behaviour of the partner is controlled. Kainz has also pointed out (1960: 129) that in the development of the child's language the imperative function is introduced at an early stage, whereas the function of representation ('Darstellung') is learned at a later time.[2]

Kainz's system of language functions ('die vier I-Funktionen', Kainz 1960: 28) comprises the following: 'die interjektive = Ausdruck, Kundgabe, die imperative = Befehl, Wunsch, die interrogative = Frage, die indikative = Bericht, Information, Feststellung' (1960: 28).

The speech act of injunction in this way is characterized as a language function of high psychological value, and we have to presume that contradictory messages — especially paradoxical injunctions — appearing in early childhood will have a very confusing effect. Watzlawick's (1967) concept of 'paradoxical injunction', has to be regarded as having a scientific connection with the 'double-bind' hypothesis developed by Bateson and his assistants in 1956. It deals with paradoxical messages, which may lead to severe disturbances of interpersonal communication if people are confronted with this kind of interaction from a very early stage of their psychological development. The concept was originally applied to the genesis of schizophrenic psychoses (Bateson *et al.* 1956); in the meantime there have been a large number of publications dealing with paradoxical messages in very different situations of everyday life (e.g. Peter 1975; Vinnai 1974; Paris 1974; Dilthey 1974; Ferreira 1960; Goeppert 1977).

Watzlawick *et al.* (1967: 194f.; 1974: 178f.) define this kind of communication in the context of their considerations on paradoxes as 'paradoxical injunctions'. In their chapter on paradoxical communication, the authors distinguish three types of paradoxes: (1) 'logico-mathematical paradoxes'; (2) 'paradoxical definitions' and; (3) 'pragmatic paradoxes', to which category belong 'paradoxical injunctions' or 'double-binds' (Watzlawick *et al.* 1967: 190–211). They also make clear (1967: 215; 1974: 199f.) that double-binds are not only contradictory but *paradoxical* injunctions.

The constituent parts of a paradoxical injunction may be summarized as follows (cf. Watzlawick *et al.* 1967: 195). The communicational frame is built up by a strong and vital interpersonal relationship that has to be characterized as complementary: i.e., the relationship is based on graduated social roles. The partner in the superior position gives a complex injunction containing an insoluble semantic contradiction. Frequently the so-called '"be spontaneous!" paradox' (Watzlawick *et al.* 1967: 199), which we all know from everyday phrases like *Cheer up!* or *Be happy!*, appears. The crucial point is that, in the pathogenic situation, the receiver of the message, being in the inferior position, will neither be able to escape from the situation nor give a comment on its absurdity because of his strong emotional dependence on his partner. His reaction will be paradoxical as well, and might correspond to the clinical picture of neurotic and even schizophrenic disturbances. If, finally, all partners are held in such a 'paradoxical game', it will be difficult to change the rules, governing this game. Watzlawick *et al.* (1967) give an example from a therapy of a married couple: 'Stripped of all ephemeral and fortuitous elements, their fights consist in a monotonous exchange of the messages: "I withdraw because you nag" and "I nag because you withdraw"' (p. 56).

The critics of this hypothesis frequently ask the question why there is not a much higher number of people showing psychopathological reactions, if it is clear that we all are surrounded by paradoxical communication in everyday life. They neglect two factors. The pathogenic effects of double-binds only come into being if they represent the predominant mode of communicational relationship from very early childhood. The second point is even more important. The linguistic structure of the double-bind can only be considered as completed if there is a corresponding reaction on the part of the receiver. If metacommunication in any form is still possible, the 'Beziehungsfalle' — as Stierlin (1959–60: 844) calls the double-bind — cannot operate, and in a strictly terminological sense, therefore, one should not speak of a double-bind. As Abeles (1976: 143) writes: 'a bind is not a bind unless it binds. The response of the subject is integral to a bind.'

Paradoxical formulations and their effects in the language of science

Coming to the practical part of my chapter, I am now going to examine some examples from earlier pedagogical literature. In 1858, the German physician and pedagogue D. G. M. Schreber proclaimed the absolute obedience of the child as a way to develop and establish his character (135f.). When parents have succeeded in getting this kind of obedience, in order to complete the chosen educational task, the *habit* of obeying has to be transformed to *an act of free will* (Schreber 1858: 135; see also Schatzman 1978: 27f.). One can formulate this more elegantly and say: 'It should be your heart's desire willingly to do what I want you to do!' In this injunction we recognize the structure of the classic double-bind that Sluzki and Verón (1971: 404) reduced to the formula: 'Be independent by depending on me'. In Schreber's conception of education, this kind of paradox is very important, and we have to remember that his son was affected by paranoia (cf. D. P. Schreber 1973), and that the history of this illness belongs to the well documented cases in the psychoanalytical literature (Niederland 1978; Schatzman 1978; Freud 1911). A modern example for this kind of 'voluntary obedience' is given in Watzlawick *et al.* 1975: 84. A mother is talking about her son: 'Ich möchte, daß Andy lernt, das zu tun, was von ihm verlangt wird, . . . aber er soll es von sich aus tun WOLLEN' (*'I want Andy to learn to do what he is asked to do . . . but he should do so of his own free will'*).

Paradoxes like that are even found in modern pedagogical compendias. There you can read, for example: 'Letzlich soll das Kind veranlaßt werden, freiwillig Gehorsam zu leisten' (*'Finally the child should be brought to obey of his own free will'*) (Starck 1971: 53); or: 'Disziplinerziehung wird ihr Ziel stets in freiwilliger Disziplin . . . sehen' (*'Disciplinary education will always find its aim in voluntary discipline'*) (Steindorf 1976: 202). If formulations like that are practised, the result may be confusing. Laing (1975: 275) speaks about 'mystification' in the sense of making an action obscure. The mystified person is no longer capable of recognizing what is *really* going on.

Schatzman (1978) reports on the opinion of J. G. Fichte on the point of 'obedience'. Children first of all have to learn to submit to their parents. This leads to the conclusion: 'Eine gewisse Freiheit müssen Kinder haben, weil ihre Handlungen ohne die freie Wahl nicht die "mindeste Moralität" haben' (*'Children must have freedom to a certain degree, because without the free choice their actions would not have "the slightest morality"'*) (Schatzman 1978: 136). The 'illusion of alternatives' (Watzlawick *et al.* 1967: 231f.) is very clear, because children do not have any opportunity to act according to Fichte's concept. If they obey simply because they fear punishment, this will be regarded as 'immoral'; if they do not obey they are 'bad' or 'ungrateful'.

The idea that stands behind the concept of 'voluntary discipline' or 'willing obedience' in our times is different. It is summarized by Netzer (1972: 71): 'vom Gehorsam zur Freiheit oder von der Fremdgesetzgebung zur Autonomie' (*'from obedience to freedom, or from the state of being dependent on other people to autonomy'*). The mental attitude of the child is characterized by perception that an injunction is necessary (cf. Netzer 1972: 71); this has nothing to do with free will but with a different state of the child's psychic development and consciousness.

Schatzman also points out (1978: 145) that D. G. M. Schreber (Schreber Senior) uses the word 'obedience' in the sense of 'freedom', and that totalitarian governments have a standpoint that is in accordance with this idea. Also belonging in the context of totalitarianism is what Langbein (1980) reports in his book about Auschwitz on the 'obedience' of the 'SS man':

> Der vom SS-Mann geforderte Gehorsam wird im 'Lehrplan für die weltanschauliche Erziehung in der SS und Polizei, erarbeitet und herausgegeben vom SS-Hauptamt' ausführlich definiert: 'Es ist ein Gehorsam, der darum besonders schwer ist, weil er aus reiner Freiwilligkeit kommt und alles verlangt, was ein Mann an Opfern hinsichtlich persönlichem Stolz, äußeren Ehren und vielem anderen, was ihm teuer ist, zu bringen vermag'. (*The kind of obedience*

> *required from the SS man is defined in detail in the 'course of instruction for the ideological education of the SS and the police, developed and published by the SS central office': 'It is a kind of obedience, which is particularly hard, because it comes from* ABSOLUTE VOLUNTARINESS, *demanding everything a man is willing to sacrifice of his personal pride, external honours, and many other things, that are dear to him.*) (Langbein 1980: 311; my emphasis)

The terrible consequences of this 'voluntary obedience' are well known.

Another example which is just as serious comes from Ritter (1936), the biographer of D. G. M. Schreber. He talks about the 'early mental education' of the newborn child:

> Alles Häßliche, Rauhe, Unharmonische muß ferngehalten werden. Vor allem unterdrücke man eigensinniges Schreien durch drohendes Klopfen an das Bettchen. (*Everything that is ugly, rude, unharmonious has to be kept at a distance. Above all one should suppress obstinate crying by beating threateningly on the cot.*) (Ritter 1936: 61)

With this formulation parents, asking a specialist for advice on educational matters, are forced to communicate in an extremely paradoxical way, for they are expected to arrive at a state of harmony by using threats. Examples taken from the books of D. G. M. Schreber and Ritter reveal an unconscious desire to dominate other persons. Another quotation which borders unintentionally on the comic serves to demonstrate this. Ritter writes about the child that is learning to walk:

> Für die Bewegung ist es wichtig, das Kind nicht vorzeitig zum Gehen oder Stehen zu veranlassen. Wenn der kleine Mensch aber selbst Lust dazu zeigt, dann GEBIETE MAN EINE STRAFFE, MUNTERE HALTUNG'. (*For the movements, it is important not to make the child walk or stand up too early. But as soon as the little person shows the desire to do so,* ONE SHOULD DEMAND AN UPRIGHT AND LIVELY BEARING.) (Ritter 1936: 62;[3] my emphasis)

I will conclude this chapter with some remarks concerning a problem I see in the field of applied linguistics. It is a conflict which might exhibit paradoxical traits, and which has to be localized between the requirements of a science planned to be interdisciplinary (i.e. applied linguistics) and the efforts of traditional linguistics to be an autonomous science. The original aims of applied linguistics were once characterized by Knobloch (1955) by the expression 'Sprachwissenschaft als Zweckforschung' ('*to carry out linguistic investigations for a practical and useful purpose*'). The programme of this discipline had already been developed and extended by Kandler (1952–53) in Bonn. Its practical nature is also emphasized in the definition of Corder (1973: 12) who writes: 'Applied linguistics is thus clearly understood as the activity of applying what is known about language . . .' This concept, of course, required collaboration with neighbouring subjects such as medicine or psychology (cf. Bülow 1981).

It is here that the problem I am concerned with arises, because even today it seems difficult — in the tradition of de Saussure's concept of a 'linguistique de la langue' (1967: 11) — to assert that linguistics has psychological or medical aspects that do not belong exclusively to the functions of a professional physician or psychologist. With so many people calling for an interdisciplinary investigation, it still happens that one is inclined to understand this project as one in which the relevant scientific disciplines coexist, and in which it is clear that the linguist does not have to get involved too much in psychological or medical questions. The following quotation is a reflection of this opinion. Scheerer-Neumann (1983) writes about the participation of linguists in the investigation of the acquisition of the graphic language code: 'Sprachwissenschaftler befassen sich mit der Sprache und der Schriftsprache *an sich*, d.h. mit dem Produkt Sprache, losgelöst vom Benutzer der Sprache, dem Menschen' ('*Linguists deal with spoken and written language in itself, i.e. they are occupied with language as a commodity, separated from the language user, the human being*') (p. 209). If this very general statement were true, there would be no basis on which a linguist might get involved in the severe problems of language disturbances (nor in those of applied linguistics in general!).

The Saussurean *langue/parole* dichotomy was adapted by the psychology of language too. In a work which, although published in 1958, still seems to be topical, Kainz makes a distinction between two 'sciences of language': The 'Sprachwissenschaft im engsten und eigentlichsten Sinne' — i.e. linguistics — deals with language as a *system*; the theory of language, or 'Sprachwissenschaft im weitesten Sinne', investigates an interdisciplinary question: the results of *all* the disciplines, engaged in the investigation of human communication are collected (cf. Kainz 1958: 270, 274). By this division of functions the conflict is indicated, because now it becomes clear what the 'real' tasks of a *linguist* are. I will mention just two examples illustrating the problem. Kandler (1955) demands, with entire justification, that the disciplines of linguistics, psychology of language and neurology should join forces in the investigation of aphasic diseases, but stipulates that, in such collaboration, the linguistic, psychological and neurological methods of consideration would have to be strictly kept apart (Kandler 1955: 281). Language is a psycho-physiological mechanism, however, and the distinction between these three methods of investigation seems, therefore, to be artificial in some cases.

In 1978 Peuser published an extensive programme for a new linguistic area, 'Patholinguistik, (cf. Peuser 1978) but in the linguistic description of the language, disturbances 'spielt die etwaige organische oder nicht-organische Verursachung der jeweiligen Störung . . . für den Linguisten keine Rolle' (*'the contingent organic or non-organic etiology of the respective language disturbance is of no importance to the linguist as an object of investigation'*) (p. 4). Let me give just one counter-example. The so-called 'normal non-fluency' (Johnson 1956: 217) of the child's speech can only be described adequately with regard to the psychological and social factors of the language development that will lead to this kind of phenomenon and also to complications. Consequently the linguist's task in this case (and in others as well) is not only to give a linguistic description but *also* to explore the reasons for a certain language behaviour. The real significance of interdisciplinary investigation can be demonstrated by an example from Bühler (1978: 111):

> Wenn die immer wieder geforderte gegenseitige wissenschaftliche Handreichung zwischen Psychologie und Linguistik Früchte zeitigen soll, so müssen die Fachmänner auf beiden Seiten den Mut aufbringen, jeder dem anderen ins Konzept zu sprechen. (*If the often-demanded mutual collaboration in scientific work between psychology and linguistics is to be productive, specialists on both sides must have the courage to discuss critically their respective standpoints in relation to scientific matters.*)

Paradoxical injunctions in magazine advice columns

As an example of 'everyday language' I am going to take those columns in magazines which offer the reader psychological advice from a specialist. Such columns are common, and many direct injunctions are given every day. Texts like those belong to 'everyday language', though they need a longer preparation time. But by contrast with scientific texts, the reader is not asking for an exact analysis of a problem but for 'good advice' that is based on everyday experience and intuition.

An increasing number of people suffer from problems that result from their environment (cf. Hellbrügge (n.d.): 101f.), especially from their interpersonal relationships. Because it may become very difficult to receive conventional therapy, columns of psychological advice offer a certain release in this situation. As Sieber (1980: 29) writes, they accomplish an important function in an anonymous society. But they also contain severe problems. How can it be possible to solve an important psychic problem by means of an exchange of letters, and what kind of psychological well-founded advice can be given in answering a question like the following one? 'Unsere Tochter (15) macht uns Sorgen. Sie tut nie das, was man von ihr verlangt . . . Ich weiß nicht mehr, wie ich mit ihr sprechen oder mich verhalten soll.' ('*We are worried about our daughter (15). She never does what we want her to do . . . I don't know any more how I should talk to her and react.*') (*Bunte* 21 (1984): 114). The possibility that paradoxical injunctions appear in the answer of the counsellor depends on the kind of the question. If there is a question about concrete problems, the answer will be concrete as well. The situation is different if the counsellor has to deal with problems of interpersonal relationship, starting from a position which is already paradoxical in a certain way. In such a situation it may happen that he makes use of generalities like: 'You have to find new friends' or 'You have to supress your anxieties'. The following examples serve to demonstrate precisely *this kind* of advice.

A woman who has great difficulties in finishing a very troublesome relationship with her partner gets the advice to do everything to experience a new love. And further on: 'leben Sie fröhlich und genießen Sie vorerst einmal Ihre Ungebundenheit' ('*Enjoy your life and your independence*') (*Freizeitrevue* 18 (1984): 85). This advice naturally has the character of a paradoxical injunction.

A man who has great problems to find a partner is advised to 'open his heart': 'Geben Sie sich ganz offen wie Sie sind und sprechen Sie ruhig von sich' ('*Act naturally, as you are, and talk about yourself*') (*Freizeitrevue* 20 (1984): 67). If the man who was seeking advice could behave in this way, he naturally would not have any problems of interpersonal contact!

Beside such generalities, reflecting a certain helplessness, there are examples of very serious paradoxical injunctions. A young woman who has just become a mother, and who is by no means getting along with her child and with the new task, gets the advice: 'Freuen Sie sich über die körperlichen und geistigen Fortschritte, die so ein kleines Wesen täglich macht' ('*Be happy about the physical and mental progress such a little child makes everyday*') (*Das Neue Blatt — Extra Aktuell* 20 (1984): 42).

A last example: a woman who is afraid that her husband deceives her, and who for that reason has tried to commit suicide, is advised: 'Versuchen Sie, die schwere Zeit durchzustehen, ohne an Selbstmord zu denken' ('*Try to get through this difficult time without thinking of suicide*') (*Das Neue Blatt — Extra Aktuell* 20 (1984): 42). About the difficulties of interpersonal relation which the couple have, the adviser writes: 'Obwohl ich nicht glaube, daß Ihr Mann vernünftigen Gesprächen überhaupt zugänglich ist, sollten Sie versuchen, ihn mit Hilfe von Bekannten und Freunden zur Einsicht zu bringen' (p. 42) ('Though I don't believe that your husband will be willing to discuss the matter reasonably, you should try to convince him with the help of friends and persons you know'). It will be difficult to follow this proposition, because one has to be convinced of its negative result.

The preliminary result of these considerations is that the general conditions of such types of 'advice' may advance the occurrence of paradoxical injunctions. The idea, mentioned above, that such a 'magazine therapy' might have an important function, has therefore to be reconsidered.

Paradoxical formulations and their possible effects in the genesis of stuttering

As a final point in my discussion I would like to consider the question of whether paradoxical injunctions play a part in the genesis of stuttering.[4] Dührssen (1976: 287) interprets stuttering as a psychogenic language disturbance, and points out that stuttering children have very often received from their parents confusing, contradictory and obviously wrong answers to their questions (p. 289).

To follow up the problem about the importance of paradoxical injunctions in the development of stuttering, I examined the short autobiographies of patients ('Selbstdarstellungen') that were collected and commented on by Westrich (1968). One has to take into consideration that these reports — their title was: 'Wie ich heute über mein Stottern denke' ('*The way I think today about my stuttering*') (Westrich 1968: 22) — have been written by the patients towards the end of their therapy. The texts therefore reflect the *content* of the therapy which in some ways reminds one of Adler's concept of neurosis. Neurosis in this way would have to be regarded as a system to maintain the security that enables the stutterer to avoid making decisions and taking actions that might cause problems (cf. Appelt 1973: 301, 303).

More important than such a theory (about which opinions may vary) is Westrich's explanation of stuttering from the point of view of communicative theory. He describes the typical conditions for the genesis of stuttering (Westrich 1968: 14). A well cared for and somewhat over-protected three-year-old child has done something which is forbidden. Called to account, he is faced with the following dilemma. Refusal to explain what has happened, as well as involving a lie, will also involve negative sanctions. An apparent escape from this situation is through what Westrich calls 'Notlösungssprechen' (p. 15) — that is, the kind of language behaviour shown by the stutterer is only *apparently* a solution to his problems. By means of his organs of speech the child demonstrates that he is willing to give a statement; but the blockage of the flow of speech or the iterations make a real statement impossible. The suttering therefore has to be regarded as 'Folge eines situativen Erlebensnotstandes' ('the consequence of a situation which the stutterer experiences as hopeless') (Westrich 1968: 15) — that is, as really paradoxical, because somebody is forced to *speak* without having an opportunity of real and effective communication.

Examples of this are found in the autobiographies mentioned above. A twenty-five-year old graduate writes: 'War ich in fremder Gesellschaft, so untersuchte ich alle Bemerkungen, die ich machen wollte, zunächst einmal darauf, wie wohl die Wirkung auf die anderen sei. Ich war stets bemüht, denjenigen, die mir überlegen waren, recht zu geben . . . Versuchte ich zu widersprechen, so setzte das Stottern ein' ('*When I was together with persons I did not know, I examined all my statements for the effect they might have upon the others. I always took care to agree with everybody who was superior to me . . . If I tried to oppose somebody, the stuttering began*') (Westrich 1968: 24f.). The communicative dilemma consists in the fact that nobody can avoid forever the risk of sometimes being alone in his own opinion. I give you another example: a sixteen-year-old pupil writes: 'Meine Mutter habe ich . . . immer als etwas herrschsüchtig angesehen; ich konnte arbeiten, was ich wollte. Sie wußte immer eine bessere Methode . . .' ('*I always considered my mother to be rather domineering. I could work as much as possible, she always knew a better method . . .*') (Westrich 1968: 26). On the next page we read: 'Ich weiß heute, daß ich zu stottern begann, weil ich die Anforderungen, die an mich gestellt wurden, nicht erfüllen wollte, obwohl ich gekonnt hätte' ('*Today I know that I began to stutter, because I did not want to carry out the orders that were given to me, though I might have been capable of doing so*'). But how can anybody react to conform with the injunction, 'Do your best, though this will never be sufficient'? A possible reaction would be to deny communication.

Further references to a possible double-bind situation in the families of the young patients can be found in an examination of often contradictory parental educational style (Westrich 1965: 24).

To summarize, one can say for the present that paradoxical injunctions seem to be important in a certain way in the everyday experience of stuttering patients. By analogy with the statements of Sluzki and Verón (1971) on neurosis, these injunctions might be reduced to the formula: 'Talk frankly, but remember that this is much too risky!'

Notes to Chapter 8

1 All translations of German quotations are mine.
2 The psycholinguistic importance of the imperative function of language is clearly demonstrated in the symptoms of aphasia. According to the law of regression, this function belongs to the speech acts that can still be carried out even in very serious cases (cf. Kainz 1960: 319, 324f.).
3 A last example from Ritter (1936: 61): 'Man erfülle kein eigenwilliges Begehren und lasse sich unter keinen Umständen von dem kleinen Erdenbürger tyrannisieren. Ebenso vermeide man es, das Kind mit 'Tändeleien' und LIEBKOSUNGEN ZU QUÄLEN' ('*You should never fulfil an obstinate desire, nor by any means let yourself by tyrannized by the little human being. Also avoid* TORTURING THE CHILD WITH TRIFLES AND CARESSES') (my emphasis).
4 It is interesting in this context that there is a version of therapeutic double-bind in which the patient is asked to stutter *intentionally*, which makes the symptoms disappear for a short time (Heidemann *et al.* 1975: 135; Watzlawick *et al.* 1975: 118f.).

References

Abeles, G. 1976: Researching the unresearchable: experimentation on the double-bind. In C. E. Sluzki and D. C. Ransom (eds), *Double-bind: The Foundation of the Communicational Approach to the Family*. New York, London and San Francisco: Grune & Stratton.
Adler, A. and Furtmüller, C. 1973: *Heilen und Bilden. Ein Buch der Erziehungskunst für Arzte und Pädagogen*. Frankfurt/Main: Fischer.
Appelt, A. 1973: Fortschritte der Stottererbehandlung. In A. Adler and C. Furtmüller (eds), *Heilen and Bilden. Ein Buch der Erziehungskunst für Ärzte und Pädagogen*. Frankfurt/Main: Fischer.
Bateson, G., Jackson, D. D., Haley, J. and Weakland, J. H. 1956: Toward a theory of schizophrenia. *Behavioural Science* 1.
Bateson, G., Habermas, J., Heinrich, D. and Taubes, J. 1975: *Schizophrenie und Familie*, (eds.) Frankfurt/Main: Suhrkamp.
Bettelheim, B. 1980: *Erziehung zum Überleben. Zur Psychologie der Extremsitu-*

ation. Stuttgart: Deutsche Verlags Anstalt.

Bühler, K. 1978: *Sprachtheorie — die Darstellungsfunktion der Sprache*. Frankfurt/Main, Berlin and Vienna: Ullstein.

Bülow, E. 1981: Interdisziplinarität, Legitimität und Finalisierbarkeit der Angewandten Sprachwissenschaft. In G. Peuser and S. Winter (eds), *Angewandte. Sprachwissenschaft. Grundfragen — Bereiche — Methoden. Festschrift für Günther Kandler*. Bonn: Bouvier.

Corder, S. P. 1973: Linguistic theory and applied linguistics. In Corder and Roulet.

Corder, S. P. and Roulet, E. (eds.) 1973: *Theoretical Linguistic Models in Applied Linguistics*. Brussels and Paris: Aimav/Didier.

Dilthey, D. 1974: Schizophrenie als Kommunikationspathologie und als soziales Delikt. *Ästhetik und Kommunikation* 15/16.

Dührssen, A. 1976: *Psychogene Erkrankungen bei Kindern und Jugendlichen. Eine Einführung in die allgemeine und spezielle Neurosenlehre*. 11th edn., Göttingen: Vandenhoeck & Ruprecht.

Ferreira, A. J. 1960: The 'double-bind' and delinquent behavior. *Archives of General Psychiatry* 3.

Freud, S. 1911: Psychoanalytische Bemerkungen über einen autobiographisch beschriebenen Fall von Paranoia (Dementia Paranoides). Reprinted in *Gesammelte Werke*, Vol. 8. London: Imago, 1948.

Goeppert, H. C. 1977: Einige Bemerkungen zur Brauchbarkeit des double-bind-Konzepts für die Beschreibung von Unterricht als spezifischer Kommunikationssituation. *Linguistische Berichte* 49.

Heidemann, B., Kellner, H. -J. and Kopf-Mehnert, C. 1975: Erste Erfahrungen mit einer Stotterangsttherapie nach Sheehan bei jugendlichen Stotternden. *Folia Phoniatrica* 27.

Hellbrügge, T. (n.d.): *Das sollten Eltern wissen. Über den Umgang mit unseren Kindern* (2nd ed.). Munich: Kindler.

Johnson, W. 1956: Perceptual and evaluational factors in stuttering. *Folia Phoniatrica* 8.

Kainz, F. 1958: Die Sprachtheorie als Verbindung von Geistes- und Naturwissenschaft. *Studium Generale* 11 (50).

— 1960: *Psychologie der Sprache*, 2nd edn., Vol. 2, *Vergleichend-genetische Sprachpsychologie*. Stuttgart: Ferdinand Enke.

— 1970: Psychologie der Sprache. In R. Luchsinger and G. E. Arnold, *Handbuch der Stimm- und Sprachheilkunde*, 3rd edn., Vol. 2. Vienna and New York: Springer.

Kallmeyer, W., Klein, W., Meyer-Hermann, R., Netzer, K. and Siebert, H. J. 1977: *Lektürekolleg zur Textlinguistik*, 2nd edn., Vol. 1, *Einführung*. Kronberg/Ts.: Athenäum.

Kandler, G. 1952–53: Angewandte Sprachwissenschaft. Name und Wesen eines kommenden Wissenschaftszweiges. *Wirkendes Wort* 3.

— 1955: Zum Verständnis zentraler Sprachstörungen. *Sprachforum* 1.

Knobloch, J. 1955: Sprachwissenschaft als Zweckforschung. *Erziehung und Unterricht* IX.

Laing, R. D. 1975: Mystifizierung, Konfusion und Konflikt. In Bateson *et al.* (eds), *Schizophrenie und Familie*. Frankfurt/Main: Suhrkamp.

Langbein, H. 1980: *Menschen in Auschwitz*. Frankfurt/Main, Berlin and Vienna: Ullstein.

Neill, A. S. 1970: *Theorie und Praxis der antiautoritären Erziehung. Das Beispiel*

Summerhill. Reinbek bei Hamburg: Rowohlt.
Netzer, H. 1972: *Erziehungslehre*. 10th edn., Bad Heilbrunn/Obb.: Julius Klinkhardt.
Niederland, W. G. 1978: *Der Fall Schreber. Das psychoanalytische Profil einer paranoiden Persönlichkeit*. Frankfurt/Main: Suhrkamp.
Paris, R. 1974: Die Grenzen des Double-Bind-Konzepts. Thesen. *Ästhetik und Kommunikation. Beiträge zur politischen Erziehung* 15/16.
Peter, H. 1975: Paradoxes Führungsverhalten. Erklärt nach der Double-Bind-Theorie. *Psychologie Heute* 11.
Peuser, G. 1978: *Aphasie — Eine Einführung in die Patholinguistik*. Munich: Wilhelm Fink.
Porzig, W. 1957: *Das Wunder der Sprache. Probleme, Methoden und Ergebnisse der modernen Sprachwissenschaft*. 2nd edn., Bern: Francke.
Psychologie Heute, special edition, 1980: *Kindheit ist nicht kinderleicht*. Weinheim and Basel: Beltz.
Ritter, A. 1936: *Schreber — das Bildungssystem eines Arztes*. Inaugural Dissertation. Erlangen.
Saussure, F. de, 1967: *Grundfragen der allgemeinen Sprachwissenschaft*. 2nd edn., Berlin: Walter de Gruyter.
Schatzman, M. 1978: *Die Angst vor dem Vater. Langzeitwirkungen einer Erziehungsmethode. Eine Analyse am Fall Schreber*. Reinbek: Rowohlt.
Scheerer-Neumann, G. 1983: Psychische Vorgänge beim Rechtschreiben: Grundlagenforschung und Anwendung. In L. Dummer (ed.), *Legasthenie — Bericht über den jugendliche. Eine Einführung in die allgemeine und spezielle. Neurosenlehre*. 11th edn. Gottingen: Vandenhoeck & Ruprecht.
Schmidt, S. J. 1972: Alltagssprache und Gedichtsprache. Versuch einer Bestimmung von Differenzqualitäten. In W. A. Koch (ed.), *Strukturelle Textanalyse*. Hildensheim and New York: Georg Olms.
Schreber, D. G. M. 1858: *Kallipädie oder Erziehung zur Schönheit durch naturgetreue und gleichmäßige Förderung normaler Körperbildung, lebenstüchtiger Gesundheit und geistiger Veredelung*. Leipzig: Friedrich Fleischer.
Schreber, D. P. 1973 (first published 1903): *Denkwürdigkeiten eines Nervenkranken*, (ed.) Samuel M. Weber. Frankfurt/Main, Berlin and Vienna: Ullstein.
Seiffert, H. 1974: *Einführung in die Wissenschaftstheorie*, 7th edn., Vol. 1. Munich: Beck.
Sieber, G. 1980: *Achtung Test. Psychologische Testverfahren — was man von ihnen erwarten darf*. Reinbek bei Hamburg: Rowohlt.
Sluzki, C. E. and Verón, E. 1971: The double bind as a universal pathogenic situation. *Family Process* 10.
Söll, L. 1974: *Gesprochenes und geschriebenes Französisch*. Berlin: Erich Schmidt.
Starck, W. 1971: *Grundfragen der Erziehung. Ein Grundriß der Allgemeinen Pädogogik*. Hamburg: Büchner.
Steindorf, G. 1976: *Einführung in die Schulpädagogik*. 3rd edn., Bad Heilbrunn: Klinkhardt.
Steltmann, K. 1976: *Unterrichten als Beruf*. Munich: List.
Stierlin, H. 1959–60: Review of A. Auerback, (ed.) *Schizophrenia* (1959). *Psyche* 13.
Ungeheuer, G. 1972: Bemerkungen zum Thema 'Umgangsspprache'. In G. Ungeheuer *Sprache und Kommunikation*. 2nd edn. Hamburg: Buske.

Vinnai, G. 1974: Sind die Befunde der psychiatrischen Familienforschung generalisierbar? *Ästhetik und Kommunikation — Beiträge zur politischen Erziehung* 15/16.

Watzlawick, P., Beavin, J. H. and Jackson, D. D. 1967: *Pragmatics of Human communication: A Study of Interactional Patterns, Pathologies, and Paradoxes.* New York: Norton.

— 1974: *Menschliche Kommunikation. Formen, Störungen, Paradoxien.* 4th edn., Bern, Stuttgart and Vienna: Huber.

Warzlawick, P., Weakland, J. H. and Fisch, R. 1975: *Lösungen — Zur Theorie und Praxis menschlichen Wandels.* Bern, Stuttgart and Vienna: Huber.

Westrich E. 1965: *Versuch einer Erfolgs- und Bewährungskontrolle an stationär behandelten Stotterern. Eine katamnestische Erhebung an rückfällig gewordenen Stotterern.* Köln-Deutz: Landschaftsverband Rheinland.

— 1968: *Der jugendliche Stotterer in seiner Selbstdarstellung. Ein Beitrag zur Psychologie menschlichen Verhaltens.* Köln-Deutz: Landschaftsverband Rheinland.

9 Jargonaphasia and schizophasia:

An essay in contrastive patholinguistics

Gunter Peuser

Introduction

Modern patholinguistic discussion, as reflected in the articles in *Brain and Language*, is not given to vast synoptic summaries of deviant language phenomena as represented by the momental work of Kainz (1969) but, more modestly, prefers to analyse and to compare individual cases or selected types of language disorder. One may therefore say that contrastive analysis is at the very core of patholinguistic methodology, whether it be the study of aphasia in different languages (see Peuser 1978) or the differential diagnosis of similar forms of deviant speech in one and the same language.

Hitherto, the method of comparing related types of basic language disorders like Broca's and Wernicke's aphasia has turned out to be very useful, shedding new light on the differences between the compared phenomena. But, as comparisons of this kind are generally based on some basic similarity, they may become dangerous, and may even impede further knowledge if the contrasted forms of language disorder are basically dissimilar; for, in this case, one is tempted to underestimate the points of dissimilarity and to overestimate the existing correspondances. (The complementary error of wrongly attributing a basic dissimilarity to similar phenomena is perhaps less likely, as our favourite pattern of thinking is to look for similarities rather than dissimilarities.)

There is, finally, another danger inherent in contrastive analysis: the abundance of characteristic traits of each of the phenomena compared may be reduced to a small set of contrastive traits or even to one main point of contrast, thus depriving the objects compared of many of their characteristics.

With this in mind we shall undertake in the following the contrastive analysis of two cases of jargonaphasia and schizophasia.

The phenomena

Schizophasia

Schizophasia, as described by Kraepelin (1896) and Bleuler (1911), is a deviant linguistic behaviour which can be (episodically) observed in certain schizophrenics. (Owing to drug therapy or due to a cultural change in schizophrenic behaviour, it seems to occur less frequently nowadays than before World War I.)

As salient points of schizophasic behaviour classical psychiatrists mentioned the famous 'Wortsalat' ('word-salad'), a witty but not very informative metaphor for distorted syntax and incoherent speech. Other frequently mentioned characteristics were lexical disorder in the form of incorrectly employed real words (semantic paraphasias) or newly coined words (neologisms), and a very elaborate style described as 'bizarr' ('bizarre') and 'verschroben' ('eccentric'). The actual linguistic discussion was opened in 1974 when Chaika — on the basis of the taperecording of a thirty-seven-year-old female and on samples recorded in the literature — published six characteristics of schizophasic language (see below).

This essentially negative catalogue, which defines schizophasia as a breakdown of linguistic rules, was extended in a later study to eight characteristics, and summarized as follows (Chaika 1982: 177):

> . . . glossomania, rhyming, alliterating, intrusions of extraneous matters, and syntactic errors of schizophrenics all proceed from a failure or inability to subordinate utterances to the requirements of sentence and topic.

Apart from defining schizophasia as a linguistic deficit due to a 'dysfunction in neurotransmission', Chaika emphasizes the unconsciousness, compulsion and permanence of schizophrenic speech. In view of this, we have to conclude that the classical as well as the modern interpretation of schizophasia coincide, in so far as it is described as a breakdown of linguistic competence. As aphasia in its generally accepted neurological definition is a breakdown of linguistic competence due to brain damage, it is only a small step to compare both disorders — or even to mix them up, calling the linguistic behaviour of schizophrenics 'aphasic' (Chapman 1966).

In 1975 Fromkin published a review of Chaika 1974, making the important point that the six characteristics of schizophasia singled out by Chaika also occur in normal speech production. We shall have to remember this when dealing with dysgrammatic features in schizophasic speech.

Jargonaphasia

Jargon, in the extensive meaning of incomprehensible speech, is characteristic of many forms of aphasia, and may be due to such different causes as articulatory disorder (dysarthric speech) or combined phonemic and lexical disorder (global aphasia or Wernicke's aphasia). It is this broad interpretation of jargonaphasia which has been adopted, among others by Lecours and Vanier-Clément (1976) in their comparison of jargonaphasia and schizophasia.

In this chapter, however, I shall deal with jargonaphasia proper, i.e. a very rare type of aphasia which is characterized by continuous semantic and/or neologistic jargon. In its uniqueness this phenomenon has been discovered and described by Alajouanine *et al.* (1952: 164):

> Contrairement aux aphasiques habituels, . . . le jargonaphasique n'a pas de façon typique les arrêts, les blocages, les efforts, les recherches. Son langage coule de source, avec l'aisance et la spontanéité du langage normal. [In contrast to the typical aphasic . . . the speech of a jargonaphasic is devoid of hesitations, blockages, the effort and stress of word-finding. By his fluency the jargonaphasic gives the impression of speaking as easily and effortlessly as normal speakers do.]

The most astonishing fact that jargonaphasics speak fluently a completely incomprehensible jargon, consisting of incorrectly employed real words (semantic jargon) or neologistic sequences of phonemes without any resemblance to real words and devoid of any meaning (phonemic jargon), has been attributed by Alajouanine to 'anosognosia', that is to say, unawareness of one's own illness. The spontaneous speech of the case described below presented a mixture of both types of jargon, that is to say, it consisted mostly of incorrectly employed German words with intermingled phonemic neologisms.

As jargonaphasics share with Wernicke's aphasics common traits of speech behaviour, i.e. severe comprehension disorder and fluent speech, they are very often considered as a subgroup and special manifestation of Wernicke's aphasia, or even as a 'transitional stage of aphasias with severe comprehension disorder' (Leischner 1979: 92). I do not share this opinion; the fact that the cases I and my colleagues observed and described elsewhere (Peuser 1978; Peuser and Temp 1981) showed only a very slow evolution from phonemic to semantic jargon, or even no evolution at all, indicates that jargonaphasia is a special type of aphasia characterized by disturbed comprehension, breakdown of self-monitoring, and fluently spoken semantic and/or phonemic jargon.

The problem of differential diagnosis

In 1976, Lecours and Vanier-Clément published a comparative description of schizophasia and jargonaphasia based on their own observation of aphasics, and on a recorded schizophasic corpus given to them by a Swiss psychiatrist. According to them, jargonaphasia is 'a deviant linguistic behaviour of which there exist several variants' and which 'belongs with the clinical picture of certain types of aphasia' (Lecours and Vanier-Clément 1976: 523). As a consequence, they included not only authentic jargonaphasia but also Wernicke's aphasia, conduction aphasia and transcortical sensory aphasia. The main intention of their paper was to demonstrate that the 'definable characteristics of schizophrenic speech' singled out by Chaika (1974) 'also belong with the jargonaphasias'. After a lot of detailed analysis and sharp observations, they conclude at the end of the paper, somewhat ambiguously (Lecours and Vanier-Clément 1976: 563):

> In summary, Chaika's characteristics Nos. 1 to 5 adequately define linguistic deviations observed in schizophasia. With the possible exception of characteristic No. 2, they also define linguistic deviations observed in the jargonaphasias. From a quantitative point of view, characteristics Nos. 2, 3 and 4 cover most of the deviant phenomena observed in schizophasia, and characteristics 1, 4 and 6 most of the deviant phenomena observed in the jargonaphasias; . . .
>
> Also from a quantitative point of view, characteristic No. 5 equally applies to certain schizophasic and to certain jargonaphasic speakers. Among Chaika's characteristics, No. 6 is the only one that does not constitute an adequate definition of phenomena observed in archetypical schizophasia.

According to this quotation, the differential diagnosis of schizophasia and jargonaphasia can therefore be made along the lines of the following checklist, which indicates nonexistence, normal occurrence (x) and frequent occurrence (xx) of Chaika's criteria:

TABLE 9.1 *Differential diagnosis of jargonaphasia and schizophasia according to Lecours and Vanier-Clément (1976).*

Deviant language parameters (Chaika 1974)	jargonaphasia	schizophasia
1 sporadic disruption in the ability to match semantic features with sound-strings comprising actual lexical items	xx	x
2 preoccupation with too many of the semantic features of a word		x
3 inappropriate noting of phonological features of words	x	xx
4 production of sentences according to phonological and semantic features of previously uttered words	x	x
5 disruption in the ability to apply rules of syntax and discourse	x	x
6 failure to self-monitor, e.g. not noting errors when they occur	x	

As the diagnostic checklist in Table 9.1 indicates, only characteristics 2 and 6, 'semantic preoccupation' and 'failure to self-monitor', unequivocally distinguish schizophasic from jargonaphasic speakers. With regard to the remaining four characteristics of Chaika's list, it is only the preference of characteristics 1 and 3 which differentiates between the groups. Criteria 4 and 5, being equally shared by (members of) both groups, are useless for differential diagnostics. This differential diagnosis must therefore be based on a statistical evaluation of the respective corpora. But as statistical data are not provided, one wonders that the authors feel sure enough to claim:

> As a rule, nonetheless, a differential diagnosis between schizophasia and jargonaphasia remains feasible on the sole basis of tape recorded samples of conversational language. (Lecours and Vanier-Clément 1976: 517)

One might speculate why such an experienced linguist as Lecours, who is without any doubt capable of distinguishing between jargonaphasic and schizophasic speakers, presents diagnostic criteria which are of little help or even misleading (see below). Can this be explained by the above-mentioned pitfall of contrastive patholinguistics, i.e. the overestimation of similarity features, or is this due to his overextensive definition of jargonaphasia as a deviant behaviour 'which belongs with the clinical picture of certain types of aphasia', including the main form and subgroups of Wernicke's aphasia?

I do not think so, for when a patholinguistic analysis of comprehension and naming is carried out, Wernicke's aphasia and schizophasia can be unequivocally differentiated. (Let us remember here that after Wernicke had in 1874 described the linguistic characteristics of sensory aphasia, logorrheic aphasics were no longer confused with schizophrenics and, consequently, were no longer sent to the madhouse.) The only plausible explanation must therefore be that Lecours's analysis of schizophasia is based on second-hand recordings, and not on patients whom he could talk to and assess.

The subsequent comparison of jargonaphasia and schizophasia will therefore be based on real cases which I examined myself, supported by the psychiatrist and neurologist Dr Temp.

The cases

Case 1 Schizophasia (Mr E)

On 10 August 1979, an apparently disorientated thirty-one-year-old man was brought by the police to the psychiatric ward of the Rhenanian Provincial Hospital at Bonn. He had been hitchhiking from Munich to Bonn but was very vague about his destination. He carried papers which showed that three years previously he had been an in-patient in a psychiatric clinic. His preliminary diagnosis was 'acute paranoid psychosis with severe thinking disorder ("word-salad", neologisms) in the context of schizophrenia'. On 11 August 1979 the psychiatrist in charge made the following report:

> Mr E is alert and completely orientated with regard to time and location. Although his thinking is severely disturbed he can satisfactorily answer questions about his personal background. During the exploration he seems to be relaxed but time and again he brusquely interrupts the ongoing conversation. His speech is fluent and intermingled with numerous neologisms. He has the feeling of being influenced by several persons, on which he does not want to comment but emphasizes nevertheless his privilege of being a free

> man and 'of breathing free air'. The normal flow of his discourse is interspersed with episodic hallucinations.

On 20 August another psychiatrist described his behaviour as follows:

> The patient has adapted well to his clinical surroundings. His spontaneous speech is not disturbed. But when he is urged to give explanations and exact descriptions, i.e. put under stress to remember and concentrate, he changes suddenly to a curiously deviant way of expression characterized by neologisms, positional change of syllables and words with an unusual meaning. The prosodic features of his speech, on the other hand, are completely normal.
>
> He seems to understand the questions and utterances of his conversational partner but is incapable of critically monitoring his own disturbed speech.

To exclude a dominant language disorder, the patient was therefore sent to the department for language and speech disorders of the Rhenanian Provincial Hospital.

During conversations with Dr Temp and the author, the patient complained again and again that he felt illegitimately imprisoned. After several weeks he escaped from the clinic and was never seen again. On 16 August Dr Temp had a conversation with Mr E, in the course of which he described the so-called 'Binet pictures' (see below). On 22 August the author performed with him a shortened version of the standard patholinguistic aphasia assessment. This examination concentrated on three critical linguistic parameters which in every aphasic are more or less disturbed: confrontation naming, sentence production and sentence comprehension.

Confrontation naming The patient correctly named forty coloured slides of familiar objects with only three exceptions: the picture of a bridge (the slide in question depicted the Golden Gate Bridge) was called 'an elongated all-sea bridge' (*eine verlängerte Allsee-Brücke*); the picture of a window was described as 'a section of a window' (*ein Fensterausschnitt*); and the picture of a wood was called 'a tree-wood' (*ein Baumwald*).

Sentence production In order to elicit complete utterances, ten slides depicting everyday situations (e.g. a woman peeling oranges in a kitchen) were shown. The purpose of these situational pictures is to assess the syntactic competence of the patient in question. Nevertheless, aphasics — as well as normal speakers — frequently give short telegraphic descriptions of the persons or objects depicted, and have therefore to be reminded to formulate 'complete sentences'. The performance of the schizophrenic was therefore quite normal when, among other things, he described the picture representing a woman standing at an ironing-board and ironing a shirt in the following way: 'an iron, an ironing-board'. But when requested to describe what the person in the picture was doing by a complete sentence, he gave a schizophasic paraphrase of the normal target sentence, namely: 'the true-ready measure by the confirmation to carry clean and dry clothes/ but also to carry them smooth and foldable, ironing assures you of' (*Die treuabfertige Maßnahme durch das Bestätigtsein saubere und trockene Kleider zu tragen/sondern sie auch glatt und faltbar zu tragen/ versichert Ihnen das Bügeln*).

This sudden leap into the schizophasic register shows in a nutshell the two outstanding peculiarities of Mr E's schizophasic style, i.e. the use of semantic neologisms (i.e. the coining of new words on the basis of existing German morphemes, e.g. *treuabfertig*) and a very elaborate style similar to legal or administrative officialese. The occasional disruption of syntactic cohesion indicated that — during his schizophasic 'excursions' — the patient had a grammatical problem which did not show in his normal conversation. A tentative normal version of this sentence could run as follows: 'The true-ready measure and the confirmation to carry not only clean and dry but also smooth and foldable clothes ironing assures you of'. It reveals that the schizophasic original is a dysgrammatical construction of the paragrammatical type. This could be interpreted as a symptom of Wernicke's aphasia, were it not for the fact that Wernicke aphasics never speak so pompously, and cannot deliberately change from normal to dysgrammatic speech and vice versa. Normal speakers, on the other hand, frequently lose the syntactic thread when formulating very long and complicated sentences.

Sentence comprehension Mr E's comprehension of spoken sentences was assessed by means of the 'three figures test' (Peuser and Schriefers 1980). But, unlike an aphasic, he performed this test faultlessly, pointing to the corresponding picture of each of the twenty instructions. This proved not only that his comprehension of spoken language was completely undisturbed but also that his level of attention and concentration was high, for even normal speakers occasionally misunderstand one or two instructions, and point to an inappropriate picture.

As each aphasic fails more or less on these tests of basic linguistic faculties, depending on the degree of his disorder, a classification of Mr E's deviant way of expression as 'aphasic' or 'aphasoid' can be ruled out.

Case 2 Jargonaphasia (Mr W)

In May 1973, Mr W — fifty-three-years-old, married, with two children, and the owner of a small factory — was in a car accident which resulted in a cranial injury with serious cerebral contusion and fracture of the right temporal and right petrosal bones. The patient suffered from right hemihypesthenia. The EEG showed pathological changes which varied from slight to moderately severe for both hemispheres.

Mr W was an in-patient in the language and speech department of the Rhenanian Provincial Hospital from 17 September to 12 December 1973. He was classified as a case of fluent, semantic/neologistic jargonaphasia. He spoke without stimulation from his interlocutor. He seemed to speak about subjects which were of great concern to him and which — of course — nobody understood. He did not explain himself by writing or by pantomime. Immediately after his accident, Mr W seems to have spoken a neologistic jargon — the people who brought him to the hospital thought he was a foreign spy speaking an unknown language. When he came to our clinic he spoke a semantic/neologistic jargon consisting of short, stereotypical sentences. This small syntactic inventory was repeated with so many prosodic and neologistic variations that the listener had the impression of hearing many different sentences. Although Mr W spoke without interruption, he did not communicate anything but the vague idea that he was very upset and annoyed. And even this information was not transmitted by verbal means but by intonation and mime. From the fact that Mr W did not use writing or pantomime, one may deduce that at this time he believed in the referential value of his speech.

When, in 1979, Mr W came to our clinic for a second time, he seemed in many respects a different person. In 1973 he had been a bit of an 'indefatigable chatterbox' who did not care about the reaction of his interlocutor. This time he was very attentive and respected the rules of communication — that is, he answered questions and fell silent when his interlocutor spoke. His spontaneous speech consisted mostly of highly stereotyped anomic speech, in which content words were replaced by pronouns, pantomime, and, occasionally, by neologisms like [ˈvaɩnəs], [ˈvaɩkəns], [mˈaxtɔs]. These neologisms had already occurred in both spontaneous speech and reading in 1973, which shows that as early as half a year after the accident his jargon had become partially lexicalized. (Stereotyped neologisms are mentioned by Green (1969) and Buckingham and Kertesz (1976).)

The systematic substitution of content words by pantomime and neologism proves that Mr W was suffering from severe anomia. The very simple, stereotypical and fragmentary sentences disguise another defect, which occasionally surfaced in the form of violations of word-order or false numerical congruence between subject and predicate. In conclusion, over the course of six years, this patient was able without therapeutic intervention to build up an efficient communication system, based on some eighty words (most of them function words) and the use of nonverbal symbolic systems. He may serve as an admirable example of the spontaneous healing capacity of the human brain which Monakow and Mourgue (1928) termed 'syneidisis'. During his second stay at our clinic, Mr W was very co-operative, so that a number of tests could be carried out The most striking feature of his lexical performance was the discrepancy between speech and writing. Whereas his oral performance — with the exception of repetition — was very bad, his graphic performance was relatively good. The fact that he repeated well on 50 per cent of the items showed a positive change in auditory comprehension as well as in his command of articulation.

His receptive performance indicated his good capacity for recognizing characteristic sounds (doorbell, car, etc.) discriminating phonemic and graphemic minimal pairs (*Tanne*/*Kanne*), showing the picture corresponding to the stimulus of a spoken or written word, and recognizing grammatically deviant sentences such as 'two boys is sitting in the room' (a complete listing of the sentences by which seven grammatical categories are tested is given in Peuser 1978). But when he was confronted with the syntactic stimuli of the token test or the three figures test (*DFT*), a dramatic breakdown of his auditory comprehension could be observed. The three figures test (see Peuser 1976; 1978; Peuser and Schriefers 1980) is a multiple-choice procedure with twenty stimulus sentences, exemplifying active, passive, affirmative and negative constructions. Mr W's score of twelve incorrect answers (out of twenty) on the DFT indicated a comprehension deficit corresponding to that of severe Wernicke's aphasia.

A comparison of these findings with the results of the clinical assessment in 1973 showed that Mr W's language comprehension had improved considerably. The same held true for his language comprehension in everyday situations. This improved comprehension went hand in hand with an improved capacity for monitoring and judging the effect of his own speech.

Text comprehension and 'concrete attitude'

The standard aphasia battery of Leischner (1974) consists of the text of a fable which the patient has to read aloud and to paraphrase:

The dog with the piece of meat

A dog stole a piece of meat at the butcher's and carried it away in his mouth.

When he ran away he came to a small river with a little bridge.

When he was crossing this bridge, he saw down in the water a second dog with a piece of meat between his teeth.

Voraciously he snapped at this dog to get the meat.

But when he opened his mouth, the piece of meat which he had stolen at the butcher's fell into the river and floated away.

The diagnostic function of this fable is not only to assess the capabilities of reading aloud and text comprehension, but also to evidence an existing disorder of 'abstract thinking' and 'abstract behaviour' which, according to Goldstein (1948), is characteristic of brain damaged patients. So, in order to verify whether the patient has grasped the deeper meaning of the fable, additional questions concerning the number of dogs and pieces of meat are asked. Unfortunately, the fact that quite a few aphasics believe that the fable is about two dogs instead of one is wrongly attributed to a reduced faculty of abstract thinking instead of to a low level of education: for, as the text does not definitely state that the second dog in the water is only a reflection, one has to know the fable and its hidden sense in order to arrive at the correct conclusion that there is only one dog.

During the months of his first stay, the aphasic read the fable aloud on various occasions, demonstrating with every new reading a characteristic slow transition from phonemic to predominantly semantic jargon (the corresponding texts are reproduced in Peuser 1978 and Peuser and Temp 1981). When, on his final examination on 5 December 1973, he was asked by the interviewer whether the story dealt with one or two dogs, Mr W answered without hesitation in his semantic jargon: 'I made only one' (*Ich habe nur eins gemacht*). What makes us believe that he really meant it was the self-assurance with which he pointed to the substantive 'dog', and the experimentally demonstrated fact that text comprehension in aphasics is better preserved than the comprehension of isolated sentences (Stachowiak *et al.* 1977).

On 16 August Mr E, the schizophrenic patient, was confronted with the fable by my colleague Dr Temp immediately after having commented on the Binet pictures. He read the text aloud fluently, with only two minor paralectic distortions. His paraphrase was quite normal and consisted mainly of literal quotations; it ended somewhat enigmatically, mentioning that the piece of meat is divided and that another creature, called 'the young one', is present. But when he was asked, 'how many pieces of meat are in the story?' Mr E answered, 'Three', and when the question concerning the number of dogs was put to him he answered, 'Four'.

How can this be explained? A patient who on 22 August complied faultlessly with the twenty difficult multiple-choice instructions of the 'three figures test' had on 16 August been incapable of grasping the meaning of a simple fable! Was it the effect of drug therapy or a transitional crisis which had faded away when I met him a fortnight after his first examination? His subsequent interpretation of the fable, darkly mentioning 'an animal which does not belong to this epoch', gives no hint that he really believed in the existence of four dogs and three pieces of meat. But as, on the other hand, the numbers given by him correspond more or less exactly to the frequency with which the words 'dog' and 'piece of meat' occur in the text, this could mean that he misunderstood the question, and consequently reacted as if the interviewer had asked: 'How many times are the dog and the piece of meat *mentioned* in the fable?' As the comprehension of the question presupposes the comprehension of the fable, this would also indicate that Mr E misunderstood the meaning of the fable, ignoring, among other things, the text-referential value of the pronoun 'he'.

If this interpretation is correct, Mr E's faulty comprehension could be a striking example of the so-called 'concrete attitude' (Goldstein 1939; 1943) which Arieti (1974: 217) describes as follows:

> There is no doubt that in many instances schizophrenics characterize themselves by being specific, concrete and unable to transcend the particular situation or set.

In the subsequent context, Arieti expresses some doubts as to whether Goldstein's theory, which is based on the observation of organic patients, also applies to schizophrenics. But our long experience with aphasic patients (see the above-mentioned text experiments of Stachowiak *et al.* (1977)) and the evidence of the present case of schizophrenia makes us wonder whether Goldstein's 'concrete attitude' might be more characteristic of schizophrenic than of aphasic behaviour.

Spontaneous speech in jargonaphasia and schizophasia

The description of Binet picture 1

The characteristics of different types of language disorder are best revealed if the speakers perform the same task, for example, talk about the same subject or describe the same picture. This procedure has the advantage that we know what the speaker in question is talking about, or should be talking about.

In order to illustrate Mr E's and Mr W's characteristics of speech, we reproduce below their description of the so-called 'Binet pictures', which form part of the standard aphasia assessment at Bonn (Leischner 1974). The subject of Binet picture 1 (see Figure 9.1) is the party game 'hide-and-seek' played by a group of persons, apparently a family.

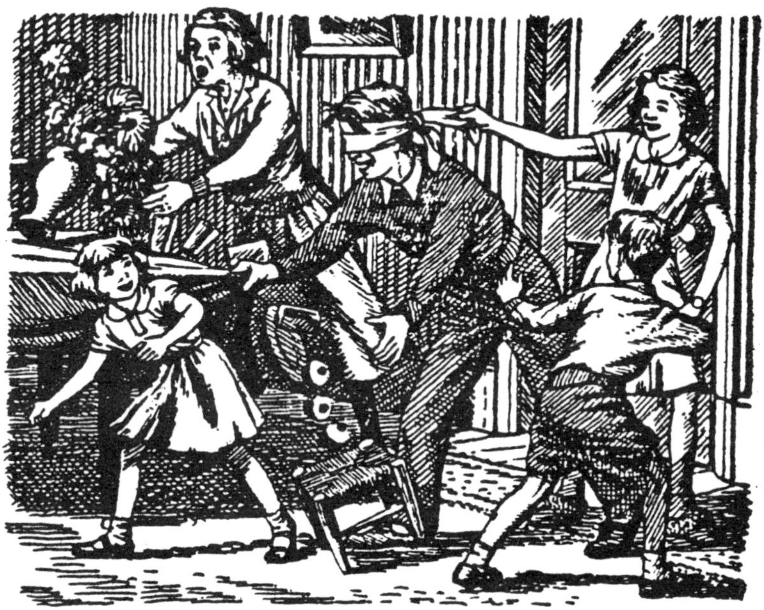

FIGURE 9.1 *Binet picture 1: 'hide-and-seek'.*

The texts given below are reproduced by an orthographic transcription which has been developed by the author (Peuser 1978) to reproduce the most important segmental and suprasegmental features of aphasic speech. The following symbols and abbreviations have been used:

I	Interviewer
P	Patient
/	normal pause (1/10–4/10 sec.)
//	long pause (5/10–5 sec.)
äh	filled pause
?	interrogative sentence

!	exclamative sentence
. . ./	open-ended sentence without lowering of voice (aposiopesis)
word	single word spoken with emphasis
/. . ./	passage omitted by the transcriber
(xxx)	incomprehensible passage
(laughing, etc.):	comment of the transcriber, or alternative interpretation of an ambiguous passage
[ ]	phonetically transcribed neologisms

The original German texts are reproduced in the Appendix.

Text 1 Description of Binet picture 1 given by the schizophrenic (Mr E)

I: I want to show you some pictures now and äh these pictures are the so-called Binet pictures which depict a specific type of situation / take your time and have a look at them and then you may describe what is going on there /

P: This picture / for example / indicates the game hide-and-seek / doesn't it?

I: Yes / and what else is happening there?

P: The hastiness of this pulled-away tablecloth and the (*original German: dative instead of nominative*) overturned tin wheeled carriage I should think / lets the (*original German: accusative*) sitting chair there with / this charmingness (*original German:* 'Holdrigkeit', *i.e. untranslatable semantic neologism*) being pulled on too coarsely and too seriously isn't it? That's all /
Hm / the man / may be the father is / blindfolded / he wants to catch the girl / but / inadvertently pulls on the table cloth /

P: Yes /

I: And what happens next?

P: Well it seems that the flower-vase is breaking into two / the flowers/ are standing without water and äh the stool is lying through the flowered (*original German: neologistic adjective derived from the verb 'blühen', 'to flower'*) blockade of the (*original German: neuter form of the article indicating that the speaker at this point has already the neuter noun 'Mädchen' instead of the feminine 'Tochter' in mind*) the daughter or the young girl isn't it? who tried to find support there isn't it? and is blocking up its way / (xxx) confidence support isn't it? this has been thus named by someone / first / (xxx) //

Text 2 Description of Binet picture 1 given by the jargonaphasic (Mr W)

I: Please pay attention now / I am showing you a picture / would you please describe what you äh what you see / just . . ./

P: Well / they are doing the (*nominative*) ['aisəntər] / with the ['ainənɔs] / isn't it? / [gə'vaigəs] / and they ['maxənt] / they ['maxəns] / they ['maxə] that/ or not? and they ['koytən dans] / they are doing that / the (*feminine*) one (*neuter*) / she does it (xxx)//

I: Well / is this a wedding?

P: (*laughing*) No no! no no no!
I: Or is it a brawl?
P: Yes / no / here / this one does it / now the ['aikəns] they are doing into the ['aikəns 'vaxtər] /
I: Or is it a game? /
P: Yes / something like that /
I: What type of game / football?
P: Here / no / that she (they) it /
I: Tennis?
P: That one does it /
I: The one (*neuter*)?
P: The one (*neuter*) does it / isn't it?
I: Or are they playing cards?
P: No no! here that here /
I: Hide-and-seek? is it hide-and-seek?
P: No / [di:t'fri:dəl 'laxən] that here must be it / must it there / or must it / and this one must it / and he really knows how to do it //

Two types of dysgrammatism

Text 2, spoken by the jargonaphasic, consists mostly of the fluently spoken semantic jargon which characterized his spontaneous speech described above; i.e. a sequence of short, nearly entirely meaningless sentences which have the following structure:

$$\text{pronoun} + \left\{\begin{matrix}\text{does, do etc}\\ \text{neologism}\end{matrix}\right\} + \text{prounoun}$$

The neologisms are minimal phonemic variations of the verb 'to do' (*machen*) or items of the small inventory of lexicalized phonemic neologisms like ['aisəntər], ['ainənɔs], which could be minimal variations of the pronoun 'one' (*einer, eine, eines*). The abundance of semantic paraphasias (i.e. inappropriately used German words) and phonemic neologisms points to the existence of anomia, which is the main symptom of aphasia. The short stereotyped sentences and occasional errors, like numerical or generic incongruence between predicate and object (*sie machen der*) or between article, pronominal subject and predicate (*die eines machen das*), indicate an underlying dysgrammatism. Intermingled with these dysgrammatic sentences are short correct idioms, e.g. 'something like that'.

When the patient denies the final question of the interviewer as to whether the depicted party game is hide-and-seek, one could deduce that he has not grasped the sense of the scene depicted. But this is contradicted by his previous rejection of false interpretations suggested by the interviewer. We have therefore to assume that, although he has a complete understanding of what the picture is about, he has probably misunderstood the expression 'hide-and-seek' owing to his disturbed comprehension of spoken speech.

On the other hand, the opening remark of the schizophrenic speaker in text 1 shows his complete understanding of the depicted scene as well as his command of the German language when he — albeit a little pompously — declares: 'this picture, for example, represents the game hide-and-seek'. Only when the interviewer insists on a more detailed description does he change to his schizophasic register which is a mixture of normal utterances and elaborated nominal constructions, like 'the hastiness of this pulled-away tablecloth', which are completely untypical of everyday speech. The fluently spoken violations of syntactic rules cannot be easily detected; they reveal themselves to the eye rather than to the ear. They consist mainly of a rupture of syntactic cohesion, which is not unusual in everyday speech. As we do not know the target sentence, the first dysgrammatical utterance of text 1 is deviant either by omission of the relative pronoun (*Die Hastigkeit . . . welche da den Sitzstuhl . . . anziehen läßt/ . . .*) or wrong position of the predicate if an embedded relative sentence was not intended (*Die Hastigkeit . . . läßt da den Sitzstuhl . . . anziehen/ . . .*). But as mentioned above, these occasional dysgrammatical lapses cannot be attributed to an underlying (permanent) dysgrammatical disorder. This is contradicted by the correct syntax of other utterances of the same text, and the patient's spontaneous speech in general. The rupture of syntactic cohesion must therefore be attributed to an occasional breakdown of psycholinguistic competence (i.e. factors like concentration and memory: see Peuser 1984), due to the effort of constructing elaborate sentences and coining complicated neologisms.

Semantic versus phonemic neologisms

In contrast to the text of the jargonaphasic, the text of the schizophrenic speaker is devoid of meaningless phonemic neologisms. Mr E's neologisms consist of correct German morphemes, and are constructed according to the rules of German word-formation. As words like *Holdrigkeit* ('charmingness'), *Blechradwagen* ('tin-wheeled carriage') and *Sitzstuhl* ('sitting-chair'), although not belonging to the normal inventory, make sense, they are to be classified as 'semantic neologisms'. With regard to the differential diagnosis of both disorders, it seems that at least our cases of jargonaphasia and schizophasia are characterized by different types of neologisms.

But these findings concerning the preference for semantic neologisms cannot be applied to all schizophrenics or all states of schizophrenia, for the literature on schizophrenia abounds in descriptions of speakers or writers creating their private neologistic lexicons. But dealing with phonemic neologisms, we cannot take into account the more or less conscious and voluntary creation of neologisms with a continuous reference (i.e. denoting one and only one phenomenon) as described by Flournoy (1900), Tuczek (1921) and others. In our context we have to consider the spontaneous *ad hoc* production of phonetic strings in ongoing speech which are absolutely meaningless i.e. without stable reference. Neologisms of this kind seem to have been uttered by the girl Renée when she was in extreme pain and despair (*Autobiography*, 1970: 79f.):

> The periods of confounding guilt persisted along with bitter moral pain and I shed tears for hours, crying 'Raïte, Raïte, was habe ich gemacht?' (What have I done?), sorrowing in my own 'language', in the meaningless, recurring syllables, 'icthiou, gao, itivare, giastow, ovede' and the like. In no way did I seek to create them; they came of themselves and by themselves meant nothing. Only the sound, the rhythm of the pronunciation had sense. Through them I lamented, pouring out the gruelling grief and the interminable sadness in my heart. I could not use ordinary words, for my pain and sorrow had no real basis.

Unfortunately, the autobiography does not inform us whether the quoted neologistic interjections were the only specimens or whether they were samples from a greater inventory; whether they were lexicalized and morphologically invariable, or minimal phonetic variations of a few basic forms, as in the case of Mr W's jargon.

As a matter of principle, everybody who is in an ecstatic or dreamy state of mind is capable of producing phonetic neologisms. But must we not distinguish between, on the one hand, the more or less voluntary productions of this kind of neo-language servicing specific expressive needs, e.g. the communication with divine authorities or the expression of unutterable pain, and, on the other hand, the involuntary output of a word production mechanism which, as a consequence of severe anomia and (temporarily) disturbed self-monitoring, has gone wild?

Let us look now at the other side of the coin. Do jargonaphasics produce semantic neologisms on the basis of standard morphemes? Yes, they do, but, to our knowledge, this does not happen in spoken but only in written jargon. Peuser (1978) described the case of a jargonaphasic woman who spoke phonemic but wrote semantic jargon on confrontation naming and dictation. The picture of a bottle of milk (*Milch*) was thus named in writing on various occasions as *Anziehr, Eintut, Wientahm*, etc. (The corresponding spoken denominations were [dɪ:], [mə'dɪ:], etc.). This discrepancy between oral and written naming which we discovered in other aphasics too (see Peuser 1978) can be explained by the situational circumstances of the graphic modality: the advantageous feedback of written language favoured the retrieval and (more or less) meaningful combination of German morphemes.

But in this context we are dealing with spoken jargon which is not characterized by elaborate semantic paraphasias or semantic neologisms but by fluently spoken semantic or neologistic jargon. Now, what is behind those fluently spoken phonemic improvisations?

The problem of neologistic speech

Jargonaphasia and the disinhibition of phonemic processes

Two conflicting hypotheses have been advanced to account for neologistic speech.

(1) Lecours and Lhermitte (1969) and Kertesz and Benson (1970) advocate the so-called 'conduction theory' of jargon, which states that neologisms are phonemic distortions of a target word.

(2) Buckingham (1977), Buckingham *et al.* (1978), Butterworth (1979), and Duchan *et al.* (1980) advance what might be called the 'anomia-theory' or 'empty-slot-filling theory' of jargon, which is based on the anomic condition of jargonaphasics described by Kinsbourne and Warrington (1963), Buckingham and Kertesz (1976), and others. According to these authors, 'neologisms appear to serve as substitutes for the root form of lexical items, when presumably these cannot be retrieved from the lexical system' (Butterworth 1979: 151). A similar statement is made by Buckingham *et al.* (1978), who suggest 'that many neologisms may also be produced during the period of time in ongoing speech when the precise word called for by the context has not yet been retrieved' (151).

With regard to the neologisms of Mr W and the other patients described in Peuser 1978 and Peuser and Temp 1981, we strongly support the second hypothesis for the following reasons. All patients suffered from severe anomia. With growing awareness of his anomia, Mr W made no effort to correct his neologisms, but replaced them by gesture and pantomime. Mrs K, the second case described in Peuser and Temp 1981, produced entire neologistic texts, which are far more difficult to explain by the conduction theory than single words.

Although in spontaneous speech and, above all, in reading aloud, we may find some phonemic distortions of target words, this strategy cannot account for the majority of the neologisms that occurred. For such a strategy to be feasible, it should be possible to recognize and reconstruct the underlying target words, at least in the case of the readings (see Lecours and Lhermitte 1969). As this is obviously not possible, what rules govern the production of neologistic jargon?

Although in Mr W's jargon there is a certain trend of lexicalization, that is to say, a tendency to reproduce the same or at least similar jargon words, most of the spontaneous neologistic structures are unstable *ad hoc* productions of a disinhibited phonological device. It was Pick (1931) who explained the literal paraphasias of fluent aphasics by the disinhibition of the intact sound-sequencing mechanism. Green (1969) observed the phenomenon of sequential repetition of various phonological segments in a jargonaphasic and referred to it as alliteration (the repetition of consonants) and assonance (the repetition of vocalic segments). These 'clang associations', which may be seen in sensory aphasics, dementias, schizophrenics and sleep talkers (Brown 1972; Cromwell and Dokeki 1968) are explained by Buckingham *et al.* (1978) in terms of a general principle of neuromuscular activity such as inhibition and postinhibitory rebound (see McKay 1970; Ohala and Hirano 1967).

Stampe (1969) holds that the principle of reduplication (the strictest form of alliteration and assonance) dominates the early period of language acquisition, thus constituting a natural phonological law which is later on inhibited by the phonotactical rules of the particular language system. It therefore seems that the neologistic productivity of jargonaphasics may be explained by the disinhibition of such processes of natural phonology as alliteration, assonance and reduplication, to which one might add the preference for CVCV structures, that is, a regular sequence of consonants and vowels which is also characteristic of glossolalic speech (Rensch 1971).

But if the neologistic output of jargonaphasics were entirely dominated by the laws of natural phonology and the principle of least effort (Zipf 1949), jargon would be reduced to a monotonous sequence of repetitive clang associations. The neologistic texts of the aphasics described in Peuser 1978 and Peuser and Temp 1981 demonstrate that this is not the case. Upon examining more closely their provoked as well as their spontaneous speech, one discovers consonant clusters and a tendency to avoid the monotony of alliteration and assonance by phonological variation. The principle of least effort and the laws of natural phonology are thus countered by a continued effort to maintain the distinctiveness of speech.

Schizophasia and the disinhibition of semantic and morphological processes

Now, which mechanism can explain the semantic neologisms of the schizophrenic speaker?

The results of the neurolinguistic assessment described above have clearly demonstrated not only that we can rule out anomia but, what is more, that the linguistic competence of Mr E is completely intact. In this case we have therefore to reject Arieti's (1974) interpretation of schizophrenia as a quasi-aphasoid state, with consequent loss or weakening of the socially established meaning of linguistic signs (connotation) and a resulting prevalence of linguistic form (verbalization). As a final consequence this would lead to clang associating 'word salad', influenced by the context and governed by the rules of natural phonology.

But we have to admit, of course, that a schizophrenic process going on for years may lead, under the combined influence of hospitalization and the administration of powerful drugs, to the kind of functional brain damage which Arieti describes. This is clearly not the case with our relatively young patient. But as our neologistic creativity is limited by the capacity of our psycholinguistic competence, it is nearly impossible to make a fresh start with every new neologism. That is to say, in all truly neologistic speech there will be a more or less pronounced influence of context, to the extent that limitation of memory obliges the speaker to re-use previously uttered morphological and syntactical models. So, even in the short text 1, we find some examples of this creative economy: the semantic neologism *Holdrigkeit* (see the second utterance of the patient) is modelled on the preceding real word *Hastigkeit*. The same holds true for the relation *Blumen — geblüht* in Mr E's last utterance.

But what really strikes us in the utterances of Mr E is not a weakening but, on the contrary, an extraordinary increase in his semantic and morphological competence. This increase of linguistic faculties has very often been observed and described, giving rise to the famous comparison of schizophasia and poetry (see, among others, Navratil 1966).

The word-production model given in Figure 9.2 is an attempt to explain this increase of semantic and morphological competence as a disinhibition of morphological rules which parallels the disinhibition of (natural) phonological rules in the jargonaphasic.

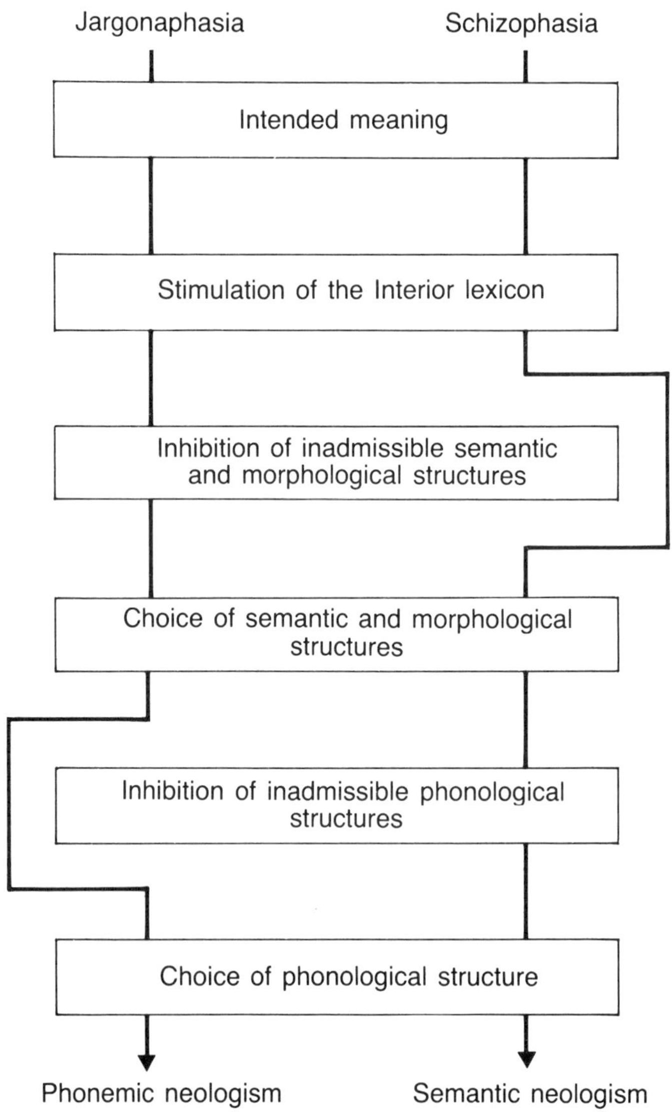

FIGURE 9.2 *The production of neologisms in jargonaphasia and schizophasia.*

As to the neuropsychological basis of this disinhibition in schizophrenics, one might speculate with Arieti (1974) that in schizophrenia we are confronted with an increased influence of phylogenetically older and anatomically deeper layers of the brain, and a corresponding release of so-called 'primary' processes, were it not for the fact that primary (i.e. primitive) thinking is better suited for nonfluent, agrammatical than fluent, paragrammatical speech, let alone the coining of new words by derivation and composition.

But the disinhibition of the normally blocked programme of word-formation in the schizophrenic speaker differs in an important respect from the disinhibition of phonological rules in the jargonaphasic. Mr E seems to be more or less in full command of his neologistic word production, whereas the jargonaphasic has lost control over his phonological device, so that the rules of natural phonology can take over.

The communicative functions of schizophasia

In assuming that schizophrenic speakers are more or less in command of their speech production, we claim with Bleuler (1911) and Lecours and Vanier-Clément (1976) that the schizophrenic Mr E deliberately and intentionally formulates what is in his mind when he looks at the Binet pictures. But as his statements are obviously far from normal, we have to ask ourselves whether there is something wrong with his selection of meaning.

By this we do not mean Mr E's mentioning a 'tin-wheeled carriage' which is not present in the present version of Binet picture 1, for the following reasons. First, we cannot exlude the possibility that — as there exist several versions of Binet pictures — Mr E was shown a picture with a pram. Secondly, if he was shown the present picture, he may have misinterpreted the plate falling down from the table as some sort of wheel belonging to a corresponding carriage.

Looking at the content of Mr E's descriptions, one must admit that Mr E has, to say the least, a tendency to over-interpret the situations depicted. This shows very clearly in his description of the third Binet picture which depicts a simple accident of everyday life: a gentleman, eager to salute a lady looking out of a window, inadvertently knocks down the little child of another lady who is passing by. Instead of giving a simple description of this event, Mr E constructs some sort of love story around these three persons, claiming that the gentleman has fallen in love with the younger lady and has consequently left the older one and their common child. According to him, this picture proves 'that it is not always the man who is let down but also the woman'.

Compared to this fiction, his 'deeper' interpretation of picture 1 (see above, text 1) is not so clearcut, but insinuates that, for at least one of the persons playing hide-and-seek, there is more at stake than just taking part in a harmless party game. In his view, the pictures seem to carry a double message: a superficial one, which he easily identifies as the party game hide-and-seek; and a deeper, hidden one, which corresponds to his private experience and his special view of the world. But this private view expressed in his schizophasic register of speech is uncovered only when the interviewer urges him to give more details, or to make a linguistic effort, i.e. to formulate complete sentences.

Schizophasia, at least in our patient, can therefore be interpreted as a reaction to communicative stress and increased demand for information by the respective conversational partner. But, contrary to the psychiatrist quoted above, who qualified this phenomenon as some sort of linguistic breakdown, we give it a more positive interpretation, qualifying it as an essentially successful linguistic effort.

In her interesting study of conversations between psychiatrists and schizophrenic patients Käsermann (1983: 144) concludes that 'the schizophrenic disposes of several variables of verbal behaviour, some of them in conformity with the expectation of the interviewer and others'. According to Käsermann, the choice of these variables depends on additional conditions such as, for example, what she calls 'invasive questioning' by the interviewer. In the light of Käsermann's findings, schizophasic reactions may therefore be interpreted as a technique to divert the interviewer and throw him off the trail. Peters and Prelle (1974) seem to follow a similar line of thinking when they tentatively define schizophasia as a verbal technique to conceal a thinking disorder. Our findings correspond to these interpretations only in so far as our patient deliberately and consciously changed from normal to schizophasic speech, and vice versa.

But the communicative function of our patient's schizophasic passages is, on the contrary, not to divert but to impress the interviewer by his deeper understanding and eloquent description of the pictures. To understand this, we have to consider that in the patient's view the interviewer is an influential personality, on whom the patient's freedom depends. In the patient's view, the whole conversation with Dr Temp on 22 August is some sort of examination, giving him the chance to demonstrate his intellectual and verbal faculties and to convince the interviewer of his normality. This is corroborated by the stubbornness with which Mr E again and again steered the conversation back to the subject of his liberty, complaining that he had been 'illegitimately imprisoned' and asking when he was going to be discharged from the hospital. If the findings of Käsermann (1983) quoted above demonstrate that schizophasic passages serve to divert the interviewer and to camouflage the patient's problems, our findings evidence that schizophasia may at least have two additional communicative functions which are closely related: the functions of persuasion and of self-demonstration.

All these functions can be helpful for the planning of therapy, the persuasive function perhaps even more than the diverting one, for if divertive schizophasia tips the interviewer off, signalling him that he has touched a sore spot, persuasive schizophasia gives insight into the problem itself by uncovering the patient's private view of the world. (The same may of course hold true for divertive passages in Käsermann's material, which, given a closer look, might turn out to be persuasive or to be divertive *and* persuasive.)

In demonstrating thus the communicative function and meaning of schizophasic jargon, patholinguistics can be helpful to psychiatry and psychotherapy in its effort to uncover the patient's problem. Linguistics, as a discipline traditionally occupied with decoding forgotten languages of the past, comes into its own in approaching the so-called 'word-salad' of schizophasia as a secret message formulated in a strange but translatable language.

With regard to the comparison between jargonaphasia and schizophasia, these findings lead us to ascertain another important difference concerning the communicative functions of both types of deviant speech; if schizophasia is intended to be either divertive or persuasive and informative, the communicative aim is frequently reached or, at least, can in principle be reached, provided the schizophasic passage is given the correct interpretation. On the other hand, the neologistic jargon of jargonaphasia is also intended to be meaningful, but it would never succeed were it not for additional situational and paralinguistic information or *a priori* knowledge, which enables the interlocutor to guess more or less correctly what the aphasic speaker wants to express. Although fluent neologistic jargon has been occasionally misinterpreted as some sort of trick designed to camouflage the patient's speech disorder, the only communicative function which can be attributed to this type of jargon is neither divertive nor informative but 'phatic'. But even this function, which serves to establish and to maintain social contact, is restricted to special types of interlocutors and special situations.

According to our previous findings (Peuser and Temp 1981), jargonaphasics maintain their fluent neologistic jargon only when they are in contact with a sympathetic interlocutor who seems to 'understand' what the patient says. Confronted with interlocutors who clearly demonstrate their lack of comprehension, the patient falls silent.

Self-monitoring and the awareness of deviant speech

In Lecour's and Vanier-Clément's checklist given above (p. 220) the awareness of one's own speech deviations (characteristic 6) is one of the two critical items which distinguish schizophasia from jargonaphasia. Unfortunately, this diagnostic criterion is not easy to handle, as it is very difficult to judge the degree of a speaker's awareness of his own speech production. First of all, Lecours himself has to concede an 'intermittent awareness' of their own speech production even to jargonaphasics (Lecours and Vanier-Clément 1976: 537):

> When one says that a given speaker is unaware of his production of deviant segments, one means that this speaker does not seem to know that his linguistic output does not make sense to the listener or, at least, that it may have a diminished or perverted communication value; in other words, the anosognosic speaker of deviant segments goes on talking as if his vis-à-vis should understand. Yet, and this may seem contradictory but we believe the observation to be valid, there often appears to be, even in logorrheic jargon, a certain level of near awareness. It is manifested, for instance, by frequent hesitations, repetitions of modalities, prepositions, etc. immediately preceding the production of a deviant segment . . .

Now, as the so-called 'anosognosic behaviour' of jargonaphasics is the most critical point in the discussion of this enigmatic form of aphasia, we gave it in our previous study a lot of attention; but the neuropsychiatric and neurolinguistic analyses of the cases described in Peuser and Temp 1981 seem to indicate that it is not anosognosia but the disruption of internal and external feedback systems that gives rise to neologistic jargon.

In March 1979, when both patients, Mr W and Mrs K, an old lady speaking fluent neologistic jargon, were at our clinic, we examined their reactions to delayed auditory feedback (DAF). Such investigations have been conducted by Alajouanine *et al.* (1964), Boller *et al.* (1978), and others, with the main result that fluent aphasics with phonemic jargon or poor repetition and/or disturbed comprehension showed no change in their speech with DAF. Our patients' reactions differed. Whereas Mr W interrupted himself, continuing with louder and slower speech, Mrs K showed no reaction at all. This clearly showed that Mr W, the patient with semantic jargon, had a relatively intact external feedback, whereas Mrs K, the patient with neologistic jargon, had a completely disrupted external feedback at the moment of speaking. Unfortunately, we do not know anything about the state of the preceding (and, as Alajouanine *et al.* (1952) rightly point out, perhaps even more important) internal self-monitoring of the patient.

Another explanation for jargonaphasics' apparent unawareness of their defective speech was proposed by Alajouanine *et al.* (1952), who compared the behaviour of jargonaphasics with the reduced self-monitoring of normal speakers during the speech act:

> Mais l'apport le plus significatif du jargon aphasique, c'est qu'il ne s'écoute visiblement pas parler. Le faisons-nous, nous-mêmes dans l'expression normale? Probablement très peu, et c'est une surprise d'entendre, retransmises par le magnétophone indiscret, les formules que nous avons, quelques instants plus tôt, prononcés, sans même avoir remarqué les termes que nous utilisions. (166). [What most impresses in jargonaphasics is their obvious unawareness of their own speech production. But how much attention do we pay to our own speech production when we are engaged in everyday conversation? Probably not very much, for it is always a surprise when hearing our own formulations reproduced by the indiscrete tape-recorder, and realize that, only a few minutes ago, we spoke without apparently paying attention to the exact expressions we used.]

These findings are confirmed by the patients' attitude toward their written production: when the intensity of the graphic feedback allowed them to control their verbal output, they recognized the faultiness of their production. Thus, what could be mistaken for anosognosic behaviour in our case of neologistic jargon is in reality the consequence of a complete disruption of external self-monitoring at the moment of speaking to what seems an 'understanding interlocutor'. Lecours and Vanier-Clément (1976) base their contention that 'schizophasic speakers are sometimes very much aware of their deviations' on the fact that schizophrenics, back to linguistic normality, may comment on their former schizophasic productions (see the example of Renée quoted above).

Even if these recorded statements may be taken at their face value, one must be doubtful if retrospective comments on one's speech production truly reflect the state of mind at the moment of speaking. In dealing with an individual's awareness of his or her own speech, one should distinguish several levels of linguistic self-control: with regard to thematic awareness, Mr E left no doubt that his interpretation of the Binet pictures corresponded to his intentions. This became very evident during the conversation on 22 August; when my colleague tried to correct him, proposing another interpretation of Binet picture 3, Mr E insisted: 'but it is also possible that my interpretation is correct', thus intimating that he was very well aware of the discrepancy between the two interpretations.

As to his syntactical awareness, we have to concede that he did not correct himself, but that, on the other hand, occasional disruption of syntactic cohesion does happen in normal speech without the speaker noting it. With regard to awareness of his lexical productions, we have to admit that choice and control of semantic features may be semi-conscious, as some expressions remain obscure. On the other hand, a speaker using the rules of word-formation correctly cannot have lost total control over his lexical output.

Towards a differential diagnosis of jargonaphasia and schizophasia

In my evaluation above of Lecours's differential diagnosis of jargonaphasia and schizophasia, I had to conclude that, of Chaika's six characteristics of schizophasic speech (which in themselves are not very consistent, as characteristics 2, 3 and 4 are very closely related), only nos. 1, 2, 3 and 6 distinguish more or less sharply between the two disorders. (With regard to nos. 1 and 3, it is only the quantitative predominance of the respective deviant feature which indicates whether the case in question is jargonaphasic or schizophasic.)

Now we shall have to look at these four criteria in the light of our own findings as described above, asking whether a reliable differential diagnosis can be based on their occurrence (nos. 2 and 6) or predominance (nos. 1 and 3) in spontaneous speech.

Characteristic 1 'Sporadic disruption in the ability to match semantic features with sound strings comprising actual lexical items' According to the speech samples given by Chaika, this somewhat awkward formulation of her checklist could be interpreted as 'occasional use of phonemic neologism and semantic paraphasia'. Lecours and Vanier-Clément (1976) are basically correct in putting forward the claim that this 'sporadic disruption' may be encountered more frequently in jargonaphasia than in schizophasia. Nevertheless, the evidence of the cases described above compels us to correct this statement in so far as it is not the sporadic but the *permanent* use of phonemic and/or semantic jargon which distinguishes jargonaphasia from schizophasia.

Characteristic 2 'Preoccupation with too many of the semantic features of a word' A simpler translation of this formulation could run as follows. As schizophrenic speakers do not subordinate their utterances to the requirements of discourse (see characteristic 5), they may be distracted by semantic features which, with regard to the respective topic, are secondary or even irrelevant (see characteristic 4). Although this behaviour is not obvious in our patient, it seems to be manifest in certain forms of schizophasia. But it is absolutely incompatible with the verbal behaviour of jargonaphasics who have lost control over the selection of semantic features. Lecours is therefore correct in concluding that the presence of this characteristic is a strong clue to the incidence of schizophasia.

Characteristic 3 'Inappropriate noting of phonological features of words' As can be judged by Chaika's speech samples, this characteristic refers to the influence of preceding context on the phonetic form of utterances (see characteristic 4).

According to Lecours, this clang-associating behaviour is more typical of schizophrenics than of jargonaphasics. Unfortunately, the cases we have described above do not fit into this diagnostic picture; the phonetic influence of the preceding context was less pronounced in the schizophrenic than in the aphasic patient (see his minimal phonetic variations of the words *machen* or *einer*). If we think of the phonemic (neologistic) jargon of the cases described in Peuser 1978 and Peuser and Temp 1981, whose productions were strongly influenced by the natural laws of repetition, alliteration and rhyming, we have to contradict Lecours and Vanier-Clément: clang-associating behaviour is much more characteristic of jargonaphasia than of schizophasia.

Characteristic 6 'Failure to self-monitor, e.g. not noting errors when they occur' This characteristic has been thoroughly discussed earlier in this chapter. With regard to our cases, we had to conclude that the schizophasic speaker was more or less consciously and intentionally producing deviant utterances (although, of course, misjudging their effect on the interlocutor). The jargonaphasic, on the other hand, was basically convinced that his speech was not adequate. His deviant production must therefore be explained by reduced self-monitoring in the moment of speaking to an apparently understanding interlocutor. That is to say, both speakers are aware in principle of their deviant speech, an awareness which may be reduced in the moment of speaking. But that, as Alajouanine *et al.* (1952) correctly point out, happens to normal speakers, too. Characteristic 6 is therefore of little use for the differential diagnosis in question.

Looking back at this evaluation of Lecours and Vanier-Clément's use of Chaika's checklist, we have to conclude that (with regard to our definition of jargonaphasia) the only hard fact which can be relied upon to differentiate jargonaphasia from schizophasia 'on the sole basis of spontaneous speech' is the evidence of predominantly and fluently spoken neologistic jargon. But why base patholinguistic diagnosis on the sole evidence of spontaneous speech? Spontaneous speech is of course a very important parameter, giving the experienced examiner decisive clues, but in concentrating his diagnostic efforts exclusively on expressive behaviour, the patholinguist would deprive himself of diagnostic parameters which have become important, among other things, for the diagnosis and classification of the aphasias.

This chapter proposes, therefore, a checklist (see Table 9.2) comprising all parameters and characteristics which are useful for a differential

TABLE 9.2 *Criteria for a differential diagnosis of jargonaphasia and schizophasia.*

Differential criteria	Jargonaphasia	Schizophasia
Focal brain damage	x	
Psychotic disorder (hallucinations, etc.)		x
Disturbed comprehension of		
everyday speech	x	
test sentences (DFT)	x	
Word-finding disorder	x	
Phonemic neologisms	x	
Semantic neologisms		x
Dysgrammatism due to defective		
linguistic competence	x	
psycholinguistic competence		x
Switching from normal to deviant speech (and vice versa)		x
Communicative function of deviant speech:		
phatic	x	
persuasive		x
informative		x

diagnosis of jargonaphasia and schizophasia. In contrast to Lecours and Vanier-Clément (see Table 9.1), all those characteristics which are shared by both speakers are omitted.

As the checklist of Table 9.2 is exclusively based on the evidence of the cases discussed in this chapter, it remains to be enlarged by the evidence of further case descriptions. But we are confident that, even in this form, it will be helpful to distinguish two forms of deviant speech which are all the more difficult to judge as they are extremely rare.

References

Alajouanine, T., Lhermitte, F., Ledoux, M., Renaud, D. and Vignolo, L. A. 1964: Les composantes phonémiques et sémantiques de la jargonaphasie. *Revue Neurologique* 110.

Alajouanine, T., Sabouraud, O. and Ribaucourt, B. de, 1952: Le jargon des aphasiques. Désintegration anosognosique des valeurs sémantique du language. *Journal of Psychologique* 45.

Arieti, S. 1974: *Interpretation of Schizophrenia*. Second Edition, New York: Basic Books.

Autobiography of a schizophrenic girl (1970). New York: New York Times Co.

Bleuler, E. 1911: *Dementia Praecox or the Group of Schizophrenias*. New York: International Universities Press (reprinted 1966).

Boller, F., Vrtunski, P. B., Kim, Y. and Mack, J. L. 1978: Delayed auditory feedback and aphasia. *Cortex* 14.

Brown, J. W. 1972: Aphasia, apraxia and agnosia. Springfield, I11.: Charles C. Thomas.

Buckingham, H. W. 1977: The conduction theory and neologistic jargon. *Language and Speech* 20.

Buckingham, H. W. and Kertesz, A. 1976: *Neologistic Jargon Aphasia*. Amsterdam: Swets and Zeitlinger.

Buckingham, H. W., Whitaker, H. and Whitaker, H. A. 1978: Alliteration and assonance in neologistic jargon aphasia. *Cortex* 14.

Butterworth, B. 1979: Hesitation and the production of verbal paraphasias and neologisms in jargon aphasia. *Brain and Language* 8.

Chaika, E. O. 1974: A linguist looks at 'schizophrenic' language. *Brain and Language* 1.

— 1982: A unified explanation for the diverse structural deviations reported for adult schizophrenics with disrupted speech. *J. Communication Disorders* 15.

Chapman, J. 1966: The early symptoms of schizophrenia. *British J. Psychiatry* 112.

Cromwell, R. L. and Dokeki, P. R. 1968: Schizophrenic language: a disattention interpretation. In S. Rosenberg and J. H. Koplin, (eds), *Developments in Applied Psycholinguistics*. New York: Macmillan.

Duchan, J., Stengel, M. L. and Oliva, J. 1980: A dynamic phonological model derived from the intonational analysis of a jargon aphasic patient. *Brain and Language* 9.

Flournoy, T. 1900: *Des Indes à la planète Mars: étude sur un cas de somnambulisme avec glossolalie*. Third edition, Paris: Alcan. Translated into English as *From India to the Planet Mars: a study of a case of somnambulism, with glossolalia*. New York and London: Harper, 1900.

Fromkin, V. 1975: A linguistic looks at 'A linguist looks at "schizophrenic" language'. *Brain and Language* 2.

Goldstein, K. 1939: *The Organism*. New York: American Book.

— 1943: The significance of psychological research in schizophrenia. *J. Nervous and Mental Disease* 97.

— 1948: *Language and Language Disturbances: Aphasic Symptom Complexes and Their Significance for Medicine and Theory of Language*. New York: Grune & Stratton.

Green, E. 1969: Phonological and grammatical aspects of jargon in an aphasic patient. *Language and Speech* 12.

Käsermann, M. -L 1983: Form und Funktion schizophrener Sprachstörungen. *Sprache und Kognition* 3.

Kainz, F. 1969: *Psychologie der Sprache* Vol. 2: *Vergleichend-genetische Sprachpsychologie*. Third edition, Stuttgart: Enke.

Kertesz, A. and Benson, F. 1970: Neologistic jargon: A clinico-pathological study. *Cortex* 6.

Kinsbourne, M. and Warrington, E. K. 1963: Jargon aphasia. *Neuropsychologia* 1.

Kraepelin, E. 1896: *Psychiatrie, Ein Lehrbuch für Studierende und Ärzte*. Fifth edition, Leipzig: Barth.

Lecours, A. R. and Lhermitte, F. 1969: Phonemic paraphasias: linguistic structures and tentative hypotheses. *Cortex* 5.

Lecours, A. R. and Vanier-Clément, M. 1976: Schizophasia and jargonaphasia: a comparative description with comments on Chaika's and Fromkin's respective looks at 'schizophrenic' language. *Brain and Language* 3.

Leischner, A. 1974: Die neuropsychologisch-hirnpathologische Untersuchung. *Archiv für Psychiatrie und Nervenkrankheiten* 219.

— 1979: *Aphasien und Sprachentwicklungsstörungen*. Stuttgart: Thieme.

McKay, D. G. 1970: Phoneme repetition in the structure of languages. *Language and Speech* 13.

Monakow, C. von and Mourgue, R. 1928: *Introduction biologique à l'étude de la neurologie et de la psychopathologie*. Paris: Alcan.

Navratil, L. 1966: *Schizophrenie und Sprache*. Munich Deutsche Taschenbücher Verlag.

Ohala, J. and Hirano, M. 1967: Control mechanisms for the sequencing of neuromuscular events in speech. *Reprints from the Conference on Speech Communication and Processing*, Massachusetts Institute of Technology.

Peters, U. J. and Prelle, J. A. 1974: Schizophasie: Verschleierung einer Sprachstörung durch Sprache? *Archiv für Psychiatrie und Nervenkrankheiten* 219.

Peuser, G. 1976: Der Drei-Figuren-Test: Ein neues Verfahren zur qualitativen und quantitativen Bestimmung von Sprachverständnisstörungen. In G. Peuser (ed.), *Interdisziplinäre Aspekte der Aphasieforschung*. Cologne: Rheinland-Verlag.

— 1978: *Aphasie. Eine Einführung in die Patholinguistik*. Munich: Fink.

— 1984: *Language rehabilitation after stroke — a linguistic model*. New York: World Rehabilitation Fund.

Peuser, G. and Schriefers, H. 1980: Sentence comprehension in aphasics: results of administration of the 'Three-Figures Test' (DFT). *British J. Disorders of Communiction* 15.

Peuser, G. and Temp, K. 1981: The evolution of jargonaphasia. In J. W. Brown, (ed.), *Jargonaphasia*. New York: Academic Press.

Pick, A. 1931: Aphasie. In A. Bethe and G. V. Bergmann (eds), *Handbuch der normalen und pathologischen Physiologie*. Berlin: Springer.

Rensch, K. 1971: Linguistische Aspekte der Glossolalie. *Phonetica* 23.

Stachowiak, F. J., Huber, W., Poeck, K. and Kerschensteiner, M. 1977: Text comprehension in aphasia. *Brain and Language* 4.

Stampe, D. 1969: The acquisition of phonetic representation. In *Papers from the 5th Regional Meeting of the Chicago Linguistic Society*. Chicago: Department of Linguistics, University of Chicago.

Tuczek, K. 1921: Analyse einer Katatonikersprache. *Zeitschrift für die gesamte Neurologie und Psychiatrie* 72.

Wernicke, C. 1874: Der aphasische Symptomenkomplex. Breslau: Cohn u. Weigert (reprinted 1974, Stuttgart: Thieme).

Zipf, G. K. 1949: *Human behavior and the principle of least effort*. Cambridge, Mass.: Addison-Wesley.

Appendix

Text 1 Description of Binet picture 1 given by the schizophrenic (Mr E): original German text

I: Ich leg Ihnen jetzt Bilder vor und / äh / das sind die so-genannten Binet-Bilder die so ganz bestimmte Situationen darstellen / schauen Sie sich erst die einen Moment an und dann schildern Sie mir mal was auf dem Bild vor sich geht /

P: Dieses Bild zeigt zum Beispiel das Blindekuhspiel an / ne?

I: Ja / und was passiert da noch?

P: Die Hastigkeit dieser weggezogenen Tischdecke und dem umgekippten Blechradwagen möcht ich bald meinen / da den Sitzstuhl mit / dieser Holdrigkeit eben zu grob und ernsthaft nich? anziehen läßt / mehr nicht /

I: Hm / der Mann / vielleicht der Vater hat / eine Binde um die Augen / möchte das Mädchen greifen / zieht aber aus Versehen an der Tischdecke /

P: Ja /

I: Und was passiert dann?

P: Ja die Vase geht wohl entzwei / die Blumen / stehen ohne Wasser / und / äh / der Hocker liegt durch die geblühte Sperre des der Tochter oder des des jungen Mädchens nich? welches dort Halt suchte ne? und ihnen den Weg versperrt / die / (xxx) Zuversicht Halt ne ? / das ist so genannt worden von einem / zuerst //

Text 2 Description of Binet picture 1 given by the jargonaphasic (Mr W): original German text

I: Nun geben Sie acht / jetzt gebe ich Ihnen drei Bilder / und können Sie mir beschreiben / was Sie / äh / was Sie da sehen / einfach . . .

P: Ja / sie machen der ['aisəntər] / mit dem ['ainənɔs] / nicht? / [gə'vaigəs] / und die ['maxənt] / die [maxəns] / die mache *das* / oder nicht / und / die ['koytən dans] / die machen das / die eines / die macht das (xxx)
I: Ja / ist das eine Hochzeit? /
P: (*lachend*) Neinein / neineinein /
I: Oder eine Prügelei?
P: Ja / nein / hier / der macht's / nun der ['aikəns] die machen in die ['aikəns 'vaxtər]
I: Oder ist es ein Spiel?
P: Ja / sowas auch /
I: Was denn? Fußball?
P: Hier / nee / das die es /
I: Tennis?
P: Der eine macht das /
I: Die eins?
P: Die eines machen das / nicht?
I: Oder ist es Karten?
P: Neenee / hier das hier /
I: Blindekuh? Ist es Blindekuh?
P: Nein / [di:t'frdəl laxen] das hier muß es auch sein / muß das da / oder muß es / und der *muß* das auch / und der *kann* das aber auch //

10 Towards an interpersonal theory of schizophrenia

Brigitte De Decker and Pete Van de Craen

Introduction

One of the most important evolutions in recent years in the field of linguistics has been the growing interest in what could generally be called communication phenomena. This is certainly due to the development of new research areas, but also to the growing importance linguists attach to extralinguistic factors involving the use and development of language in general. These factors, such as cognitive growth, the role of interpersonal interaction and various other social (i.e. strictly nonmentalistic) factors, have created new fields of interest for linguists.

It is no surprise, then, to learn that the Second Mons Conference on Language and Language Acquisition put forward the notion of 'contextual linguistics', which aims for the simultaneous study of language and context (see Löwenthal *et al.* 1982). Prior to this, Hymes (1973) pleaded for a 'socially constituted' linguistics, Yngve (1975) mentioned 'human linguistics' as a new field of research, and Vanek (1979) suggested a holistic approach, while one of the authors of this chapter favours a 'social linguistics' (see Van de Craen 1982). The latter approach pursues a research view which looks at communication as a means of building up linguistic knowledge. Furthermore, the idea is fostered that the experience of communication itself shapes (inter)personal behaviour and thus affects personality. In other words, there can be no competence without the dynamic experience of communicative performance. In addition to this, it is recognized that interpersonal communication is dominated by social values which can only be studied by taking into account both the content and the meaning of the interaction processes. Epistemologically, it is presumed that the meaning of the communicative act in an interaction process can be studied by means of a hermeneutic methodology based on the personal history and experience of the participants. In this way, (verbal) communication may be regarded as the actualization of internalized interpersonal behaviour, which in itself is a product of previously experienced interaction.

At the University of Brussels (Vrije Universiteit Brussel), at least three fields of research are being explored by means of this theoretical approach. These areas include urban multilingualism, language and education, and the language use of schizophrenics. The present chapter pertains only to the latter. In the first section of this chapter the Gricean maxims with reference to conversations with schizophrenic people will be discussed; in the second part, attention is focused on aspects of lateralization; while in the third an attempt is made to relate communicative behaviour and lateralization processes using Sullivan's concept of anxiety. It is argued that this approach may lead to new views on the origin of the schizophrenic syndrome.

Communicative behaviour of schizophrenic people

Abnormalities of behaviour are often described and interpreted in terms of disturbances of communication. Rationality of communication could indeed be a clue to the success of workable interaction, i.e. the success of getting meaning across. Meanings are developed from sorting out experiences, and through communication with others. Successful communication with the self and with others implies a continuous process of correction by others as well as self-correction. In this way information about the self, the world, and the relationship of the self to the world is constantly updated, and leads to the acquisition of what could be called 'appropriate' interaction patterns. Acquisition of these techniques increases the individual's chances of mastering life. Successful communication, therefore, becomes synonymous with adaptation and adjustment to life itself. Whenever an individual is confronted with a conflict situation, this will be reflected in the individual's behaviour, including his verbal communicative behaviour.

Before going into the distorted language use of schizophrenics, we will look at the general conditions applying to logic in conversation in terms of the theoretical framework developed by Grice (1975). Grice argues that at each stage of a conversation, certain possible conversational moves can be excluded as being conversationally unsuitable. He formulates a general principle which participants are expected to observe: the 'Cooperative principle'. In this chapter we assume this co-operative principle. We claim that the lack of co-operation in schizophrenic discourse distorts the communication and consequently hinders the therapeutic process. If we attempt to analyse the events taking place in the interaction between patient and therapist, and the efforts directed at influencing the patient by means of psychotherapy, we arrive at the conclusion that the problems fall into the realm of communication as a co-operative activity. Small wonder most people, and even therapists, find it hard to 'co-operate' with schizophrenic patients. Let us now consider transaction 1.*

Transaction 1 T = therapist
P1 = patient, female fifty years of age

T: and how long have you been working there?
P1: but it's just a bottom sleepin' here I'm going to cover it, you can see mate, I say it's just a bottom sleepin' here nobody anymore isn't it lady you can see that nobody sleeps here anymore . . .
T: tell me, J, how long have you been working there?
P1: I'm not J, anymore, mate, it's just a bottom that's lyin' here
T: but how long have you been working for these people?
P1: I don't know maybe a year or . . . maybe nine years

Grice's principle of co-operation can be summarized as follows: 'Make your conversational contribution as is required, at the stage at which it occurs, by the accepted purpose or direction of the talk exchange in which you are engaged' (Grice 1975). It is argued that in transaction 1, the patient violates the co-operative principle, i.e. she refuses to accept the direction given by the therapist, namely to talk about her work. By repeating his question three times, the therapist forces a certain co-operation upon the patient so that she can hardly deny it, even though she shows a certain unwillingness to follow the therapist's directions. The schizophrenic person hereby indicates that she is too busy with her own thoughts. The patient's non-cooperative attitude is characteristic of her noncommittal behaviour. The evasive answers form an avoidance strategy used to escape certain threatening and compulsive situations, in this case the conversation with the therapist — who nevertheless aims at eliciting a meaningful reaction from his schizophrenic interlocutor, since his only possibility of helping the patient to maintain an ordinary relationship lies in breaking through her stereotyped behaviour and idiosyncratic, self-centred utterances, possibly by confronting her with events, objects and persons in her environment. Without co-operation from the patient herself, the therapist finds himself confronted with an almost impossible task. However, schizophrenic persons do not always 'opt out of the

* The original Dutch material has been translated by the authors.

conversation' and out of the co-operation principle as drastically as in this case.

A number of extracts from conversations with schizophrenic speakers will be examined, illustrating a violation of what Grice calls the maxims of conversation. Grice distinguishes four categories, each maintaining more specific maxims and submaxims. They are called Quantity, Quality, Relation and Manner. The maxim of quantity relates to the quantity of information that is provided, and includes the following submaxims:

- Make your contribution as informative as is required
- Do not make your contribution more informative than is required

Let us consider the following transactions with schizophrenic speakers in which the maxim of quantity is not properly applied in the Gricean sense.

Transaction 2 P2 = patient, female thirty years of age

P2: my mummy is very upset, yes (*laughs*)
T: nothing to laugh about
P2: no
yes, it's sad (*laughs*), it's sad the owl said, and he looked at his young and it was an owl itself
T: I didn't get that
P2: (*repeats the expression*) don't you understand? I don't either anymore and I won't say it again, you know, I'm going to eat my apple to store vitamins for telling stories, otherwise I'll crumble to pieces

Transaction 3 P3 = patient, male thirty-six years of age

T: You haven't been taken into hospital just for no reason have you?
P3: I don't know
T: what went wrong then?
P3: I don't know (*irritated*), I was discharged no longer than one hour eh, this guy comes up to me and says it, yes, he says, you have hypnotized the doctor, I say, yes, I can't do that, you know (*laughs*), then he says I hypnotized the doctor, where he got that I don't know, you know

Transaction 4

T: what I don't understand in your story, is your relationship towards this second Christ?
P3: well I had to submit myself, I was the elder, just like Christ who was born from the family of David, something like that I suppose

Transaction 5

P1: that I'm nobody anymore
T: how long have you been here now?

P1: I'm not here yet, mate
I'm not here
I'm just a bottom that's lyin' here
you can see that I'm not here
T: an' where are you now?
where are you now, just tell me
P1: I don't know anymore, it's just a bottom
that's lyin' here lady
you can see nobody anymore, no J to be seen,
just a bottom

In transactions 2, 3 and 4, the schizophrenic speaker's conversational contributions lack sufficient information to be comprehensible to the therapist. In transaction 5, the over-informativeness and redundancy of information is confusing in that it is liable to result in an apparently autistic monologue primarily governed by one stock phrase: *I'm not here yet, it's just a bottom that's lying here*. In transactions 2, 3 and 4, the patients attempt to answer the therapist's questions, but in a way they fail to do so, since the information given is somewhat confusing and certainly not as informative as is required for the purpose of the exchange. In transaction 5, the patient's ontological insecurity becomes the touchstone for all her linguistic performances. The patient remains conceptually and ideationally disconnected. In this conversation we are confronted with a transformation of anxiety into communicative strategies, namely a withdrawal from the interaction participant, in this case the therapist. All interaction processes must be interpreted in what we might call a context of security. The patient's idea that she is not really there, that she is just a bottom lying there, represents a protective device against the experience of anxiety, failure . . . Instead of saying I'm insecure, I'm anxious, I'm in pain, the patient claims that she does not exist and that all of her actions are insubstantial. If in 'normal' conversation an interlocutor were to be confronted with this kind of over-informativeness and redundancy, he would look in vain for some particular point in this over-informativeness. However, in the case of schizophrenic conversation, the therapist may draw the conclusion that the constant repetition of similar information is certainly not a side-issue of the conversation — as is often the case in normal speech — but in fact is used as a communicative device to protect the patient against painful interactions and to moderate the strong negative feelings towards the self.

If we turn to the following maxims of conversation we find that, especially in schizophrenic conversation, the submaxims of the four Gricean maxims overlap, in that, for example, a schizophrenic speaker who in an interaction violates the maxim of quantity, i.e. to be informative, also fails to obey the maxim of manner, i.e. to be perspicuous.

The second maxim, that of quality, has one supermaxim: 'Try to make your contribution one that is true' and two submaxims:

- Do not say what you believe to be false
- Do not say that for which you lack evidence

This category is a very hazardous one, especially in the case of schizophrenic discourse. The schizophrenic speaker seems to deny the fact that human relations are multipolar phenomena. He assigns himself to a role, and takes the liberty of ignoring the strong determination of roles by a mutual relationship. This distortion seems to make a schizophrenic person unaware of his impact upon others, although he maximizes the coercive aspects of the messages of others upon him. The state of anxiety prevents the schizophrenic person, first, from receiving messages correctly and, second, from interpreting information which he already possesses. Consequently, the schizophrenic builds up a distorted model of himself and of the world. It is then extremely difficult for the nonschizophrenic interlocutor to decide what is 'true' and what is 'false' in the schizophrenic's world. As Maher claims: 'if the patient tells us that he is the brightest man in the hospital . . . smarter than the superintendent, we might not be so inclined to query the processes by which he came to this conclusion', whereas 'a patient who believes that his children are plotting to kill him for his money may well be disbelieved because his inference seems to be unlikely to the clinician' (Maher 1966: 7). Transactions 6 and 7 are examples of the constant doubt of the schizophrenic speaker as to the validity of his statements, and of his unwillingness to relate something which he is not convinced is true.

Transaction 6

T: (*after the refusal of the patient to finish his story*) so you're making us curious
P3: yes, could be
T: would you like us to ask: 'what is it?'
P3: no (*silence*) it isn't meant that way
T: and yet, you have difficulties talking about it?
P3: yes, I don't know if it's correct, you know

Transaction 7

P3: yes, I don't know if it's right, you know and moreover, I've said it before, you know, if it's God the Father, you know, I'd rather sit with the devil (*laughs*)

In these transactions the speaker displays a certain avoidance strategy. Under the pretext of ignorance, he avoids talking about his actual problems. Evidence of this is also found in the numerous 'conversation-stoppers' such as: *if it's God the Father you know, I'd rather sit with the devil.* On the whole, Grice's maxim of quality and his demand for truth and honesty in a conversation cannot easily be transferred to schizophrenic conversation. Notions such as truth and falseness are not easily applicable to this kind of communication, in that schizophrenic speakers do not necessarily hold the same values and the same frame of reference as 'normal' speakers do. For, as argued by Ruesch and Bateson: 'such a statement as "The word cat stands for a certain small mammal" is not either true or false. Its truth depends upon agreement between the speakers that it be true. In terms of such agreement they understand each other; or where disagreement occurs they will meet with misunderstanding' (Ruesch and Bateson 1951: 212). So, when a patient says *I'm not here, it's just a bottom lying here*, it is obvious that such a remark must be interpreted on a different level of communication. It is quite irrelevant to decide whether the utterance is true or false. What is important is to know why the patient is so persistent in using this expression throughout the conversation. Perhaps she wants to make the interlocutor aware of her problems, which she cannot formulate in a different way. If so, we are confronted with the tragedy of a schizophrenic speaker: by clinging to metaphores and symbolic manifestations, the schizophrenic speaker expresses a number of deeply rooted and symptomatic experiences in order to make performance possible. But at the same time, the metaphoric and symbolic language use exclude the patient's conflictive experiences from public communication and render them inaccessible to others.

The last two Gricean categories — Relation, which consists of one single maxim: 'be relevant', and Manner: 'be perspicuous' i.e. avoid obscurity, ambiguity — in a way overlap with a number of the maxims already discussed. Transaction 8, for instance, illustrates that metaphoric language use renders the schizophrenic communication obscure and difficult to interpret for the therapist:

Transaction 8

P2: Jesus doesn't like you to help me

T: no? how come?
P2: because he was too upset earlier when I . . .
when I became ill
it's terrible, you know, he always threatens me with death because he has forgotten . . .

In schizophrenic conversation it often happens that when a patient starts communicating with another patient or with his therapist, the mere act of communicating can carry the statement 'we are communicating'. In fact, this may be the most important message that is sent and received. The question of relevance of the messages is not always in order at this point of communicative behaviour. Haley, in *Strategies of Psychotherapy* (1963), illustrates this by giving an example of a verbal exchange between two schizophrenic speakers who seem to be ignoring each other's speech. Yet they are communicating. It seems that human beings 'make conversation' rather than accept the message which would be implicit in silence, namely, we are not communicating. This message would provoke anxiety, not in the least because it implies rejection.

In this section we have tried to indicate the logic of schizophrenic conversation. Ignoring the maxims of conversation is justified in the context of the schizophrenic person's fundamental problems. It is argued that the task of the interlocutor in the therapeutic interview is to accept the schizophrenic's symtoms in terms of their communicative function. It is chiefly Sullivan (1953) who has emphasized the interpersonal, communictive function of the 'schizophrenic symptom'. By finding out how and what the patient is trying to communicate, how he/she is behaving in interaction, we hope to gain a deeper insight into and a better understanding of the interactional dimensions and complex mechanisms which drive the schizophrenic individual towards isolation, self-estrangement and anxiety. We will now consider schizophrenics from an entirely different angle, emphasizing certain cognitive and physiological aspects of the syndrome.

Communicative behaviour and lateralization processes

Scholars like Mead, Dewey, Sapir and Sullivan in the United States, and Bühler and Piaget in Europe have formulated hypotheses which might appear similar to the basic thinking of what we have called social linguistics. In recent years evidence has become available that these hypotheses, which are social in nature, are backed up by biological and physiological findings. This development has opened up new ways of thinking, directed towards a possible fusion between social and biological phenomena previously thought to be unrelated. Studies of cerebral organization in connection with cognitive styles are chiefly responsible for this new development.

It is by now a well known fact that the functions of the right and left hemispheres are different and at the same time complementary. Most right-handed adults have a left hemisphere specialization for language, time-related functions and so-called propositional thought, while the right hemisphere specializes in spatial relations, Gestalt perception, and so-called appositional or compositional thought (see Hardyck 1976; TenHouten 1982). The way these hemispheric functions are separated or laterilized suggests a connection with cognitive styles. Compare, for instance, so-called 'field-dependent' persons with 'field-independent' persons, i.e. persons who take a social-intuitive approach to problems and those tending to display a much more intellectual and relational approach. Field-dependent persons do not seem to be left-laterilized but rather 'laterally differentiated', i.e. they 'tend to use the hemisphere most appropriate to the task at hand' (TenHouten 1982: 30). Of course, this raises the question as to where this difference originates.

One answer is that some cultures foster interaction styles favouring one or other particular occurrence of cognitive styles. In this connection TenHouten (1982) mentions the case of Mexican Americans who live in a 'dualistic culture' because their Mexican side requires a field-dependent mode while their American side requires a field-independent mode. Hence the idea of 'bicognitive thinking' which could contribute to a bicultural identity. The important deduction to be drawn from this is that hemispheric functioning and laterilization are influenced by the exposure to certain forms of interaction which are purely social in origin. Or, as TenHouten puts it: 'the structure of social dominance influences the development of thought and contributes to its structure' (TenHouten 1982: 50).

The macro-level functioning as described above has, of course, also got a micro-level counterpart influencing individual development. Reviewing the literature of language acquisition, Bates (1979) mentions no less than twenty-two groups and subgroups of intracultural differences in style involved in first language acquisition. Although not all of these styles have been proved to have a physiological correlate in the form of hemispheric functioning — mainly because they have not yet been studied in detail — it should be clear that modes of interaction and communication might be responsible for these differences.

Let us now turn to theories of communication in connection with schizophrenia. One of the most influential hypothesis regarding communication in general and the pathology of communication in particular is, of course, Bateson *et al.*'s (1956) idea of double-bind. Double-bind is first and foremost a communication syndrome involving conflicting messages due to a disregard for the unity of interaction, the latter term stating that communicative behaviour implies a unity between what people say, how they act and what they outwardly show. Furthermore, it is hypothesized that a state of schizophrenia may be induced by recurrent patterns of the double-bind syndrome.

Prior to Bateson's work, Sullivan had formulated his interpersonal theory of schizophrenia stressing the influence of interpersonal experience during the maturation process as well as the importance of environmental living conditions (Sullivan 1953). Living conditions may evolve in such a way that a state of anxiety appears, ultimately leading to schizophrenia. This actually means that communicative and/or emotional conflicts either during the first years of childhood or later in life, e.g. during the development of peer group relationships, may lead to a state where persons seem to break with the generally accepted way of acting as a social being.

One of the syndromes that is widely discussed in this respect is the notion of 'thought disorder', i.e. the use of speech described as ranging from circumstantial to complete incoherence (see Rochester and Martin 1979). Rochester and Martin found striking differences between patients diagnosed as thought-disordered and those diagnosed as not, especially in some formal aspects of language such as the use of structural elements and the presence of relatively high proportion of generic groups in interviews. These results are explained by relating them to hemispheric lateralization. Following Shimkunas (1978), Rochester and Martin suggest that schizophrenics diagnosed as thought-disordered have an overexcited left hemisphere functioning 'in parallel with a potentially highly arousable hemisphere' (Rochester and Martin 1979: 193). Thought-disordered schizophrenia is thus seen as an

> asymmetrical dysfunction in cortico-hemispheric integration. Over-excitation of the left hemisphere during the actute stage disrupts effective verbal-conceptual reasoning and focal attention information processing. Right hemisphere overexcitation during chronicity intensifies perceptual-emotional mediation, potentiating narrowed attention to subcortically stimulated imagery in the context of behavioural withdrawal. During acute stages of schizophrenic disorganization, left-hemisphere verbal-temporal information-processing strategies break down, seeking compensation in right-hemisphere perceptual-emotional mediation. The right hemisphere's orientation toward simultaneous processing potentiates increased attention to temporally immediate environmental cues. (Shimkunas 1978: 227–8)

Evidence for this hypothesis comes basically from research into split-brain patients as originated by Sperry and his colleagues (see Sperry 1968). By disconnecting the right hemisphere (commissurotomy) Sperry found that both hemispheres kept on functioning, albeit separately. Moreover, this state goes unnoticed by the patients. Earlier studies had already revealed differences in affective reaction in the two hemispheres following amytal injections (see Galin 1974 for a review). This points both to different hemispheric tasks and also to the fact that the dissociation of experience in normal people may induce a state of cerebral organization not unlike that seen in commissurotomy. By describing the potential results of a double-bind situation on both hemispheres, Galin (1974) has explicitly drawn attention to this. Suppose a mother says, 'I am doing it because I love you dear', but that her face shows, 'I hate you and will destroy you'. Since both hemispheres have different tasks, the left will take care of the verbal cues and the right of the nonverbal ones. However, 'the two hemispheres might decide on opposite courses of action: the left to approach and the right to flee . . . the left hemisphere seems to win control of the output channels most of the time, but if the left is not able to "turn off" the right completely, it may settle for disconnecting the transfer of the conflicting information from the other side' (Galin 1974: 576). But even if the right is cut off, it may continue to lead a life of its own and may ultimately interfere. Hence the hypothesis 'that in normal, intact people mental events in the right hemisphere can become disconnected functionally from the left hemisphere (by inhibition of neuronal transmission across the corpus callosum and other cerebral commissures) and can continue a life of their own' (Galin 1974: 574–5).

In addition to split-brain research, a growing number of experimental studies show a connection between schizophrenia and hemispheric dysfunctioning. On the whole, two kinds of evidence are produced. First, it seems that right-handed schizophrenics generally show a dysfunction of the left hemisphere and, second, some sort of interhemispheric disturbance takes place. The latter conclusion is corroborated by measurements of the corpus callosum showing 'a widening in the schizophrenic group of that portion of the corpus allosum lying between the genu and the splenium' (Schweitzer 1978: 983). Whereas in normal patients the dysfunctioning of one hemisphere is compensated by the other, schizophrenic people seem to lack this ability. This has prompted Gur to speak of the triple disability of schizophrenics regarding hemispheric organization, namely 'by having a dysfunctional left hemisphere, by failing to shift processing to the right, and by an overactivation of the dysfunctional hemisphere' (Gur 1979: 273).

Since we are mainly interested in communication and the use of language, we should also bear in mind the role of the right hemisphere in language processing. In the last decade the right hemisphere has been brought into prominence, and is no longer regarded as superfluous with regard to language production. Gardner has pointed out that people deprived of the use of the right hemisphere use a kind of mechanical language lacking 'the holistic integration of feelings, situational cues, and interpersonal relations' one would expect in normal conversations (Gardner 1974: 296). Deprivation of the use of the left hemisphere, on the other hand, leaving the right hemisphere in charge, leads in contrast to a kind of holistic language use, stock phrases and word pictures.

This reasoning leads to the deduction that so-called thought disorder and communicative syndromes are grounded on lateralization processes or, in other words, that certain conditions such as anxiety may influence a person's 'hemisphericity' (Smokler 1979) and hence his communicative and personality style. By the same token this hypothesis, which points at interpersonal factors causing at least some forms of schizophrenia, also shows the close interaction between social and biological factors. Consequently, this may open new ways of looking at language in general, and schizophrenia in particular.

Communicative behaviour, personality and schizophrenia

Let us start with a fairly typical case study.

J is an unmarried right-handed woman, born in 1933, the second of five children of a family with a history of epilepsy and alcoholism. Her two younger brothers and elder sister are married. After her father's death in 1967 she continued to live with her mother and elder sister, both epileptics, at her parents' farm. Her mother is described as a violent, aggressive woman, who treated her children very strictly. Ten years before she died completely senile in 1978, she started drinking. J now lives alone with her sister. J was made to start working at the farm at the age of fourteen. But at twenty-nine, while still living with her parents and in spite of their bitter disapproval, she started working at a factory. After some years of heavy working she was able to buy out her brothers and sisters so that she became the sole owner of the farm and the surrounding small piece of land. In 1963 she suffered a nervous breakdown and she is reported to have attempted suicide twice. After this first contact with psychiatric hospitals it took until May 1976 before she was again admitted to hospital. She was showing aggressive behaviour and incoherent speech a state apparently due to a conflict with neighbours about the sale of an adjacent piece of land. The ensuing problems caused her to be readmitted the following year. This time she was feeling depressed instead of aggressive, threatened to commit suicide and was again speaking incoherently. After her mother's death (February 1978), followed immediately by the death of her mother's sister, she collapsed again. She began to speak incoherently again, expressed her wish to die and actually staged a suicide attempt. Since then she has frequently been admitted to hospital and eventually she had to stay there permanently.

This very anxious woman feels that everything has been taken away from her and that 'they' are now trying to take away her properties, too. Her sister feels that J might as well come home 'to work' since improvement does not seem to occur. In 1982 extensive recordings of conversations with the therapist were made often in the presence of one of the authors. One typical interaction is the following.

T: J.
J: *I'm nobody any more*
T: How long have you been here?
J: *I'm not yet here*, mate, *I'm not here,*
it's just a bottom that's lyin' here
you can see I'm not here
T: where are you then?
tell me where you are
J: I don't know any more, *it's just a bottom that's lyin' here*, lady, you can see, *nobody any more nobody any more, no J any more, a bottom*
T: How's your sister?
J: I don't know, mate, I'm telling you, *only a bottom that's lyin' here, nobody any more, she is not here*
T: Where does your sister live, now?
J: (gives name of the street and number)
T: O yes: Does she live there by herself?
J: Yes
T: You used to live with her, didn't you?
J: Yeah, I used to live with her, yeah
but here nobody sleeps any more
T: You've been living together there, with your mother, too,
I thought, haven't you?
J: Yeah, with my mother, yeah, my mother I have . . . Mind you, she died
T: Yes
J: She died
T: Did you cry a lot?
J: Yes, I felt very badly
T: Yes
J: She was a good woman, *but nobody sleeps here, any more but a bottom*, don't you see that, lady, that *nobody sleeps here any more*?
T: Tell me, J, . . .

J: *I'm not J any more*, mate
T: When did you, . . .
When did the troubles start?
J: It's been lasting for years now
T: For years?
J: Yes, but *nobody sleeps here any more*,
you can see clearly enough that *a bottom sleeps here* . . .

In contrast to the impressive number of studies on lateralization and language in aphasic patients, we have no knowledge of studies looking into the relationship between hemispheric dysfunction and language and communication phenomena in schizophrenics. We even lack the beginnings of an answer to basic questions such as to what extent hemisphericity influences communicative behaviour and vice versa. Yet examining conversations with schizophrenic people shows similarities with aphasic speech that are often amazing.

Peuser (this volume) has compared jargonaphasia with schizophasic speech. However, in the conversation above, no use is made of word-salads or neologisms as in schizophasic speech. With reference to communicative effectiveness, it is still possible to describe this speech as neologistic because of the repetition of the phrases *I'm nobody any more, (it's) (only a bottom) that's lyin' here*, and *nobody sleeps here any more*. These phrases can be considered neologistic with respect to the Gricean maxims of conversations, as has been demonstrated in the first section of this chapter; but this constant repetition of stock phrases is also a reminder of some kind of receptive or jargonaphasia, although it is of course true that this speech is not entirely unintelligible or empty of meaning. Instead, one could say that the meaning lies in the special way the message is communicated: the denial of her own existence by means of the stock phrases is in fact an indication of her anxiety and her overall mental situation.

Let us relate this case to lateralization. If an emotional state such as anxiety is capable of influencing a person's hemisphericity, one would at least expect traces of this in speech and/or communicative behaviour. If the left hemisphere is overactivated, as is evidenced by a growing body of literature, one would expect impairments of so-called propositional thought, and thus an impairment of analytical abilities in favour of Gestalt utterances. It is difficult to say anything about J's thought here, but it is clear that she has trouble answering questions in a straightforward way. Of course, there is still the possibility that she *chooses* not to answer them, but is not one of the characteristics of schizophrenia the lack of choice in behaviour, thought and speech? This lack of choice may well be provoked by the state of overexcitation of the left hemisphere, resulting in a rather uncreative, 'automatic' speech, in this case full of stock phrases, with few initiatives, and rather empty from a communicative point of view.

What are the reasons for this dysfunction of the hemisphere, and why is it that not all schizophrenic people seem to suffer from it? Let us start answering the latter question. It seems from the literature on the subject that most, if not all, right-handed schizophrenics seem to suffer from some kind of impairment of the left hemisphere (see Walker and McGuire 1982 for a review) and also from compensatory mechanisms possibly affecting the right hemisphere (cf. Schweitzer 1982). As for the first question, which incidentally is not answered in the medical literature, we may again refer to Sullivan's anxiety concept. This states that personality will be greatly affected by any state of anxiety. But this state of anxiety not only influences outward behaviour, it also deeply affects organized structures in the brain such as cerebral hemispheric functioning. Two important inferences can be drawn from this line of thought. First, outward experience may influence inner structures in such a way as to cause severe impairments in their functioning and, secondly, internally organized structures are only stable with respect to a certain stage of equilibrium. If the state of equilibrium changes, the overall organization changes in a search for a new equilibrium.

Towards an interpersonal theory of schizophrenia

It now seems possible to bring together what were previously thought to be unrelated observations. On the one hand is Sullivan's predominantly social concept of anxiety and, on the other hand, recent observations with respect to hemisphericity. It is hypothesized that the internalization of interpersonal experiences in some people leads to a dramatic distortion of behavioural and physiological equilibrium. A certain kind of communicative behaviour is one indication of this. A number of theoretical advantages are linked with this approach.

First, this way of looking at schizophrenia presents an opportunity to bring together the medical and the social paradigms. If cerebral organization, or any other physical functioning for that matter, can be impaired by outward experiences resulting in a state of anxiety, it should not come as a surprise that pharmacological treatment can at least temporarily reduce the effect of certain dysfunctions. However, this treatment will not be sufficient for cure in the traditional sense of the word. Secondly, schizophrenia can no longer be regarded either as a disease or as something purely social. The existence of so-called hereditary schizophrenia can now be seen as also resulting from interpersonal interaction patterns, since anxiety patterns are much more likely to be produced in a schizoid environment than in a nonschizoid one. Thirdly, the interpersonal hypothesis as stated here is open to empirical testing. This is a great step forward with respect to both the pharmacological and the social approach, since neither approach was able to draw conclusive inferences as far as the nature of schizophrenia is concerned. The study of communicative behaviour coupled with handedness, aspects of memory, eye movements and lateralization should be able to shed new light on the schizophrenic syndrome. Fourthly, the interpersonal approach not only contributes to the study of schizophrenia but is also valuable for the development of the social sciences in general. In this way the interpersonal theory of schizophrenia is a contribution to the development of a dynamic interactive social theory.

References

Bates, E. 1979: *The Emergence of Symbols*. New York: Academic Press.

Bateson, G. 1973: *Steps to an Ecology of Mind*. London: Granada.

Bateson G., Jackson, D., Haley, J. and Weakland, J. 1956: Towards a theory of schizophrenia. Reprinted in Bateson 1973.

Cole, P. and Morgan, J. (eds.) 1975: *Syntax and Semantics*, Vol 3: *Speech Acts*. New York: Academic Press.

Galin, D. 1974: Implications for psychiatry of left and right cerebral specialization. *Arch. Gen. Psychiatry* 31.

Gardner, H. 1974: *The Shattered Mind*. New York: Vintage Books.

Grice, H. 1975: Logic and conversation. In P. Cole and J. Morgan (eds), *Syntax and Semantics*, Vol 3.

Grossman, R., San, R. and Vance, T. (eds.) 1975: *Papers on the Parasession on Functionalism*. Chicago: Chicago Linguistic Society.

Gur, R. 1979: Cognitive concomitants of hemispheric dysfunction in schizophrenia. *Arch. Gen. Pscyhiatry* 36.

Haley, J. 1963: *Strategies of Psychotherapy*. New York: Grune & Stratton.

Hardyck, C. 1976: A model of individual differences in hemispheric functioning. In H. Whitaker and H. Whitaker (eds), *Studies in Neurolinguistics*, Vol. 3.

Hymes, D. 1973: The scope of sociolinguistics. In R. Shuy (ed.), *Sociolinguistics: Current Trends and Prospects*.

Löwenthal, F., Vandamme, F. and Cordier, J. (eds.) 1982: *Language and Language Acquisition*. New York: Plenum.

Maher, B. 1966: *Principles of Psychopathology: An Experimental Approach*. New York: McGraw-Hill.

Rochester, S. and Martin, J. 1979: *Crazy Talk*. New York: Plenum.

Ruesch, J. and Bateson, G. 1951: *Communication: The Social Matrix of Psychiatry*. New York: Norton.
St Clair, R. and Von Raffler-Engel, W. (eds.) 1982: *Language and Cognitive Styles*. Lisse: Swets & Zeitlinger.
Schwartz, S. (ed.) 1978: *Language and Cognition in Schizophrenia*. Hillsdale, NJ: Erlbaum.
Schweitzer, L. 1978: Abnormalities of cerebral lateralization in Schizophrenia patients. *Arch. Gen. Psychiatry* 35.
— 1982: Evidence of right cerebral hemisphere dysfunction in schizophrenic patients with left hemisphere overactivation. *Biological Psychiatry* 17 (6).
Shimkunas, A. 1978: Hemispheric asymmetry and schizophrenic thought disorder. In S. Schwartz (ed.), *Language and Cognition in Schizophrenia*.
Shuy, R. (ed.) 1973: *Sociolinguistics: Current Trends and Prospects*. Washington, DC: Georgetown University Press.
Smokler, I. 1979: Cerebral lateralization and personality style. *Arch. Gen. Psychiatry* 36.
Sperry, R. 1968: Hemisphere deconnection and unity in conscious awareness. *American Psychologist* 23.
Sullivan, H. 1953: *The Interpersonal Theory of Psychiatry*. New York: Norton.
TenHouten, W. 1982: Social correlates of cerebral lateralization: a neurosociological approach. In R. St Clair and W. Von Raffler-Engel (eds), *Language and Cognitive Styles*.
Yngve, V. 1975: Toward a human linguistics. In R. Grossman *et al*. (eds), *Papers on the Parasession on Functionalism*.
Van de Craen, P. 1982: Social linguistics: an outline for interactional linguistics on hermeneutic foundations. Dissertation, Vrije Universiteit Brussel (written in Dutch).
Vanek, A. 1979: The holistic theory of human communication. *Papers in Linguistics* 12 (3/4).
Walker, E. and McGuire, M. 1982: Intra- and interhemispheric information processing in schizophrenia. *Psychological Bulletin* 92 (3).
Whitaker, H. and Whitaker H. (eds.) 1976: *Studies in Neurolinguistics*. 3 Vols. New York: Academic Press.

11 Some effects of supportive psychotherapy on texts written by schizophrenics

Klaus Schonauer and Gerd Buchkremer

Schizophrenia and cohesion as constructs

Experimental research work on schizophrenia is the attempt to explain a construct by means of additional constructs. In order to focus our attention on this epistemological starting point we would like to quote a popular German reference book of psychology:

> [A construct is a] designation for hypothetical categories for comprehensive descriptions or explanations of behavior in relation to a *specific frame of concepts* (model). Constructs refer mainly to those *hypothetical states or processes* which cannot be *developed* directly, but only *by* supposed causes or effects, or only by *broad classes of indicators*. (Translated from Drever and Fröhlich 1971: 163; our italics.)

This definition could be applied to the concept of schizophrenia and most of the medical, psychological and linguistic concepts which have been used to treat, to observe or to interpret psychotic language behaviour. It also fits 'cohesion'. 'Cohesion' is a concept developed by Michael Halliday and Ruqaiya Hasan, and described in detail in *Cohesion in English* (1976). Like many constructs concerning psychotic behaviour (e.g. 'filter deficit', 'response interference'), the term itself has been adopted from physics. The specific 'frame of concepts' to which cohesion refers is modern text linguistics. As a construct it was designed to answer the question, 'What makes a text a text?'

In the introductory chapter of *Cohesion in English*, Halliday and Hasan offer the following definition:

> Cohesion occurs, where the interpretation of some element in the discourse is dependent on that of another. The one presupposes the other in the sense that it can not be effectively decoded except by recourse to it. (Halliday and Hasan 1976:4)

Following a stratificational theory of language, they call cohesion a 'relational' concept which is based on semantic and lexicogrammatical ties between one cohesive element and another — usually preceding — element in the discourse, to which we shall hence refer to metaphorically as the 'anchor element'. Cohesion involves both 'meaning' and 'wording'.

In developing the concept of 'cohesion', Halliday and Hasan rely mainly on offering very instructive examples. In terms of the definition of constructs quoted above, this means that they set up 'broad classes of indicators'. They dêtermine five main categories and nineteen subcategories of cohesion.

In Table 11.1 we have listed one subcategorical example for cohesive ties between independent clauses for each of the main categories. All examples are constructed ones, and as they are meant to give a survey they are quite simple. In the first example the cohesive element is a pronoun which refers to a nominal group in clause A as anchor element. In the second example the cohesive element replaces the anchor element, a noun, which occurs in clause A. In the next example a gap has to be filled with the complete verbal phrase stemming from clause A. In the fourth example a conjunction implicates an adversative relation between the two clauses. In the last example the cohesive element and the anchor element are lexically related, because one element can be seen as superordinate to the other.

Applications of the cohesion concept

Waldemar Gutwinski (1976), another student of the cohesion concept, claims that cohesion is much more exact and clearcut than the related concept of coherence as it is used in rhetoric and composition theory and — we should add — in psychopathology: Since the work of Eugen Bleuler the construct of schizophrenia has been disjunctively affiliated to the concept of coherence. 'Looseness of associations' and 'circumstantiality' were among the basic classes of indicators which Bleuler used to develop the construct of schizophrenia. One or two years before the publication of Halliday and Hasan 1976, Jim Martin, a linguist, and Sherry Rochester, a psychologist, became interested in the concept of

TABLE 11.1 *The five main categories of cohesion, with constructed examples for some of their subcategories.*

Category	Subcategory	Clause A	Clause B
	(other possible subcategories)	preceding referent, 'anchor element'[a] italicized	items referred to, cohesive element italicized
1. Reference	1.1 *Pronominal* (Demonstrative Comparative)	'What's new about *uncle Herbert*?'	'*He*'s going to be 69 next week.'
2. Substitution	2.1 *Nominal* (Verbal Clausal)	'Herb, which *robe* can I wear at the concert hall tonight?'	'Well, the little pink *one* might suit Debussy.'
3. Ellipsis	3.3[b] *Clausal* (Nominal Verbal)	'*Has* Gertrude ever *been to Acapulco*?'	'No, but some of Herb's colleagues have ——.'
4. Conjunction	4.2. *Adversative* (Additive Causal Temporal Continuative)	*Herbert dreams about flying to Acapulco with Gertrude.*	*But* she constantly refuses to climb an aeroplane.
5. Lexis	5.3 *Superordinate* (Same item Hypo/synonym General item Collocation	'Isn't it Gertrude's *birthday* today?'	'Well, she says it's only her diamond *jubilee* as a nonsmoker.'

[a] The expression 'anchor element' is not used by Halliday and Hasan.
[b] Classification numbers of the subcategories chosen as an example follow the original coding scheme from Halliday and Hasan (1976: 333–8).

cohesion through personal contact with Gutwinski. They applied the concept of cohesion to experimental research on schizophrenic discourse. Rochester and Martin (Rochester *et al.* 1977; Rochester and Martin 1979) examined the amount of cohesive ties and the distribution of their main categories in texts that had been produced in standardized contexts by so-called 'normal' speakers and by speakers which had been diagnosed as schizophrenic. To specify the notion of cohesion in schizophrenic discourse, they introduced a new construct: thought disorder. Those speakers who exhibited at least some of the indicators of this construct — measured by Robert Cancro's (1969) 'index of formal signs of thought disorder' — were examined in a separate subject group. Some of Rochester and Martin's central results were the following:

1 In all subject groups, the amount and the distribution of cohesion changed considerably with different contexts (interview texts and spontaneous reproductions of a short story).
2 All subjects used cohesive ties when producing spontaneous texts. Differences between subject groups were considerably smaller than differences between contexts.
3 Analysis of the amount and distribution of cohesive ties can be performed with interrater reliability scores of between 87 and 100 per cent.
4 Both 'thought-disordered' (TD) and 'non-thought-disordered' (NTD) schizophrenic subjects constructed significantly fewer cohesive ties between the independent clauses of their texts than 'normals' (N).
5 For TD schizophrenic subjects in interview texts there was a nonsignificant tendency to rely less on conjunctional cohesion (fourth category), and more on lexical cohesion (fifth category).

Method of the study

Our own experimental work followed both Halliday and Hasan's theoretical framework and its appliction to schizophrenic discourse worked out by Rochester and Martin. We examined seventy texts which had been produced by thirty-two speakers diagnosed as schizophrenic, and by ten speakers who had never shown any symptoms of psychosis. To separate 'thought-disordered' and 'non-thought-disorded' schizophrenic speakers we used a 'thought disorder score' based on nineteen selected items taken from the 'questionnaire for the assessment of psychological states' designed by the German Committee on Methods and Documentation in Psychiatry (AMDP).[1] As we used a different instrument to measure thought disorder, strictly speaking we applied a different construct to separate subject groups from that used by Rochester and Martin. The total amount of our text corpus was 1,172 independent clauses, 12,659 words, 3,026 cohesive ties. The situational context of all texts was a cartoon task. All subjects were asked by the interviewer to tell a story represented in a four-image cartoon sequence. For a special reason we chose two cartoons which are reproduced on page 270.

The two cartoons were chosen to have considerably differing contents but, at the same time, similar cognitive difficulty. As we were particularly interested in the effects of psychotherapy on cohesive structures, all schizophrenic subjects were asked to produce one text *before* attending a

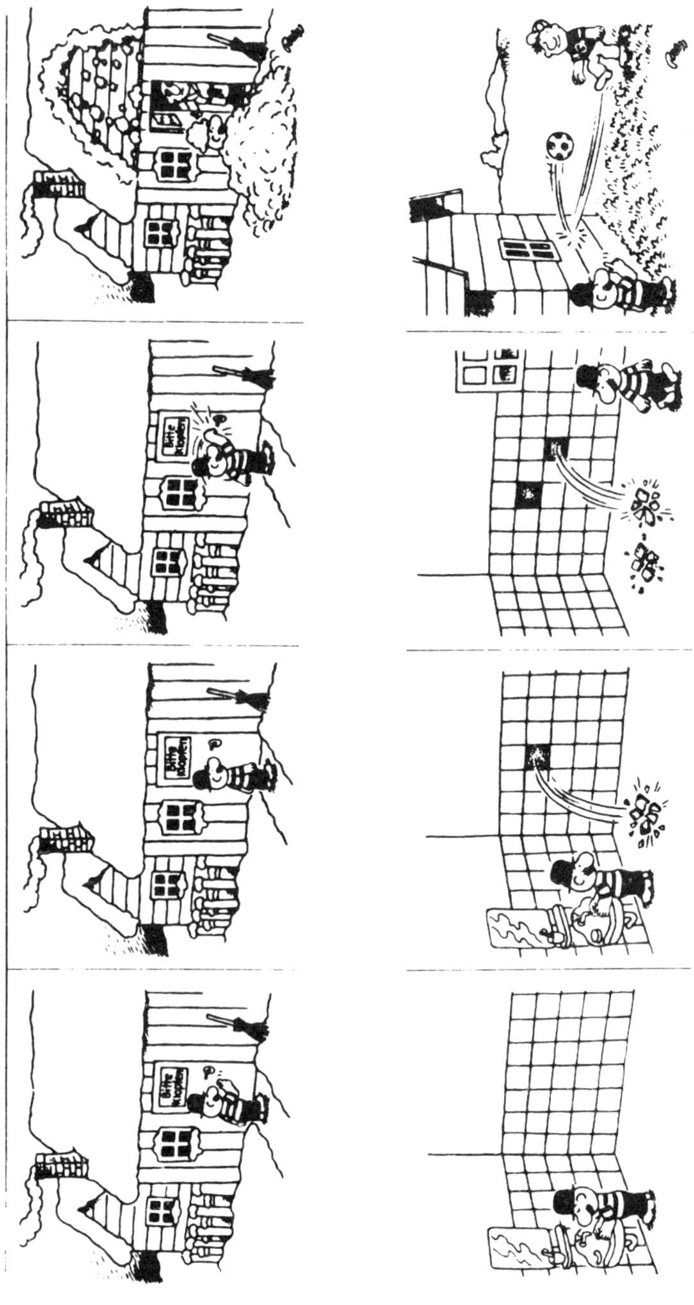

FIGURE 11.1 *Cartoons used for the interviews.*

three-month psychotherapy programme and one text thereafter. Consequently our experimental design was a combination of transversal and longitudinal analysis which we have outlined in Table 11.2.

TABLE 11.2 *Distribution of examined texts among subject groups and their chronological relation to psychotherapy.* The duration of the psychotherapy for both TD and NTD subjects was approximately three months. The statistical procedures were Scheffé Test and LSD Test for the transversal study and t-Test for connected samples for the longitudinal study.

Time 24 + 24 = 48	Group 26 + 30 + 14 = 70 TD	NTD	N
Before	14 subjects, 1 text each = 14 texts	18 subjects, 1 text each = 18 texts	4 subjects, 2 texts each 6 subjects, 1 text each 14 texts
During	2 subjects leave psychotherapy	6 subjects leave psychotherapy	
After	12 subjects, 1 text each = 12 texts	12 subjects, 1 text each = 12 texts	

Transversal study: 70 texts
Longitudinal study: 48 texts

For the transversal study (i.e. of differences among groups), all 70 texts that had been produced were examined with no regard to their chronological relation to psychotherapy. These 70 texts were made up as follows: 14 + 12 = 26 texts produced by 'thought-disordered' schizophrenic speakers; 18 + 12 = 30 texts produced by 'non-thought-disordered' schizophrenic subjects; and 14 texts produced by so-called 'normals'. Performing the longitudinal study (i.e. looking for differences in time) we considered only those 24 subjects (= 48 texts) who attended the complete psychotherapy programme. Otherwise the statistical procedure of 't-Test for connected samples' would not have been applicable. By chance, these 24 schizophrenic subjects were distributed equally among the two schizophrenic subject groups. Sex, age and cartoon tasks were distributed fairly equally among the groups, but the groups were not matched for intelligence, socioeconomic status or premorbid adjustment.

All schizophrenic subjects were outpatients of the psychiatric department of the University Medical School at Münster. They were not paranoid, and most of them had overcome the peak of their psychosocial crisis. The most important aim of the psychotherapy programme was to support them while entering a process of stabilization, and to improve their individual skills in coping with social stress factors (see Fiedler and Buchkremer 1979). Most of them received neuroleptic medication, and were able to modify the dosage in cooperation with the therapists. One of the present authors, Gerd Buchkremer, was supervisor of the psychotherapy programme. He conducted most (sixty-seven out of seventy) of the interviews. He was also therapist in a group of neurotic patients from which six out of ten of the 'normal' subjects came. The other four 'normals' were college students. The other author, Klaus Schonauer, performed the transcription procedure and cohesion analysis without having met the subjects, and consequently without knowing the subject group actually analysed (with the exception of three texts produced by 'normals' who were interviewed by Schonauer before he performed the cohesion analysis).

Results of the study

Transversal results

As Table 11.3 shows, our transversal study confirmed Rochester and Martin's finding that schizophrenic speakers set up fewer cohesive ties

TABLE 11.3 *Average number of cohesive ties per independent clause.* LSD-Test: N differs significantly from both TD and NTD at p = 0.05 level. Scheffé-Test: N differs significantly from NTD at p = 0.05 level, but not from TD.

Groups	Cohesive ties per independent clause
TD (n = 26 texts)	2.4898
NTD (n = 30 texts)	2.3352
N (n = 14 texts)	3.1488

when producing a text than do 'normals'. Depending on the statistical procedure employed, these differences were significant at the 5 per cent level between 'normals' and both schizophrenic subject groups (LSD-Test) or only between 'normals' and 'non-thought-disordered' schizophrenic subjects (Scheffé's Test). In contrast to our preliminary hypothesis, TD subjects produced slightly more cohesive ties than NTD subjects. The analysis of cohesive ranges led us to a similar surprise. As the 'cohesive range' of a text, we defined the average number of independent clauses between cohesive elements and their corresponding anchor elements. If we take the clauses from Table 11.1 as a text, and if we determine that the underlined items in the right columns were the only cohesive elements occurring in the text (which is actually not true), the cohesive range of this text would be exactly 1.0, because cohesive elements and their corresponding anchor elements always occur in neighbouring clauses.

Table 11.4 shows that in TD texts we found the broadest cohesive ranges of all subject groups, although the differences were very subtle and in no case significant. This clearly contradicts our preliminary hypothesis, because we had expected that schizophrenic speakers would rely mainly on immediately neighbouring items while producing a text. Instead, our schizophrenic subjects established cohesive ties in their texts which were at least as broad as those of the so-called 'normals'. The interpretation becomes even more complicated if we consider the strongly significant negative correlation (with a Pearson p value of 0.014 and a correlation factor of −0.411) between thought-disorder scores and cohesive ranges which was found in the TD subject group, but not in the NTD subject group. This means that, although there was a tendency for the TD subjects

TABLE 11.4 *Average number of independent clauses covered over by each cohesive tie* (= 'cohesive range'). LSD and Scheffé Tests yield *no* significant differences among subject groups.

Groups		'Cohesive range'
TD	(n = 26 texts)	2.6032[a]
NTD	(n = 30 texts)	2.5157
N	(n = 14 texts)	2.5192

[a] For TD-subjects—and *only* for this subject group—there was a significant (Pearson p = 0.014) negative (Pearson r = −0.411) correlation between 'cohesive range' and 'thought-disorder score'.

with high thought-disorder scores to set up narrower cohesive ranges — as indicated by the negative correlation — the average values among all TD subjects were even higher than the average values among NTD subjects. It also means that, inasmuch as the high-scoring TD subjects produced narrow ties, the low-scoring TD subjects produced compensatory broader ties.

Longitudinal results

A possible explanation for the contradictions outlined above may be found when we consider some results of the longitudinal study. We see in Table 11.6 that, as far as thought-disorder is concerned, the TD subjects may have benefited more from the therapy than NTD subjects. We have to say 'may', because the 'before and after' differences were not significant. Table 11.5 gives some confirmation for this supposition. It lists the before and after differences for the amount of cohesion in its right column and for cohesive ranges in its left column. The right column shows that in both schizophrenic subject groups the amount of cohesion increased considerably. The p values very near to 0.05 indicate in both cases that these differences are due to systematic and not to casual variations,

TABLE 11.5 *Longitudinal results.* Pre- and post-therapy mean values of 'cohesive range' and the number of cohesive ties per independent clause. p = t-Test probability (connected samples) of accidental differences. *p-levels lower than 0.05* are usually defined as significant.

	'Cohesive Range'			Cohesive Ties per Independent Clause		
Groups	Before	p	After	Before	p	After
TD (n = 24 texts)	2.2886	0.015	2.9402	2.1418	0.053	2.6738
NTD (n = 24 texts)	2.5172	0.948	2.4981	2.1974	0.049	2.6251

TABLE 11.6 *Pre- and post-therapy mean values of 'Thought-Disorder Score' as designed for the purpose of this study.*

Groups	Before	After
TD (n=12 subjects)	10.33	7.00
NTD (n=12 subjects)	1.50	3.00

and that there is some justification in interpreting them as an effect of psychotherapy. (Nevertheless we must not forget that there were still some uncontrolled or unparallelized variables involved, as we pointed out in describing our experimental method.) The left column shows that only the thought-disordered schizophrenic subjects improved their cohesive range to an impressive extent after the therapy. This result is consistent with the negative correlation between thought-disorder scores and cohesive ranges in this subject group only. Consequently it leads to the supposition that the specific deficit or the specific particularity of schizophrenic discourse pointed out by several research groups concerned with cohesion, coherence and related concepts such as Salzinger's 'immediacy hypothesis' — (Salzinger *et al.* 1964; 1970; 1978) seems to be more related to the construct of thought-disorder than to the more general construct of schizophrenia.

We have pointed out mainly those statistic results which showed significant differences between schizophrenic and nonschizophrenic speakers, as was suggested by our interpretative procedure. We should not forget to emphasize that there were no such differences in many of the other analysed variables, and that schizophrenic speakers do in our view, construct 'normal' (whatever that means) texts. An important aim of our study was the attempt to show that schizophrenic speakers may benefit from supportive psychotherapy also as far as their general linguistic competence is concerned. We tried to emphasize that the gathering of experimental data and the interpretative accumulation of that data in order to achieve empirical results are two different steps. At the outset, we quoted a popular definition which states that the development of constructs involves 'broad classes of indicators'. Working with indicators is mainly a semiotic problem.

Finally, we would like to remark that the type of indicator traditionally preferred by medical researchers, which is called a 'symptom' and which Thomas Sebeok (1979: 100) defines as an 'obligatory, automatic, non-arbitrary sign', is probably not the most suitable one for understanding schizophrenic discourse.

Note to Chapter 11

1 The AMDP (= Arbeitsgemeinschaft für Methodik und Dokumentation in der Psychiatrie) Questionnaire for the Psychiatric Assessment of Psychological States consists of 100 different items. We chose the following 19 items because *in our view* they could serve as 'broad classes of indicators' in order to describe the construct of thought disorder:

Item 9 (Auffassungsstörungen), Item 10 (Konzentrationsstörungen), Item 11 (Merkfähigkeitsstörungen), Item 12 (Gedächtnisstörungen), Item 13 (Konfabulationen), Item 15 (gehemmtes Denken), Item 16 (verlangsamtes Denken), Item 17 (umständliches Denken), Item 18 (eingeengtes Denken), Item 19 (Perseveration), Item 21 (Gedankendrängen), Item 22 (ideenflüchtig), Item 23 (Vorbeireden), Item 24 (Gedankenabreißen), Item 25 (inkohärentes/zerfahrenes Denken), Item 26 (Neologismen), Item 55 (Gedankenausbreitung), Item 56 (Gedankenentzug), Item 57 (Gedankeneingebung).

Clinical raters assessed values between 0 and 3 for each item and each schizophrenic subject. The individual's sum of all items we arbitrarily called 'thought-disorder score'. The rating procedures were performed twice: the first time before the subject's attendance at the psychotherapy programme, the second time immediately afterwards. A schizophrenic subject was classified as 'thought-disordered' if his or her pre-therapy score exceeded 5. The highest possible score was 57, the highest score assessed for a subject was 25.

References

Cancro, R. 1969: Psychological differentiation and process-reactive schizophrenia. *Journal of Abnormal Psychology* 74.

Drever, J. and Fröhlich, W. D, 1971: *Wörterbuch zur Psychologie*. Munich: Deutscher Taschenbuch.

Fiedler, P. A. and Buchkremer, G. 1979: Differentielle Psychotherapie bei Patienten mit schizophrenen Störungen. In F. Reimer, (ed.), *Verhaltenstherapie in der Psychiatrie*. Weinsberg: Weisenhof/Kunow.

Gutwinski, Waldemar 1976: *Cohesion in Literary Texts*. The Hague and Paris: Mouton.

Halliday, M. A. K. and Hasan, R. 1976: *Cohesion in English*. London: Longman.

Rochester, S. R. and Martin, J. 1979: *Crazy Talk: A Study of the Discourse of Schizophrenic Speakers*. New York and London: Plenum Press.

Rochester, S. R., Martin, J. R. and Thurston, S. 1977: Thought-process disorder in schizophrenia: the listener's task. *Brain and Language* 4.

Salzinger, K., Pison, S. and Feldman, R. 1970: The immediacy hypothesis and response-produced stimuli in schizophrenic speech. *Journal of Abnormal Psychology* 76.

Salzinger, K., Portnoy, S. and Feldman, R. 1964: Experimental manipulation of continuous speech in schizophrenic patients. *Journal of Abnormal and Social Psychology* 68 (5).

— 1978: Communicability deficits in schizophrenics resulting from a more general deficit. In S. Schwartz, (ed.), *Language and Cognition in Schizophrenia*. New York: Erlbaum.

Sebeok, T. A. 1979: *Theorie und Geschichte der Semiotik*. Reinbek: Rowohlt.

12 The analysis of dialogues with a schizophrenic patient

Marie-Louise Kaesermann

Introduction

The work presented here is part of a project which initially started with the question whether observable speech oddities of schizophrenics could be understood as strategies to avoid verbal exchange on specific irritating subjects. Answering such a question presupposes definitions (1) of specific schizophrenic speech oddities, and (2) of what is meant by a 'strategy'. In what follows I am going to concentrate on elaborating the first primarily methodological point.

The problem of research into schizophrenics' verbal behaviour

It is already commonplace knowledge that the verbal behaviour of at least some of the people diagnosed as schizophrenics is bizarre. But, despite this, no-one seems to be quite able to describe the *exact* nature of this weirdness: 'We are faced with the paradox that while we recognize schizophrenic language when we see it, we cannot define it' (Lorenz 1961: 28). Instead of trying to find reliable and valid *descriptions* of this class of behaviour the vast bulk of research starts from a loose definition of 'deviance' as difficulties with the *meaning* of language, then singles out one specific aspect of meaning establishing verbal operations (e.g. handling of syntactic restrictions), and sets out to test which hypothesis could best explain observed differences between schizophrenics and controls.

The tendency in today's research into schizophrenic verbal behaviour is to explain it as a sign of information-processing problems (e.g. Schwartz

1982). But according to this new and sophisticated form of the old thought-deviance explanation, the deviant verbal behaviour of schizophrenics is only an epiphenomenon of processes which are not specifically related to the knowledge and use of language: And it is my contention that — even if it ultimately should turn out that schizophrenics' verbal behaviour is best explained in terms of an information-processing deficit — it is premature to try to gather the respective evidence. How could one possibly be successful in finding a pertinent explanation for a class of phenomena which in itself is not clearly described?

One aspect of the problem of defining *what* is in need of an explanation is the question of specifity of the relevant behaviour. Everybody concerned with the analysis of schizophrenics' verbal behaviour should have some reason to assume that what he is working on is really characteristic of this population. As we all know that diagnostics in this field is of only very limited worth (e.g. Stephens 1978), we should be able to provide for alternative means of systematic identification of the relevant types of behaviour.

The work to be presented here has to be seen against this background. It is not primarily aimed at explaining *why* schizophrenics talk the way they do, but is thought of as preparatory to the ultimate answer of this question.

The problem of the description of schizophrenics' verbal behaviour

The task of description cannot be tackled in a straightforward manner, for there is no description as such. First one has to decide what it is one wants to describe. In this case it is not just verbal behaviour as such, but verbal behaviour which is thought to be deviant in its meaning-transmitting function and the occurrence of which contributes to the person involved being differentially diagnosed as schizophrenic. Thus the task of description presupposes dealing with two problems, namely, the problem of deciding about the meaning-transmitting function of speech and the problem of deciding about deviance. Each will be considered in turn.

For the speaker, handling the meaning-transmitting function of speech amounts to trying out solutions to the task of how one best gets another person to understand what one wants to convey. Knowledge of linguistic means (phonology, syntax, semantics, pragmatics) is prerequisite to solving this problem. However, communicating successfully demands more than adding up these devices: it is an achievement which integrates all of them in the service of some communicative intention. In the case of schizophrenics' verbal behaviour, there is evidence to suggest that the alleged oddities of speech arise, not from problems with any of the specific linguistic devices, but from problems with their integration: it is the communicative act as such which strikes one as being deviant. 'Schizophrenics are sometimes difficult to understand . . . [they] often ignore the pragmatic *rules underlying conversation* . . . Naturally . . . this makes them hard to follow, but it does not reflect on their language competence — only on their performance. Schizophrenics' speech is disturbed, but their language competence appears intact' (Schwartz 1982: 588 my italics). As Ruemke (1941) had already observed when he tried to define the so-called 'Praecox-Gefühl': 'Die Störung betrifft etwas, was die Relation zwischen den Menschen bestimmt' ('The deviance concerns something which determines the relationship between people'). Therefore, to be able to describe this kind of communicative deviance in any detail one should have access to a model of communicative exchange. After treating the problem of deviance I will introduce such a model in this chapter.

A persons's — normally a psychiatrist's — intuitive assessment of a schizophrenic's difficulties with meaning transmission must rest upon an implicit body of knowledge (rules) about the average, normal course of dialogues. Conceptually speaking, diagnosing deviance implies the use of some standard against which the behavioural unit in question is measured. A standard governing dialogues can be thought of as comprising all the relevant bits of knowledge one has to take into account in order successfully to transmit meaning, as well as the ability to register failures and to correct them (Kaesermann 1980). Actually occurring deviations from this model could be identified if the analyser could make systematic and explicit use of at least part of an average speaker's tacit knowledge about dialogues.

Summing up the two points, one is led to assume that the description of the bizarre speech of schizophrenics has to rest upon a model which prescribes the average way of interactively transmitting meaning, and which therefore provides a basis for an exact description of the ways in which a schizophrenic's speech deviates from it. It is to be expected that some of the types of deviance grasped in this way are ubiquitous, and perhaps only a few are specifically related to the schizophrenic condition. Perhaps it is not even one single type of deviance. To find out about specificity one has to compare the patterns of deviance in different diagnostic groups (including so-called normals). To be useful, however, such a comparison has to be based upon a systematic intersubjectively shared instrument of description. In what follows, the structure of such an instrument/model is outlined and then the kind of analysis established on such a background is demonstrated in detail.

Before this task is tackled, it should be remembered that the idea of looking at schizophrenic's (verbal) behaviour from an interactive or communicative point of view can also be found elsewhere. First, there is the work of the Palo Alto group (e.g. Bateson *et al.* 1956; Bateson *et al.* 1969; Watzlawick and Weakland 1977; 1980) which rests on the strong assumption that a certain pattern of communication acquired in early childhood (the so-called 'double-bind' situation) is causing schizophrenia or — in a lesser form — is typical in families with children developing schizophrenia. From what has been said so far, it should be clear that stating the necessity of a model of communicative exchange for the analysis of a schizophrenic's verbal behaviour does not imply any hypotheses as to the cause(s) or developmental prerequisites of schizophrenia[1] but is motivated solely by the conviction that it is communication rather than language itself which is actually disturbed in the schizophrenic's case. Secondly, there are authors (e.g. Leodolter 1975) who — with or without adhering to the communicative causation hypotheses of schizophrenia — start from the same conviction, and base their description of the schizophrenic's deviant verbal behaviour on explicitly stated systems of rules of conversation/communication. What I shall propose here corresponds to this type of work in so far as it also assumes and makes explicit certain facts about dialogues (e.g. Searle 1969; Grice 1975; see also Kaesermann 1983). However, as will become clear presently, it is at the same time much simpler in terms of the number of rules or conversational maxims it takes into account and more ambitious with regard to their empirical anchoring in concrete interaction.

A communication model: some aspects of the interactional transmission of meaning

One possible view of meaning, as an interactional process of mutual achievement of understanding, has been formulated above. Such a conception, which has been elaborated in detail elsewhere (e.g. Kaesermann 1980; 1983; Foppa 1984) rests on two important assumptions. First, an utterance is primarily conceived of not so much as a unit with certain given *structural* properties, but as one which has a function within the process of production of meaning. An utterance is seen as instrumental in achieving some communicative goals (e.g. the goal to make oneself understood, or the goal to make the addressee react in the desired manner). Generally speaking, an utterance is conceived of as a formulation of a set of underlying communicative intentions. Secondly, one can assume that it is the relationship between what speaker A expected his interlocutor B to understand and/or do and what B *really* understood and/or did after interpreting A's utterance, A_1, which is controlling the (verbal) reactions of speaker A after the interchange A_1 — B: if he feels himself misinterpreted or neglected in any other way he will — provided he still sustains his initial intentions — intervene correctingly in A_2.

The depicted sequence of three consecutive utterances A_1 — B — A_2 of two speakers is the minimally required unit of analysis if one claims to model the interactional constitution of meaning (see also Foppa 1983). However theoretically convincing this may be, the model developed thus far defies empirical practicability because of some flaws associated with the concept of correction. The empirical claim to rely on A_2 as an index of whether utterance B was or was not an adequate realization of A_1 (involving grasping the 'meaning' of what speaker A said) has to take into account two problems. First, only if speaker A is thought of as being an *ideal* speaker is it legitimate to assume that corrections will occur whenever B's verbal reaction deviates from the expectations associated with A_1 For different reasons, though, such an assumption does not seem to be opportune: e.g. the ability of speaker A to spot in B even the slightest deviation from the expectations formulated in A_1 presupposes extremely lucid and well defined intentions underlying A_1; and even if, for speaker A, the underlying intentions are at least partly defined at the moment of utterance, he can either find B's reaction hopeless and give up, or he can be irritated by B's reaction to such an extent that he loses track of what he initially wanted to achieve. This last possibility of speaker A's non-ideal reaction in A_2, is particularly obvious in a dialogue with a psychotic person. It is mainly for this reason that there has to be a way of judging the possible deviance of B independently of whether or not A_2 is a correction. Secondly, even if one chooses to disregard the fact that an average speaker does not meet the requirements for ideally leading a dialogue, there remains the problem of the identification of a given utterance — A_2 — as either a correction or a non-correction. Besides the most obvious possibility of A_2 being a repetition of A_1, in a case where B did not grasp the meaning of A_1, there are presumably numerous but as yet unknown types of correcting interventions. These can probably be identified not by some inherent features of A_2 itself, but only by taking into account the functional relations within the respective unit of analysis. If one wants to adhere to the model outlined above, one has to deal with these two problems in a way which finally provides methods for identifying failures and corrections occurring in a dialogue between non-ideal interlocutors.

The essence of the method to be elaborated presently can be expressed as follows. If it were possible to explicate in a sufficiently detailed manner what speaker A intends his utterance A_1 to achieve (in terms of a set of expected possible reactions in B), then it would be possible to judge whether a given utterance B lies within this range or deviates from expectation, and, in the latter case, should be corrected by speaker A's utterance A_2. Furthermore, if it were possible to detail in which way the observed utterance B deviates from the expected one, it should also be possible to forecast how such a deviation should ideally be counteracted by A_2. Finally, it would be possible to compare the observed A_2 with such an expected A_2 and, therefore, to assess whether or not the former is to be considered as a correction. The rationale of the foregoing is to make some informed assumptions about what ideally should happen in a dialogue, and to use these expectations as a framework within which actual utterances may be judged as to whether and to what extent they meet the respective requirements.

The relevance of the model for the analysis of schizophrenics' verbal behaviour

In an average dialogue the roles of A and B may be arbitrarily assigned to the two interlocutors. It is even possible to exchange roles. In the case of the analysis of dialogues with a schizophrenic person which aims at a specific description of deviances occurring in the schizophrenic's utterances, it seems reasonable to assign role A to whoever talks with the schizophrenic in role B, because B represents that part within the unit of analysis for which there exists a standard (a predicted set of acceptable reactions) against which possible deviances can be judged and described in detail. But such a methodological convenience in itself does not answer the question of whether looking at dialogues with a schizophrenic from the point of view of the model is fruitful at all. For this, one has to turn to some substantial considerations. That is to say, one has to find out whether there exists an aspect of communication which is particularly difficult to deal with for a schizophrenic person. If one tries to list the functions an utterance A_1 can have (e.g. being understood, expressing and inducing emotions, making clear one's opinion about various things), it is the information-seeking function of an utterance which seems to be most problematic for the schizophrenic (e.g. Avenarius 1966). Confronted with the task (which could be formulated in an A_1) of providing information on specific subjects (e.g. the contradiction between reality and some delusional thoughts), the schizophrenic person seems bound to deviate from an average communication pattern.[2] Therefore, a relevant aspect of communication with a schizophrenic person could be grasped if it were possible to incorporate the information-seeking function into the model described so far. Note that the selection of this function cuts across traditional linguistic categories. Grasping the information expectation of one's interlocutor involves every aspect of linguistic knowledge.

Modelling the communicative exchange of information

In specifying the proposed model in order to implement the information-seeking function of utterances one can proceed as follows. There is at least one easily identifiable linguistic form, namely the question (except in its rhetorical variety), which serves this function in speech. A question can be seen as a 'given-new' structure (Clark and Haviland 1977) where the 'new' part can be seen as an empty space which has to be filled or specified by the addressee's answer. If one assumes that the interrogator himself, in posing a question, is quite clear about what kind of reaction from the addressee would form an adequate realization of his expectations, then he should be able to judge an actually occurring answer against his expectations. The result of such a comparison yielding the assessment of adequate answers, as well as of occurrence and type of discrepancies, should control the occurrence and type of a correcting intervention.

The possibility of using this question—answer—rection—specification of the A_1 — B — A_2 unit in the analysis of concrete dialogues depends on whether it is possible:

(a) to assign concrete questions (A_1) to specific types of given new structure and to predict on this basis the set of expected appropriate answers (B_e);
(b) to find a differential description of types of discrepancies (B_o), and to predict on this basis the type of expected correcting interventions (A_{2e}); and
(c) to specify criteria for comparing actually occurring reactions (A_{2o}) with the predicted ones.

The list of tasks to be solved does not include predicting the course of dialogues after an appropriate answer. This is not because to follow such a thread would be impossible, but because this aspect is not focal in dealing with discrepancies. For similar reasons I am going to concentrate on an elaboration of the first two points, only occasionally hinting at the third one. As the main aim of this chapter is to propose an instrument for describing occurring discrepancies, it does not deal with the question of how the schizophrenic's partner is affected by the schizophrenic's manner of speech.

The analysis of concrete dialogues with a schizophrenic patient

The material to be analysed here stems from a single case study of dialogues, and consists of seven interviews (each lasting half an hour) between a male schizophrenic long-term patient and an experienced psychiatrist. The criterion for the selection of the patient was — besides his being diagnosed as schizophrenic — the presence of topics (everyday as well as illness-related ones) which he presumably did not like to have discussed. It was assumed that mentioning these topics — which were established on the basis of a written doctor's report and of the oral report of the staff — would promote the patient's deviant verbal behaviour. The seven sessions took place every other day within a two-week period. They were taped and videotaped for the nonverbal aspects of communication (Kaesermann *et al.* 1984). The first and seventh interview were intended to be neutral in content, while for the remaining five the psychiatrist was asked to talk about one or more of the irritating topics (for example, the patient's experience at work or his delusional thoughts about religion). Apart from being obliged to indicated which utterances he believed to be particularly invasive (for technical details see Kaesermann 1983), the psychiatrist did not have to follow any other instructions. The patient was correctly told that the interviews were aimed at getting to know him better, and to learn about dialogues, but that they would not have any consequences for him (for example, on his work situation or his stay at the clinic). The effects of this setting on the occurrence of speech oddities in general, and of some selected speech parameters, are reported elsewhere (Kaesermann 1983; Alberti and Kaesermann 1983).

The identification of types of questions and the definition of sets of expected answers

Another way of saying that a speaker, in uttering a specific question, has a limited set of expectations as to what would form an appropriate answer is to state that a question (in contrast to, say, a statement) restricts the set of possible (verbal) reactions of the addressee in a systematic way. For the data analyst, then, the empirical task is first, to define the type of restrictions which are provided by a specific question, and secondly, to construct the set of possible answers. As will be clear presently, such a subclassification of the total set of questions, although using formal criteria as a means of identification, aims at differentiating the information-seeking function by defining different types of question/answer formats.

A question (identified by the formal features of an interrogative sentence) restricts the range of possible (verbal) reactions in two important ways. First, by a question (as opposed to a statement) the addressee is obliged[3] to react verbally in a way which allows for the inference that he is aware of the task-character of his partner's utterance. Making a reply to a preceding question does not imply having correctly understood what one is expected to do. In terms of answering a question as filling or specifying an empty space, this means only that, to be identifiable as a reply, the addressee's utterance does not need to be a thoroughly appropriate filler of the empty space of the preceding question. As long as there is no other utterance in the context which could be thought of as a frame of reference, it is seen as a reply, however deviant it may be as a specific answer. Nor is it implied that, having understood the preceding question, the addressee should also be willing to comply in solving the given task: an explicit rejection (e.g. *I don't want to tell you, because this doesn't concern you*) presupposes an awareness of the task-character, and therefore is to be seen of as a reply.

The empirical decision of whether a given utterance following a question is to be considered as a reply (R) is made as follows. For each given pair of question (A_1) — consequent utterance (B), the analyser puts himself in the position of an interpreter. He assesses

(a) whether it is possible to establish any connection between the utterance and the preceding question; if this is not the case, the utterance is judged to be a nonreply (NR). Characteristic examples of NR are the 'Vorbeireden' (talking at cross-purposes) of the schizophrenic, as well as simultaneous speech. If any connection can be established, the analyser must go on to decide

(b) whether it is possible to find yet another interpretative connection with one of the utterances of the preceding context. If this is the case, the utterance is judged to be ambiguous as regards its status as a reply (R?); if it is not the case, the utterance is judged to be a reply.

This method capitalizes on the average speaker's ability to grasp and interpret the functional status of an utterance in a given context. Although this kind of potential forms the basis of the assessments just described, one does not need to rely solely on this intuitive knowledge, but can resort to a set of explicit criteria of cohesion (Halliday and Hasan 1976; Wykes and Leff 1982) which can be used to legitimize the identification of utterances as either (R), (R?) or (NR).

The second kind of restrictions given by questions results from a functionally (as opposed to formally) motivated subdivision of the total set of questions according to the type of empty space they contain. If one thinks of a question (a 'given-new' structure) as consisting of an empty space (the 'new' aspect) as well as of an (explicit or implicit) *instruction* to the addressee on how to proceed with an empty space, the problem of identifying different types of questions amounts to:

(a) deciding about how to proceed by identifying a given empty space, and
(b) defining criteria for the identification of a given kind of instruction, as well as
(c) determining how to proceed with questions which do not seem to be accompanied by any (explicit) instruction.

Each of these problems will now be dealt with in turn.

(a) By determining what constitutes the empty space in a given question, one can proceed as follows. In the case of simple and alternative yes/no questions and questions with a performative verb (e.g. *Could you tell me more about X?*), the empty space is considered to be that part of the question which is implied when the question is minimally asserted or denied (e.g. *Did he come? Yes/no (he did (not) come*, or *Could you tell me about this new book? Yes/no (I can('t) tell you about this new book*). A given instruction (see below) has to be executed on the verbatim implications of what this minimal assertion/denial test yields. In the case of *wh*-questions and alternative *wh*-questions, the empty space is implied by that part which can be replaced by an X (e.g. *Who came? X came*).

(b) In the analysed corpus,[4] four types of explicit and therefore obligatory instructions on how to proceed with an empty space can be distinguished by formal criteria. As these instructions define what kind of information with reference to a given empty space should be given, it is possible to infer which formal characteristics an appropriate answer must have in order minimally to provide the required content.

Demands of expansion/specification (E)

A_1: Können Sie mir etwas über den Alltag auf der Abteilung erzählen?
(Could you tell me something about the daily routine on the ward?)
(III 2, 1)[5]

A_1: Ich have gehört, dass die Psychiater äh sagen: Ja äh der Herr X, der soll selber mehr von sich sagen. Und äh wie erleben Sie das?
(I have heard other psychiatrists say: yeah, Mr X he should be more spontaneous in telling things about himself. And how do *you* experience this?)
(III 4, 4)

Demands of expansion are formally marked either by a speech act verb (example 1) or by a *wh*- doing combination (example 2) which cannot be filled by an elliptical selection (see below). A third type of demand of expansion is given by questions without such markers (usually multiple paraphrases) which (for syntactic and/or semantic reasons, i.e. resulting ambiguity) cannot be answered minimally by *yes/no* or elliptically. The identification of this latter type does not rely on formal markers of the given question but on hypothetical continuation of the dialogue.

The set of possible answers to this type of question consists of:

(a) a (positive) execution of the instruction (e.g. for example 1: *yes* + an unlimited amount of new information with reference to the empty space 'daily routine on the station'); and
(b) a (negative meta-) rejection of the execution of the instruction (e.g. for example 1: *no* + a legitimation of the rejection). It could be a matter of debate whether such an adjunct should be thought of as optional or obligatory. Where a minimal *no* answer would be ambiguous (e.g. *could you tell me whether the train has already left?*), an adjunct (e.g. *no, I can't* or *no it hasn't*) is necessary. Also, there are social conditions of obligation: within an assymmetrical dyad, the lower-level interlocutor is probably obliged to legitimize rejections. If he avoids fulfilling this obligation, he is bound to be confronted with an additional question (e.g. *Why don't you want to tell me?*). In the concrete analysis of dialogues, such minimal responses are considered neither as appropriate nor as violating but as neutral with regard to expectation.

Concrete B utterances following an E, provided they have the status of a reply, are compared with these answer formats and judged to be either conformant, neutral or deviant from the expectation.

Demands of selection (S)

A_1: Wie lange waren Sie dort, wieviele Tage waren Sie dort, im Urlaub?
(For how long were you there, for how many days were you there, on holiday?)

(VII 4, 7)

A_1: Wie geht's denn?
(How are you then?)

(V 1, 2)

Questions of this type presuppose certain facts (e.g. example 1: that the patient had been on holiday and that holidays have a certain variable duration) and demand of the addressee a selection of the alternative(s) which hold(s) true. Formally, they are marked by a *wh-* pronoun (*who, when, what*, etc.). For some questions marked by a *wh-* pronoun, however, it cannot be decided whether they have to be identified as demands of selection or as demands of explication, because they can be interpreted either way (e.g. example 2 can be understood either as a demand of explication of one's health condition or as a demand of selection of qualification like *good*). With regard to possible answers, therefore, one has to assume that the choice of E answers is as appropriate as the choice of S answers.

The set of possible answers to this type of question consists of:

(*a*) a selection of the correct item(s)/value(s) on the presupposed variable (e.g. for example 1: a minimally elliptical answer like *for four days* or *I don't remember exactly: six or seven days*); and
(*b*) a rejection of the given task (e.g. for example 1: *I am not going to tell you* + a legitimation of the rejection).

Concrete B replies following S are compared with these answer formats and judged as to whether they fit them.

Demands of verification (V)

A_1: Und wer macht die Farbmuster, wer, machen, tun Sie die selber ausdenken?
(And who creates the patterns of colour, who, do you create them yourself?)

(I 4, 13)

A_1: Und was gibt es, nen kleinen Teppich, oder gibt es n'Handtuch?
(And what is it going to be, a small carpet, or is it going to be a towel?)

(I 4, 4)

Questions of this type presuppose some facts, select one (or more) possible alternative(s) within this range, and submit this conjecture to verification. (With respect to example 1 given above, this means that the fact that there is a set of possible alternative creators of colour patterns is presupposed, and one of the possible alternatives is selected for verification.) In uttering a presumably contrafactual conjecture, a speaker is able to provoke an explicit disagreement in his partner. This conversationally interesting use may be particularly opportune when conversing with a person who does not like to speak a lot and therefore tends to provide only the minimally required information. Formally, these demands are marked by a combination of a *wh-* question (of the E or S variety) and a (simple or alternative) *yes/no* question.

The set of possible answers to this type of questions consists of:

(*a*) a verification of the given conjecture (minimally by uttering *yes* or, in the case of the alternative *yes/no* question, by repeating the correct alternative *yes/no a carpet*); or a rejection of the conjecture combined with an alternative selection or expansion (depending on the *wh-* part involved) of the correct item (e.g. example 1: *No, (it is) the occupational therapist*). The adjunction of the correct alternative is obligatory because a minimal *no* answer would not cover up the *wh-* expectation of the question. However, for the same reason not every possible adjunct (i.e. *no* + a legitimation, in example 1: *no, I've no talent for this at all*) meets the given requirements;

(*b*) a rejection of the given task with or without legitimation, depending on how one has decided to proceed about the question of optionality. Note that every V question requiring a minimal *yes* answer can be thought of as a V+(Sel(L)) or V+(E(L)) where the additional selection or expansion is optional.

Demands of consensual validation (CV)

A_1: Na, das wird sich auch wieder legen, hm?
(Well, that's going to get better soon, isn't it?)

Questions of this type are primarily aimed at gaining support for the speaker's opinion about something. Formally, they are marked by the absence of an inversion as well as by some tag forms.

The set of possible answers to this type of question consists of:

(a) an utterance of support (minimally *yes*) or of disagreement + formulation of the addressee's own opinion about the same thing (e.g. example 1: *no, I don't believe it does.*) It does not seem possible to mark disagreement by a minimal *no* answer because a speaker in uttering a CV does not expect dissent. So, even if this unexpected answer version occurs, nevertheless he somehow has the right to know why;

(b) a rejection of the task.

In sum, the four types of instruction can be distinguished by specific formal markers as well as by the hypothesized continuation of dialogue. The set of possible answers consists in each case of either a fulfilment or a (legitimized) rejection of the task given by the instruction. For an answer to count as adequate, it has to contain minimally that amount and type of information which is necessary and sufficient for an interpreter's identification of it as an unamiguous, noncontradictory and presumably true fulfilment or rejection of the relevant instruction. The forms used to solve such a task can vary within these restrictions: you can convey your consent by uttering *yes* as well as by uttering *surely*, or even by using some indirect statement. There can be more information in an answer than the amount asked for by the question. This additional information can be conveyed, for example, by *surely* instead of *yes*. To deal with this aspect of the information-seeking paradigm in a systematic way would be possible. For the given purpose, however, utterances are treated as adequate regardless of whether they contain just the necessary and sufficient information or whether they contain also some additional information.

I turn now to a discussion of how to assess sets of possible answers for questions without any (explicit) instruction. After we have identified all the questions in the corpus which belong to one of the four types characterized by an explicit instruction, there remain a number of questions which can be understood as (simple or alternative) *yes/no* questions in so far as they can in principle be minimally answered by *yes, no* or *I don't know*, respectively. Answering *yes/no* questions by *I don't know* is linguistically possible. However, it is not clear under which social circumstances such an answer has to be complemented by a reason. Deciding about this issue would require a theory of uncertainty which cannot be provided here.

Questions of this residual category do not seem to bear any instruction how to proceed with their respective empty space because they are devoid of any of the formal markers previously mentioned. However, it is feasible to deal with the problem of formulating sets of acceptable answers to these questions if one proceeds by what I would like to term the 'minimal-answer-version test'.

(*a*) After having defined the given empty space, one has to decide whether minimal *yes* and minimal *no* respectively would be possible, in so far as using them would not result in contradiction, nor in ambiguity or untruth (as far as this can be judged at all). If one of the minimal versions violates one of these conditions, there has to be an adjunct which shows either an awareness of that fact or even corrects for it, as in the following examples

B:	Ja, es war beides recht.	Yeah, both of them were OK
A_1:	Beides recht?	Both of them OK?

B_e: **no*
no + obligatory adjunct compensating for arising contradiction (e.g. *no, I was just mistaken*)

(IV 7,5)

A_1:	Kommt das immer wieder vor oder ist das sehr selten, dass das kommt?	Does it happen again and again or does it very rarely happen at all?

B_e: **yes/no*
yes/no + obligatory disambiguating adjunct (e.g. *yes/no again and again*)

(VII 10,6)

(*b*) For the possible minimal versions, one has to decide whether, with respect to the demands of the question, they would convey sufficient information. If one rightly or wrongly assumes that there is such a thing as, for example, an implicit demand of expansion, then it is obvious that a minimal *yes* as an answer would not be sufficient, provided one also assumes that implicit instructions have the same power of obligation as explicit ones. However, as I am not certain whether or not there exists an unequivocal solution to the problem of identifying implicit instructions (whether because of lack of pertinent criteria[6] or because such questions are inherently ambiguous as regards instruction), I proceed by judging occurring minimal versions as *neutral* to expectation.

(*c*) There still remains the question of how to proceed with non-minimal answers (answers with an adjunct) in cases where a minimal answer would have been at least neutral to expectation. It can be demonstrated empirically that providing *more* than minimal information does not necessarily lead to an appropriate answer:

A_1:	Hat die das gemerkt, dass Sie sich verliebt haben in sie, war das auf Gegenseitigkeit?	Did she realize you had fallen in love with her, was it a mutual thing/ emotion?
B:	Jaja, aber nume n es Jahr, da bi n i äbe furt, nach I.	Yes yes but just for a year then I went away, to I (*name of town*).

(V 13,6)

The occurring adjunct is irrelevant with regard to the given empty space (*yes/no she did (not) realize I had fallen in love with her*) and therefore such an answer, though not minimal, cannot be judged to be adequate. It is perhaps less of a problem to realize the inappropriateness of a given adjunct when you see it. The question, however, remains of how one can define or forecast the range of appropriate adjunct solely on the basis of a given question. As a possible solution I propose the following proceeding. For each question one has to determine what kind of questions a speaker still could ask after the given question had been answered minimally (e.g., for the given example: *Yes.—How did you recognize it?* and *No.—Why not?*). The content of the hypothesized answers to these hypothesized additional questions is what an actually occurring adjunct should contain in order to count as appropriate.

In sum, leaving open the question of whether the residual category of formal *yes/no* questions could still be subdivided according to implicitly given instructions, I propose to define the set of their respective possible answers by the application of the 'minimal-version test'.

The description of occurring answers (B_0) and the prediction of the type of correcting intervention (A_{2e})

The set of actually occurring utterances (B, in this case the schizophrenic's verbal reactions) can be subdivided into three groups: instances which conform to one of the predicted possible answers; instances which are neutral as regards expectation; and instances which do not belong to either of these groups, and which are therefore considered to be deviant in one way or the other. This last group consists of B utterances which either violate the restrictions given by a question (NR, R?) or the ones given by a specific type of question (R which is deviant in some way). As it is this last group which is of focal interest here, I am not going to dwell long on the other two. While it can be asserted that, with regard to A_{2e}, conformant B answers should not be followed by any repetition of A_1, it is an issue in its own right to systematize a more differentiated prediction of the positive features of the expected speaker reaction. Solutions within this realm will presumably depend on how one treats this issue of surplus information given by a specific answer, as well as on how one goes about larger ('thematically' defined) units of dialogue. With regard to the neutral B answers, one can assume that all the information they convey is correct but that they presumably contain too little of it. Therefore, as a rule A_{2e} should be aimed at eliciting the missing information, and this could be done by adding a specific question (a question with an explicit instruction like *could you tell me more about it?* or *whom did you meet there?*). Again, it is a separate question of how to formulate conditions under which this principle would be modified (e.g. there are social conventions as to if and who is allowed to ask specific intimate questions).

There remains the group of B utterances to be dealt with which are, by definition of the model, to be considered as deviant. To substantiate my initial claim about a systematized description of verbal deviance, I cannot stop at assessing (dichotomously) the occurrence of deviance but have to try to show how exactly these utterances are odd. There are numerous, in my opinion, unsatisfactory ways to solve this task (e.g. by classifying on the basis of phonological, syntactic or semantic errors). Instead, there is one way dictated by the proposed model (i.e. by its information-seeking implementation) which can be considered to be more to the point. If basically a speaker expects his partner to deal correctly with the informational aspect of his questions, then a differential description of deviance should specify in which ways one can fail to fulfil that expectation. To be able to grasp types of failure, one has to recall the structure of demands given by a question: the addressee is asked, by presupposing some given information to execute an (explicit) instruction on an empty space in order to produce an answer with certain canonical features (e.g. it has to be understandable, unambiguous, noncontradictory, fitting to truth and reality, etc.). Given this background, failures can occur at each point singly or in combination, and I shall proceed to give examples of such failures.

(*a*) *Failure of the task as a whole* is assessed if it is not possible to find any connection between a given answer and its preceeding question (in example 1, this case coincides with NR) and if there is a certain connection, not simply between a given question/answer/pair but also to some other utterance in the preceding context (in example 2, this case coincides with R?)

(*1*)	A_1:	Wie lange sind Sie jetzt schon hier in der Klinik, Herr X?	How long have you now been here at the clinic, Mr X?

	B:	Ja, ich bin gerne unter Menschen, ja also ich, ich, aber ich kann mich nicht so äussern.	Oh, I like to be with people, that is I, I, but I have difficulties expressing myself.

(I 7,4)

(2)	A_k:	Sie hätten lieber, wenn das Obstbäume wären?	You would prefer them, if they were fruit-trees?
		(...)	(...)
	A_1:	Glauben Sie, dass Sie da nen Einfluss drauf nehmen könnten, was für Blumen auf die Station kommen? Könnten Sie da Einfluss drauf nehmen?	Do you think that you could have any influence on what kind of flowers will be brought to the ward? Could you have any influence on it?
	B:	Ja, (*wenn das X waeren*), da hätt mes schöner.	Yes (*if they were X*) then it would be more beautiful.

(III 10,2)

Confronted with this kind of failure, the speaker should in A_{2c} react essentially with a repetition of the initial question A_1. Such a repetition could either be a verbatim version of A_1 or a version which is introduced by some meta-comment (e.g. *no, what I mean is...*, or *yes, but what I meant to ask is...*).

(*b*) *Failure to correctly treat given information* is assessed if presuppositions are changed (example 1), if they are negated (example 2) or if they, instead of the given empty space, are verified and expanded (example 3):

(*1*)	A_1:	Freuen Sie sich, wenn die kommen, oder haben Sie eher's Gfühl, ist es Ihnen nicht so lieb?	Do you like them to come or do you feel, don't you like it really?
	B:	Ja, mängisch han i s Gfüehl, si wölle mi lieber nid.	Yes, sometimes I feel they don't really like to have me.[7]
(2)	A_1:	Was würden Sie denn machen, wenn jemand käm und würd sagen: Jetzt hab ich genug von dem Qualm?	What would you do then, if somebody came and said: Now I am really fed up with your smoke?
	B:	Nei, das seit kenne.	No, nobody says this.

(III 7,3)

(*3*)	A_1:	Wenn Sie irgendetwas stört, was, was Sie gerne geändert hätten, was machen Sie dann? Auf der Abteilung? Wenn irgendetwas Ihnen auf die Nerven geht? Was machen Sie dann?	If you are bothered by something that, that you would like to have changed, what do you do then? On the ward? If something gets on your nerves? What do you do then?
	B:	Ja, das isch eigetlich d J, wenn sie brüellet, de chunnt sie eim uf d Närve. Ja, ja, ja.	Well, it is really J when she screams then she gets on your nerves. Yes, yes, yes.

(III 10,7)

Confronted with this kind of failure the speaker should react by re-establishing the initial distribution of given and new information, and by asking again for information specifying the given empty space. This is not exactly the same task for a negation (there, one probably has to proceed by assuming some contrafactual givens, e.g. in example 1, *yes, but if someone complained; what would you do?*) and for an elaboration, where one can reinforce the initial question with regard to the actual specification of the given (e.g. in example 2, *yes, exactly, that's a good example and what do you do in this case?*).

(*c*) *Failure to recognize correctly the empty space* is assigned if the answer implicitly or explicitly transforms the empty space given by the question by substituting some derivative of it (example 1):

(*1*)	A_1:	Wie ist es jetzt eigentlich mit Ihnen, Herr X: Ham Sie vor, dass Sie äh mal wieder mit ner Arbeit beginnen? Wie stellen Sie sich das vor?	How is it now in your case, Mr X. Do you plan that you eh to start work again sometime? What do you think about it?
	B:	Ja, das chönnt ig scho, ja.	Yes, this I could really do, yes.

(II 2,4)

In the above example, the empty space (*yes/no I do (not) plan to start work again*) is substituted by the derivative (*yes/no I can(not) start work again*). By this transformation, the reference to mental activity concerning future work is deleted, and is therefore no longer something to be discussed. By transformation of the empty space, any part may be deleted, or substituted (e.g. the question about a habit may be answered by reference to a specific event in the past; the question about what something means when it occurs may be reversed and answered by reference to what it does not mean), or new parts may be added.

Confronted with this kind of failure, the speaker should react by repairing the transformation. In the case of example 1 above, this could be done by asking for the missing/deleted part of the empty space (e.g. *do you sometimes think about it?*).

(d) Failure to execute correctly takes place if a given instruction is mistaken for another one (e.g. if there is a verification in place of an expansion explicitly requested; if there is a selection of, for example, a place instead of a description of a person (example 1); or if a given empty space, instead of being verified or negated, contains some additional information where it is doubtful whether it holds true (example 2); or where the addition countermands what had been verified before (example 3).

(*1*)	A1:	Was war denn das für ne Frau?	What kind of woman was she then?
	B:	Aebe, i dere Glasfabrik.	Well, just in that glass-factory.
			(V 13,4)
(*2*)	A_1:	Fällt Ihnen das schwer, jemanden anzusprechen von den Pflegern oder von den Schwestern? Jemand Neues, den Sie gar nicht kennen, zum Beispiel? Um zu sagen: Ich möcht jetzt raus. Macht Ihnen das Mühe?	Is it hard for you to address somebody from the team? Somebody new, for example, somebody whom you don't know at all. And to say: I would like to go for a walk. Do you find it hard to do so?
	B:	Nei, das macht mer nid Müeh, nei... wün igse kenne dert	No, I don't find it hard, no... because I know people there
			(III 9,2)
(*3*)	A_1:	Tun Sie sich da selbst, selbstbefriedigen, selbst erleichtern?	Do you masturbate then, relieve yourself?
	B:	Bis jetz scho, ja, aber jetz mach ig s de nümm.	Up to now, yes, but from now on I won't do it.
			(II 8,6)

A simple way to state what is happening here is to say that a given empty space is minimally reacted to by being verified or negated (in so far as being neutral to expectation). Instead of a consequently possible expansion in the case of a verification, however, there is an addition of information which is either marginal, or irrelevant, or even false or contradictory with regard to the implied and therefore specifiable proper empty space. If one assumes that a speaker within the information-seeking paradigm pursues the strategy to get to know more about a defined empty space (this 'more' being a verification or even a verification-based expansion), then he is in a good position either if the addressee (spontaneously, in the case of the residual *yes/no* category, or in executing an explicit instruction, in the case of E) reacts by providing an expansion or if he reacts minimally. For in the latter case, the speaker can easily continue the dialogue by adding some specific explicit questions. However, he is in a less comfortable position if he is confronted with an expansion-like verification, because then the possibility of asking for a proper expansion of the given empty space depends on the possibility of somehow disregarding the additional distracting information. While this may not pose too many problems for an alert speaker in cases where the distracting information is marginal or irrelevant (example 1) it is a little bit more difficult in cases where the distracting information is presumably false (as in example 2, where a speaker could react by stating his disbelief or by confronting the addressee with obvious discrepancies); and it does seem to be almost impossible in cases where the additional information annuls the existence of the primarily verified empty space (example 3). It is possible that this latter kind of *failure* is a candidate for identification as a specifically schizophrenic reaction.

(*e*) *Failure correctly to select features of the answer* is assessed if from the form of the answer it is not possible to arrive at an unambiguous interpretation (example 1), or if the answer, being a correct execution of a given instruction on a given empty space, does not meet one or more of an answer's required canonical attributes (example 2, 2a, 2b)

(*1*)	A_1:	Sie stöhnen so, tut Ihnen das sehr leid, dass Sie's nicht gemacht haben, die Kochausbildung.	You are moaning now, do you regret it a lot that you didn't start with it, with the training as a cook?
	B:	Ja, i wär glich hie glandet, nid, öb ig jetz Choch gsi wär oder nid…	Yes, I would have landed in here regardless of whether I had been a cook or not…

(IV 5,2)

Because a possible conjuction ('yes, *but*', 'no, *moreover*') is left out and it is not clear whether the *yes* is meant as a correct or incorrect assertion or just as a signal—'I got the question and am going to answer'—this answer remains ambiguous with regard to the empty space (*yes/no I do(not) regret that...*).

(*2*) A_1:	Können Sie mir da n bissl was erzählen davon (von den Ferien)	Can you tell me then a little bit about it (about the holiday)
B:	Ja, wir gingen in den äh, in, nach, nach, äh, nach dem, wir sind gelaufen hinauf bis zum Wasserfall nach der Engstligenalp.	Yes, we went on the eh, on, to, to eh to the we walked up to the waterfall on the Engstligenalp.

(VII 3,5)

This answer is deviant because it violates a canonical format of narration which would begin by stating the place of the holiday (e.g. *We were in Adelboden for X days and there was...and...*).

(*2a*) A_1:	Sind Sie schnell, kommt Ihnen schnell der Schlaf, oder verlieren Sie die Uebersicht über die, über die Arbeit, oder was ist der Grund?	Are you often, does sleep quickly overcome you, or do you lose control over the, over the work you do, or what is the reason?
B:	Ja, das isch eh das isch wäg de n Ouge, nid, wäg däm Gseh, nid. I gseh nämlech z schtarch, nid, ig, nid, ig gseh so starch, de chan i äuä nid viel...	Yes, that is eh that is because of my eyes, you see, because of my sight, you see. I see too strongly, you see, I, you see, I see so strongly then I probably cannot much...

(II 4,5)

(*2b*) A_1:	Ja doch, gibt schon Leute, die's angeht?!	But yes, there are people whom it bothers?!
B:	Ja, villicht mit ere andere Istellig, ja, dass das vorchunnt, ja.	Yes, perhaps with a different attitude, yes, that this happens yes.

(III 13,1)

In both of these answers the patient violates the canonical requirements of an answer in using words and phrases (*my eyes, my sight, I see too strongly, attitude*) which denote aspects of his psychotic experience and which cannot be clarified throughout the series of interviews. Beside failing a correct execution of an instruction by verifying and subsequently countermanding an empty space, this kind of failure seems to be a specifically schizophrenic reaction.

As regards possible speaker reactions to failures of this kind, it seems to be quite easy to find a disambiguating intervention (example 1) or an intervention which compensates for missing information (example 2, e.g. by specifically asking *Have you been in Adelboden?*), as long as the structure of the reality referred to is accessible to the speaker. However, if this condition is not fulfilled (examples 2a, 2b) the speaker is either forced to ask some meta-questions (like *How do you mean 'attitude'?*) or to leave the field altogether because a simple repetition of his initial question is hampered by the fact that he has already got an *answer* which is clearly recognizable as such. In both cases, therefore, he is forced to leave a given subject-matter.

It remains to be mentioned that in a given question/answer/pair there may occur a combination of two or more failures. It is still an open question as to how one deals with this fact with regard to forecasting A_{2e}.

Conclusion

Against a background of a psychopathologically anchored definition of schizophrenics' difficulties with speaking and of a communication model which allows the specification of some characteristic aspects, this chapter has outlined an instrument for the development of the description of deviances which occur in dialogues between a schizophrenic patient and a psychiatrist. The recognition of types of deviances within the given model depends on an assumed structure of the task to be solved when answering questions (or, more generally, when reacting to communicative demands or requests). This structure allows forecasting reactions which are conformant, as well as identifying and describing differentially the ones which have to be considered as nonconformant with a set of given expectations.

The main result of this research so far is that it is possible to develop an instrument which combines formal and functional criteria, and by which the total set of dialogue sequences can be categorized (see Figure 12.1). Furthermore, some aspects of what one might call the implicit knowledge of an average speaker about *dialogues* has been made explicit (e.g. the attributes of a canonical answer). Substantial results on the schizophrenic's reaction will be reported elsewhere (Kaesermann, 1986). Suffice it here

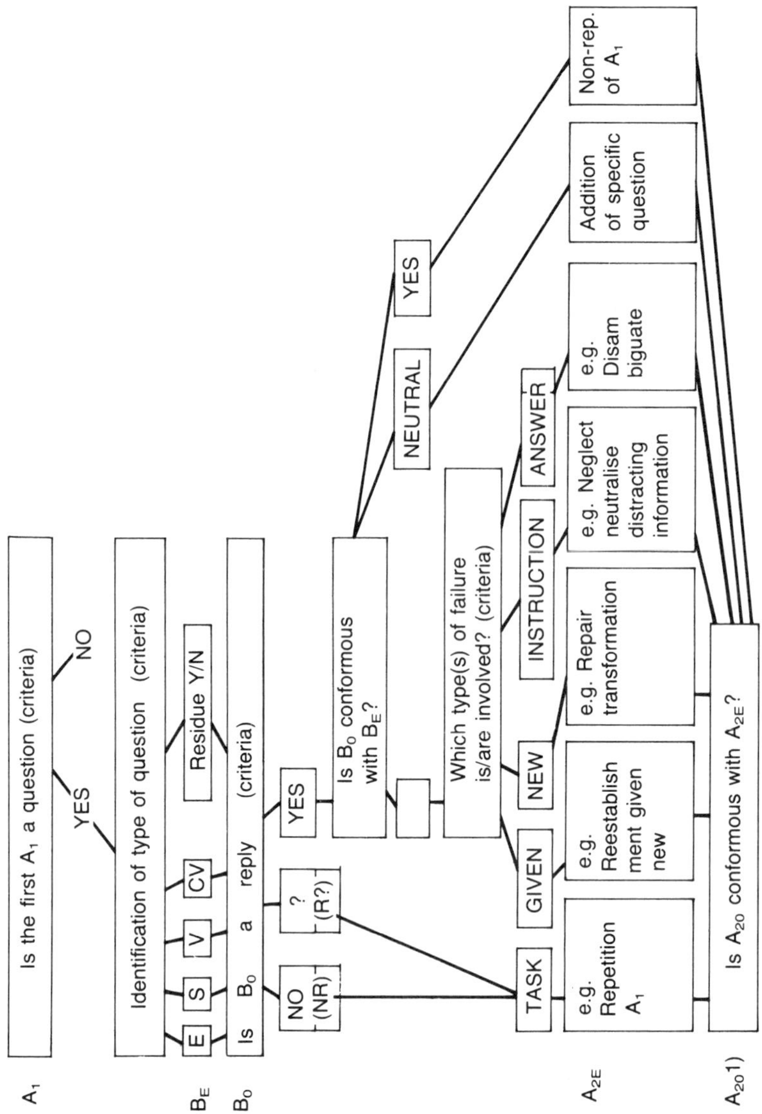

1) A_{20} is A_1 of the following A_1 – B – A_2 sequence.

FIGURE 12.1 *Schematic review of steps of analysis.*

to state that an impressive amount of the schizophrenic's reactions are nondeviant. This is corroborating evidence for statements found elsewhere (Schwartz 1982; Rochester 1978). Besides the evidence that the occurrence of deviant reactions obviously depends on the irritating quality of the subject-matter discussed, the impact of the conditions (e.g. extent and type of context, dialogue partner) which may control the type of deviance differentially has not yet been systematically investigated.

It remains an open question as to which of the defined and identified failures are specific to schizophrenia; two possible candidates have been mentioned. To find out about specificity, one should compare similar dialogues of different diagnostic groups. Moreover, it is not clear whether the observed behaviour is specifically related to schizophrenia only, or also to the situation of a quite strongly structured interview. There is some anecdotal evidence from less structured dialogues which shows that uncanonical reactions are much more likely to appear in such contexts.

In tackling the problem of deciding about specificity one would create the prerequisites for the ultimate testing of hypotheses aimed at explaining the relevant observations. If one also took account of how the schizophrenic's interlocutor is affected by the former's way of speaking, one would perhaps be able to answer the question about the strategy character of the observed failures.

A last remark concerns the model as such: in its given form it cannot yet deal with bigger thematic units; but I think that an elaboration of the concept of the empty space will help to transform its actual sequential-additive form into a hierarchical one, which will be better fitted to modelling real dialogues.

Acknowledgement

I would like to thank Andreas Altorfer, Beat Brauchli and Klaus Foppa for having spent time discussing various parts of this paper.

Notes to Chapter 12

1 For a review and evaluation of this research, see Angermeyer 1978 and Hirsch 1979.

2 There are several hypotheses which could explain such a phenomenon: actual cognitive disorganization, triggered by emotion-loaded contents leading to a verbal breakdown; tapping a cognitively unstructured domain; avoidance of emotional upset by trying to digress. It is my contention, however, that a

falsification of any of these hypotheses must rest upon a detailed description of the types of deviance involved.

3 For a sophisticated elaboration of the problem of obligations of verbal requests from the *speaker's* point of view the reader is referred to Herrmann 1982: 120–6. For the present discussion, it seems sufficient to assert the obligation character of questions, and to proceed to take a closer look at the interactional effect these obligations have on a *hearer*, and how they may be identified empirically.

4 As Snell-Hornby (1984: 13–18) independently, for a different material and from a different point of view, arrives at roughly the same classification of questions, there is reason to believe that the system proposed here is not just an idiosyncratic aspect of the given dialogues.

5 Examples are drawn from the corpus of the seven interviews; the bracketed numbers refer respectively to interview, page of transcript, and instance on that page.

6 A possible criterion for the identification of an implicit V is whether, for a given *yes/no* question one can find any *wh-* question for which the given *yes/no* question is a possible answer. The objections that such a construction is possible for each question, or that for any question there are numerous possibilities, can partly be refuted by reference to contextual restrictions.

7 In this example the problem arises because of a confusion about the German personal pronouns for second person singular (*Sie* 'you') and third person plural (*sie* 'they'). One could conjecture that this is not a specific problem of the schizophrenic, but stems from the fact that he, as an originally Swiss German-speaking person, is conversing with a High German-speaking psychiatrist. But then one would have to explain why the patient does not always get confused over the possible interpretations of these homophonous forms.

References

Angermeyer, M. 1978: 20 Jahre Double Bind: Versuch einer Bilanz. *Psychiatrische Praxis* 5.

Alberti, L. and Kaesermann, M. L. 1983: Funktion des Sprachcodewechsels bei einem chronisch schizophrenen Patienten. *Sprache und Kognition* 3.

Avenarius R. 1966: Ueber Grössenwahn und Sprachverwirrtheit. *Nervenarzt* 8.

Bateson, G., Jackson, D. D., Haley, J. and Weakland, J. H. 1956: Toward a theory of schizophrenia. *Behavioral Science* 1. Translated into German in J. Habermas, D. Heinrich and N. Luhman, (eds.), *Schizophrenie und Familie*. Frankfurt; Suhrkamp, 1969.

Clark, H. H. and Haviland, S. E. 1977: Comprehension and the given-new contract. In R. O. Freedle, (ed.), *Discourse Production and Comprehension*. Norwood, NJ: Ablex.

Foppa, K. 1983: Neue Methoden zur Analyse sprachlicher Interaktion I. In H. Werbik, (ed.), *Beiträge zum Symposium 'Analyse von Handlungen: Kommunkative Prozesse und Interaktion'*. Erlangen: Institute of Psychology, University of Erlangen-Nürnburg.

— 1984: Redeabsicht und Verständigung. *Manuskripte* 23(84).

Grice, H. P. 1975: Logic and conversation. In P. Cole and J. L. Morgan, (eds.), *Syntax and Semantics*, vol. 3: *Speech Acts*. London: Academic Press.

Halliday, M. A. K. and Hasan, R. 1976: *Cohesion in English*. London: Longman.
Herrmann, T. 1982: *Sprechen und Situation*. Berlin: Springer.
Hirsch, S. R. 1979: Eltern als Verursacher der Schizophrenie. *Nervenarzt* 50.
Kaesermann, M. L. 1980: *Spracherwerb und Interaktion*. Bern: Huber.
— 1983: Form und Funktion schizophrener Sprachstörungen. *Sprache und Kognition* 3.
— 1986: Das Phänomen der sprachlichen Inkohärenz in Dialogen mit einem Schizophrenen. *Sprache und Kognition 3*.
Kaesermann, M. L., Altorfer, A. and Schultheiss, M. 1984: Die Bedeutung des nonverbalen Verhaltens in Dialogen mit einem schizophrenen Patienten. In E. Aebi, P. Hartwich and D. Stille, (eds.), *Video in Psychiatrie und Psychotherapie*. Berlin: Platane.
Leodolter, R. 1975: Gestörte Sprache oder Privatsprache: Kommunikation bei Schizophrenen. *Wiener Linguistische Gazette* 10–11.
Lorenz, M. 1961: Problems posed by schizophrenic language. In H. Vetter, (ed.), *Language Behavior in Schizophrenia*. Springfield, Illinois: Thomas.
Ruemke, H. C. 1941: Das Kernsymptom der Schizophrenie und das 'Praecoxgefüehl'. *Nederlandse Tijdschrift voor Geneeskunde*, 4516–21.
Rochester, S. R. 1978: Are language disorders in acute schizophrenia actually information processing problems? *Journal of Psychiatric Research* 14.
Schwartz, S. 1982: Is there a schizophrenic language? *Behavioral and Brain Sciences* 5.
Searle, J. R. 1969: *Speech Acts*. London: Cambridge University Press.
—1971: *Sprechakte*. Frankfurt: Suhrkamp.
Snell-Hornby, M. 1984: Statements, questions, and directives. *Pedagogical English Grammar* 6, Series B, paper 100/6.
Stephens, J. H. 1978: Long-term prognosis and followup in schizophrenia. *Schizophrenia Bulletin* 4.
Watzlawick, P. and Weakland, J. H. 1977: *The Interactional View*. New York: Norton.
—1980: *Interaktion*. Bern: Huber.
Wykes, T. and Leff, J. 1982: Disordered speech: differences between manics and schizophrenics. *Brain and Language* 15.

13 On the problem of accessibility in conversations with schizophrenic people[1]

Diek Van Bijsterveld

The central problem considered in this chapter is 'accessibility'. Before one can have a conversation at all, one has to get access to the chosen participant: one has to announce an intended conversation one way or other. This is a call for access on the level of interaction. Once the access on the level of interaction is settled, speakers will have to get access, at the level of topic, to each of the propositions which compose the topic. The vehicle for getting access is coherence; if speakers' utterances are not coherent, however, the possibility of restoring coherence is less problematic than the persistent problem of getting access, once it is clear that there *is* a problem of access. For access to be achieved, several preconditions have to be fulfilled: to get access to the interaction, one has to be available for the interaction. To get access to a topic, one has to specify sufficiently the propositions which compose the topic.

There is a problematic aspect to entering into a smooth conversation with a schizophrenic conversation partner: it is equally problematic for the schizophrenic participant himself. For instance, if a conversation partner wants a previous proposition specified, a simple sub-sequence like *what do you mean?* is rather obvious. But suppose that is not understood either, so that the reaction to the question cannot be recognized as such? The small patterns like sub-sequences are in themselves very common, but there is a risk that a nonschizophrenic conversation partner may have to use them too much. To prevent the conversation starting to irritate his partner, he will have to resort to other techniques, which might become very difficult for the schizophrenic participant to interpret as relevant.

I shall focus on four techniques which the nonschizophrenic participants use in order to fulfil the preconditions which are apparently necessary to continue the conversation. The very problem of access is displayed in the frequent use of those techniques. A conversation can then turn into a ritual dance, irrespective of what the theme or intentions of the partners are. 'Making' the conversation, keeping it going, can become the issue on the surface instead of remaining on a deeper level of what a conversation is about, as is the case usually.

Preliminaries

Several types of studies on language and schizophrenia

There is a long tradition of interest in language and schizophrenia, mainly because a disruption or a disturbance of speech has been considered an indication of a disorder of thought. The tradition of research starts more or less with the assumption that the 'language disorder' might provide information about the disorder in thought: research in this area has focused on the syntactic and semantic structures of sentences of schizophrenic speakers. The data was collected through experiments, such as Chapman *et al.*'s (1964 and 1976) multiple-choice tests on the meaning of ambiguous sentences. Tests of understanding of proverbs were carried out, as well as experiments on sensitivity to syntactic sentence structure (Carpenter 1976; Gerver 1967). All these studies found a certain degree of difference between schizophrenic groups and nonpatient groups in the carrying out of the tasks set, but none of these differences was significant enough to warrant the conclusion that there was a definite case of language disturbance which is part of the condition of schizophrenia.

In 1970 Salzinger formulated his so-called 'immediacy hypothesis', according to which schizophrenic speakers are able to connect only immediately adjoining sentences coherently, which leads to their incoherence in any longer production of text. Since then researchers have also been concentrating on monologues. These monologues have been judged on their coherence, sometimes indirectly via the Cloze procedure, where each *n*th word was systematically left out and had to be reconstructed, in some experiments by nonpatients, in others by schizophrenics (Salzinger *et al.* 1970; Salzinger and Feldman 1973; Portnoy 1973). Another method was to disconnect all sentences of a monologue and then have it reconstructed, as was done by Rutter (1979).

These researchers mostly found that it was more difficult to reconstruct monologues of schizophrenic than of nonpatient or other control groups, but there were contradictory findings as well. The results of the various types of research might well be due to the fact that 'language'—and consequently language disturbance—is considered an isolated phenomenon and not an interactional activity. Very few investigators have paid attention to the discourse problems which may arise in conversations with schizophrenic people. I shall discuss some aspects of that type of research next.

Towards an interactional approach of the language use of schizophrenic people

Rochester *et al.* (1977) emphasize that the 'listener's task' in a conversation with a schizophrenic participant is a very difficult one. This conclusion, however, is derived from the analysis of the utterances of the schizophrenic speakers, as described in Rochester and Martin's later (1979) study. Since they used judges who were not participants to point out the disrupted parts of the typed-out interviews, their study is not really an analysis of interaction. Chaika (1974) and Fromkin (1975) also concentrate on the discourse problems of the schizophrenic speaker. Chaika mentions, for instance, 'idiosyncratic' utterances as typical for schizophrenia, while Fromkin argues that such utterances are merely 'slips of the tongue', because they are not uncommon even amongst people 'working at the White House'. Both Chaika and Fromkin seem to overlook the fact that there is always the possibility of asking for clarification of an 'idiosyncracy', or anything else the addressee has not understood. Whether a participant in a conversation actually chooses to make such a request depends of course on his judgement of the relevance of that particular phase of the conversation. But if he asks for clarification he will probably find his addressee taking his own words as a 'slip of the tongue' as well, in some way or another, and not as something containing a degree of reality for him beyond that.

Surprisingly little attention has been paid to the way in which the nonschizophrenic partner reacts to the 'idiosyncratic' talk of the schizophrenic participant in the conversation. It may be conjectured that the reactions of the nonschizophrenic participant co-structure the conversation. Ideas that cross our minds during a conversation are usually not brought out; and if they are, we motivate the action with expressions like *that reminds me of*, etc. That kind of interactional activity is rarely seen in a schizophrenic participant in a conversation. But even if a speaker does not classify his 'slips of the tongue' as such, the reaction of the addressee (e.g. correction, acceptance, paying no attention) may become vital for the structure of the conversation.

An interesting point may very well be the difficult task of the listener as Rochester indicated. But in a conversation all participants are speakers and listeners as well, of course. Therefore an analysis of what happens in a conversation with a schizophrenic and a nonschizophrenic participant cannot be restricted to an analysis of the utterances of the schizophrenic speaker. For that reason I shall deal here mainly with the utterances of the nonschizophrenic participant, in order to achieve a firmer grasp on that difficult task.

Data

Two types of conversation were collected. The first one was a 'free' conversation: participants having coffee together and no instruction about a set topic that could serve as an agenda. The second type, however, did have an agenda: the nonschizophrenic participant was asked to try to stick to the topic as much as possible. This topic was something of concern in the daily life of the schizophrenic participants of which the nonschizophrenic participants did not know very much. The schizophrenic participants were all familiar with it, and therefore the information they could give was 'real' information for the nonschizophrenic partner.

It is a serious problem in the research of language and schizophrenia that results are difficult to compare, schizophrenia being rarely defined as a term (Wykes 1980). In this study, therefore, all schizophrenic participants were selected on the basis of their diagnoses according to the criteria of Diagnostic Statistical Manual III (1980). The schizophrenic participants had lived in the hospital for at least seven years. The nonschizophrenic participants were a psychiatrist and a layman. Each of the latter two had a conversation with each of the schizophrenic participants twice: once without and once with an agenda. However, since a diagnosis does not give information on the intensity of the symptoms, nor on the precise nature of those symptoms, there was an interview, and a Brief Psychiatric Rating Scale (BPRS) was completed by two psychiatrists after each conversation.

All participants were invited for the conversations. This implies that the conversations were organized, and not collected via participant observation, for instance. This method evades the methodological problem that speech should be collected in a natural setting, if a study of natural speech is to be made. On the other hand, there were good reasons for deciding against the method of participant observation: none of the schizophrenic participants was very talkative on the ward. Most of them could not be expected to take the initiative. Moreover, the most natural setting of conversations for the schizophrenic participants was via appointments. As a matter of fact, I found that it was very unusual to invite them to 'drop in and have some coffee'. The only one who accepted my invitation was rather disturbed to find that I did not have any other reason for the invitation than to chat with him, that there was no special purpose, and that I had no intention of switching on the tape. The invitation 'to have a conversation' was acceptable for an appointment, and making an appointment was the natural thing to do.

For the nonschizophrenic participants it was less natural, at least at first. I always asked some questions afterwards, e.g. whether the tape-recorder has bothered them or distracted them. Uninvited by me, they always told me whether they had experienced the conversations as being 'difficult' or 'easy'; never once when they reported that the conversation had been 'difficult' did they say that they had noticed the tape. All conversations and some of the BPRS interviews were audiotaped and transcribed.

If a conversation has at least one or two set topics, these can be considered as an external 'task' which participants can fall back on. They can use them as means of restructuring and reorganizing the conversation when it has become very difficult, and they can use them as an excuse for the difficulties they help to create. Such excuses are not available in the free conversations, except where they talk because I asked them to do so. (And indeed, in every conversation it is the nonschizophrenic and not the schizophrenic participant who falls back on this 'task' once or twice, after very long silences for instance. This, however, is not my main concern here.) I shall focus only on the free conversations in this chapter, for reasons that will become clear later, although I will refer sometimes to the BPRS interviews and the agenda conversations as well.

For symbols used in the transcriptions, see Appendix 1 to this chapter.

On accessibility

Two levels of accessibility

There is nothing new in saying that people try to be 'good' participants, and in doing so try to create a 'coherent' conversation. That does not mean that 'good' or even 'coherent' can be considered as an external standard which requires all kinds of rules to be followed. It does mean that there must be an 'internal' standard, that is to say internal for each conversation, which leads to the experience by participants of a conversation as 'good' or not.

The fragments that will be discussed in this chapter are all parts of conversations which were evaluated, as subsequent reports showed, as 'difficult' or 'impossible'. This has to do with accessibility as a problem in connection with structuring the conversation. I shall discriminate here between a level of interaction and a level of topic. In the reality of a conversation there is no such sharp distinction, of course.

Before one can have a conversation at all, one has to get access to the chosen participant; one has to announce an intended conversation one way or another; one has to make sure that the intended partner is not involved in some other activity, for instance. This is a call for access on the level of interaction. Once the access on the level of interaction is settled, speakers will have to get access, at the level of topic, to each of the propositions which compose a topic.

This is a more complicated problem, because this problem involves the *degree* of access, while the problem of access on the level of interaction is not a matter of more or less. Usually there is no 'degree of interaction'. Later on I shall show, however, how difficult the problem of access on the level of interaction can become for a nonschizophrenic participant with a schizophrenic partner.

Frame incongruence

Accessibility at the topic level is related to differences in frame of reference of participants. 'Frame of reference' alludes to the knowledge and beliefs about the world which people have. A speaker reveals his frame of reality with any proposition. Let us assume a speaker said: *I dreamed I was the emperor of China*. He would reveal that it was a dream, and that, according to his frame of reality, one can very well dream of being emperor of China. He also shows the assumption that his addressee may have dreams in which he can be anything that he could not be in 'reality'. If his addressee answers: *Well, tell you what, I am the emperor of China*, it would present the first speaker with the problem of how to go on, now that his supposedly congruent frame of reality was not quite so congruent after all. Whatever he does it will be related to the incongruence of frame of reference: he can only opt for a direct or a more indirect way of talking about it.

A speaker can, for instance, decide to accept frame incongruence fully, as in the next fragment from a BPRS interview between a psychiatrist and a schizophrenic man who often mentions that he is the emperor of China:

Psychiatrist: How are things going on in the world, you know, I can't keep up with that,

Patient: Well, there is a lot of rumour in China, finance doesn't work well. I want to have my passport.

The psychiatrist uses the presupposed inaccessibility of the patient's frame of reference as a motivation for his question. He thus establishes the inaccessibility in an indirect way, as if it is a well known fact of life and need not necessarily be an insurmountable problem of incongruence of frames of reference. It is structured in such a way that it need not become the focus of the discussion. The psychiatrist's question might just as well have been about a subject in a paper he had not yet read about. At the same time the question suggests the inaccessibility to a certain degree: he may not need total access. Now this may be because this fragment stems from an interview that was to be about complaints of the schizophrenic participant. And, as the emperor of China does not complain about being the emperor of China, this may have functioned as 'small talk', at least at this point of the conversation.

The next fragment shows a different approach:[2]

A: What of China?
B: I'm *em*peror of China

Here, A's question poses the frame incongruence: apparently A tries to get access to B's frame, demonstrating this incongruence in a very direct way at the same time.

Whatever form or strategy a speaker uses, once the fact of frame incongruence has been established—no matter the degree of directness—he has to cope with it. The problem then is, in which way and at what level the problem of access is handled in conversations that were subsequently reported as difficult by the nonschizophrenic speaker.

Preconditions

In interaction, each participant shows a preference for a certain reaction of his partner in his utterance. Whether the given reaction was indeed in accordance with the preference of the previous speaker is for him to demonstrate in his next turn. The activity of making a conversation is an activity of interpreting and at the same time of showing a preference in doing so (Franck 1979). One cannot always know or give the preferred reaction, so there may be a delay (Pomerantz 1978) before it is forthcoming. Weijdema *et al.* (1980) call such a delay in the main sequence of turns a sub-sequence. They are interested in sub-sequences in particular because sub-sequential talk shows explicitly the preconditions for a preferred reaction that otherwise would have been fulfilled. They formulate different classes of preconditions which were not fulfilled at the moment of the sub-sequence. I shall mention only those that are of some importance for the fragments to be discussed.

The first precondition, then, is the precondition of availability:

A: Could you spare me a minute?
sub-sequence { B: Just a second, have to get this fixed first
A: Okay, I'll wait }
B: All right then, what can I do for you?

B's initiative for the sub-sequence demonstrates that the precondition of availability is not fulfilled on his part. After the delay, the problem of getting access for A on the level of interaction is solved. Another precondition concerns the proposition of the utterance. What has been said and was not understood can be asked about; a participant can demonstrate the need for more detailed specification of his partner's proposition that way. This precondition is 'relative', in Weijdema *et al.*'s term, which means that it does not concern each and every utterance, but depends on the knowledge of the participants. On the other hand Weijdema *et al.* distinguish 'absolute' preconditions, which concern any utterance, like the precondition of availability mentioned above, and the precondition of audibility.

This last is seen in the next fragment from one of the free conversations (see also p. 313).

B: (...) then I will catch fish for the food—for the money, and also—ehm feast the eyes
sub-sequence { A: ice?
B: feast the eyes }
A: feast the *eyes*, *yes*, (1) yes (1), well, that's gr*ea*t, really!

A starts the sub-sequence *ice*? and shows that *ice?* functions as a preference to fulfil the precondition of audibility, as can be seen from A's next turn: A confirms that the precondition has indeed been fulfilled by means of the repetition of B's former reaction. It can also be seen in this fragment that, after the precondition has been fulfilled by B, there is still a problem to be solved. It is still not quite easy for A to go on.

Sympathizers

The picture presented so far shows that participants in a conversation have to get access, both on the level of interaction and on the level of topic. To warrant access, preconditions have to be fulfilled: of concern here are the absolute preconditions of audibility and—on the level of interaction—the precondition of availability; on the level of topic the precondition of proposition/specification.

The problem of getting access, then, is the problem of trying to get these preconditions fulfilled. As can be seen in the fragment above, this may be not at all easy. I shall now discuss four techniques which the nonschizophrenic participants used as a preface for fulfilling a precondition. I call them 'sympathizers':
Interactive Repetitions: these are reactions, in which (part of) the former utterance is repeated literally;
Minimal Responses, like *hm*, *yes*: often functioning as continuers in a conversation;
Response Cries: they are 'cries' of sympathetic identification with what has been said.
Evaluations: they evaluate the partner's utterance(s) in such a way that they evaluate the emotion of what has been said.

Analysis

Four techniques of sympathizing

First I shall discuss the four techniques separately, with the aid of some fragments from the free conversations which were reported afterwards as 'difficult' or even 'impossible to keep going'. In the fragments, A is the nonschizophrenic speaker, B the schizophrenic participant. All fragments are excerpts from different conversations. Having discussed the techniques, I shall turn to longer fragments in which these four techniques of sympathizing function as options to get access at different levels: in one fragment, access to interaction is the main object (hence the precondition of availability); in the other, it is the access to the topic which is the main object (hence the precondition of proposition/specification). The shorter fragments were transcribed using 'play notation'; the longer ones using 'partiture notation', because overlaps and pauses are crucial here.

In the free conversations there is talk about daily life in the hospital: about food, as in fragments 1 and 4, about the use—and shortage—of money, and about how to go back to 'society'. In fragment 1, the schizophrenic speaker first initiates the topic 'food in the hospital', and then says:

(1)

	1	B:	and I invested. (*softly*) it must have been 6000 guilders
	2	A:	how much?
	3	B:	8000 guilders fish
→	4	A:	g*ee*! (.) what do you have with fish?
	5	B:	didn't get any!
	6	A:	what do you have with fish, did you do something with fi=
	7	B:	=invested!
	8	A:	yes,

(2)

	1	B:	they're after my money
→	2	A:	yes
	3	B:	have to buy clothes, after all
→	4	A:	sure, sure, yeah

(3)

	1	B:	well, I don't mean those 9 y*ea*rs for the cure, what we are doing
→	2	A:	no?
		B:	*now*
→	3	A:	what we are doing *now* (.) yeah yeah (1) all the same for the cure again (.) hm
	4	B:	well, all the same for the cure, but very m=quite a lot
→	5	A:	yes
	6	B:	(*laughing*) I never went through so much! such a lot!
→	7	A:	(*laughing*) god! you can say that again!
	8	B:	ehm-*YES*, never went through so much!
→	9	A:	gee! god! well, that's quite—ehm quite a good sign isn't it,
	10	B:	yes I feel it=feel it too, you know
→	11	A:	*yes*. you feel it too.

(4)

	1	B:	and then I will sail all the seas of the world, then I will catch
	2		fish for the food=for the money, and also—ehm feast the eyes
	3	A:	ice?
	4	B:	feast the eyes
→	5	A:	feast the *e*yes, y*e*s, (1) yes (1) well, that's gr*e*at, really! a great
→	6		plan!

Interactive repetitions. According to Weijdema *et al.* (1982) Interactive Repetitions (IR) are a kind of sub-sequence: they are repetitions of what the partner said. They can have various functions, but one of them is always 'acceptance' when the intonation is affirmative, as in: fragment 3, line 3: what we are doing *now*; fragment 3, line 11: *yes*, you feel it too; fragment 4, line 5: feast the *eyes*, *yes*.

Besides 'acceptance', there is the interactional function of taking the turn and, because there is no 'real' topical contribution, the IR functions as continuer, displaying a delay of a possible topical contribution. Line 5 in fragment 4 and line 3 in fragment 3 illustrate the point:

A: feast the *eyes*, yes, (1) yes (1), well, that's gr*ea*t, really! a great plan!

A: what we are doing *now* (1) yeah yeah (1) all the same for the cure again. (.) hm

The short silences after the IRs are not taken up by the schizophrenic speakers; they are taken up by the nonschizophrenic participants via the *yes* and *yeah yeah*. Then there is a short silence again in which the nonschizophrenic participant in both cases tries to hand the next turn to the schizophrenic speaker, and again the latter does not respond, so the former has to continue himself. At that particular moment there does not seem to be a possibility of continuing on the topical level for either participant. (Note that in these fragments all participants are different, so it is not a matter of personal style.)

Even if there can be acceptance of *feast the eyes*, now that the precondition of audibility is fulfilled, at least some precondition on the proposition has not been fulfilled in fragment 4, line 5. In fragment 3, line 4, A continues after the second short silence with a second IR which was the other component of B's former utterance:

B: well, I don't mean those 9 y*ea*rs for the cure, what we are doing *now*
A: no? what we are doing *now* (.) yeah yeah (1) all the same for the cure again (.) hm
IR1 a b IR2 a b

After this second (partial) IR a short silence (a) follows and a minimal continuer (b) as well; so we can see here this small pattern even within the turn.

In my opinion the use of IR as a continuer on the level of interactional organization functions as a technique of trying to get access to the partner's topic.

Minimal responses. What is usually called a minimal response, e.g. *yes, huhuh, hm,* is a very difficult thing to describe. Its precise functions are not at all easy to grasp. I want to distinguish here between those that are merely continuers and those that are in a way sympathizers; in other words, between those that have a clear interactional function and those that have the interactional function of organizing the present speaker's turn, mixed with an empathic agreement with what has been said.

fragment 2, line 2: yes
fragment 2, line 4: sure, sure *yeah*
fragment 3, line 3: (.) yeah yeah (1)
fragment 5, line 5: feast the *e*yes, y*e*s (1)

As I mentioned above, the turn after the short silence is taken by the nonschizophrenic participant; the intonation, however, is such that the *yeah, yes* and the somewhat prolonged *yeah* could also function as repetitions of A's own display of acceptance. So, by emphasizing the acceptance component of the conversation at this point, this response also functions as an emphasis on continuing. Since, after these minimal responses, there is that short silence again, this silence may show that at least the nonschizophrenic participant's urge to continue is not shared by the other, schizophrenic, participant.

Response cries. I borrow this term from Goffman (1981). He describes the function of response cries, provided they are not self-talk but meant for someone else, as follows: 'as it were out of sympathetic identification, and as a sign of fully following the exposition'. Examples are:

fragment 1, line 4: g*ee*!
fragment 2, line 4: sure, sure
fragment 3, line 7: god! you can say that again!
fragment 3, line 9: gee! god!
fragment 4, line 5: that's gr*ea*t, really!

There is something quite different in these response cries, though. Consider Goodwin's (1984) remarks on them: they seem to function as prefaces to assessments. Being interested in assessments, Goodwin found that some of them were what Goffman called response cries, displaying empathy. In the short list above, all the utterances could be like the ones Goodwin described as prefaces.

But if we return to the short fragments, the same does not apply. They function differently. Compare for instance fragment 1, line 4:

A: gee! (.) what do you have with fish?

Here, after the short silence which demonstrates that the response cry also functions as a continuer, the nonschizophrenic participant asks for proposition specification contradicting his previous empathy. Empathy presupposes emotional access to what has been said. But how can one show this, if there is this proposition one did not quite understand? That there is some lack of understanding can be seen from what follows after the short silence: *what do you have with fish?*.

Atkinson and Heritage (1984) found in their material, provided by social workers who visited families, that displaying empathy was used by social workers to ask questions, for instance, about how things were going in the family. Atkinson and Heritage argue that there is a contradictory element in using empathy while performing an institutional activity.

In the fragments above, however, there was no such institutional job to be done. There was not even an external agenda in these free conversations, apart from the activity of having a conversation. So response cries in this material could not be used for closing a previous topic, or for closing *and* prefacing an 'institutional' topic. The topic at hand is all there is for the participants, and being sympathetic will not solve the problem of (in)accessibility. In displaying this kind of empathy (even if the intonation is very sympathetic), which is then followed by a question which reveals a lack of understanding, one only demonstrates more clearly the problem of inaccessibility.

Evaluations. As I mentioned above, speakers can evaluate their partner's utterance in such a way that they judge the emotional value of what has been said:

fragment 3, line 9:

8 B: ehm—yes, never went through so much!
9 A: gee! god! well, *that's quite—ehm quite a good sign isn't it*

fragment 4, lines 5–6:

5 A: feast the *e*yes, y*e*s, (1) yes (1) well, that's gr*ea*t, really! *a great plan*!

Those evaluations are a kind of IR, in that they repeat part of what was said; but the repetition is rather the interpreted emotional 'colour', so that it shows the partner how the emotional value of his utterance has been interpreted. In that respect, evaluations have to do with accessibility. Unlike response cries, where this emotional interpretation is vague, an evaluation gives a more explicit interpretation. And, like response cries, evaluation is a very delicate technique, because it means interpreting part of something that has been said while the exact proposition was not clear. In that way all three techniques are different strategies of attempting to get the precondition of proposition/specification fulfilled. Consequently these techniques are techniques of getting access to a topic; frame incongruence is displayed in the process. Because of the humouring effect of the sympathizers, there seems to be a repair function at the level of interaction as well. Even if the preferred reaction is not given by the schizophrenic partner, the interactional level must be guarded by the nonschizophrenic participant.

I now want to turn to two longer fragments, which quite aptly show how the struggle for access is lost. In the first fragment, the non-schizophrenic participant attempts to gain access at the level of interaction; in the second, the frequent use of sympathizers does not solve the problem of access at the level of the topic.

Inaccessibility at the level of interaction. The following fragment is representative of the whole conversation, although the conversation itself is not representative of the material I have; after about ten minutes the nonschizophrenic participant commented that 'it was impossible to go on'. The fragment stems from the first part of the conversation; B speaks in a very slow and sad voice:

(5)

1 B: they are grouching you better be in Arnhem
2 A: oh no you don't like that

3 B:
4 A A*rn*hem. how=what of Arnhem? (2) did you live in Arnhem, (4) have you *been*

5 B: ((*whispers*)) grouching too much grouching
6 A: in Arnhem? (2) but then *you*'re

7 B: ((*whispers*)) grouching grouching grouching
8 A: not grouching, are you? what are they speaking

9 B: ((*whispers*)) grouching grouching grouching((coughs)) (2) grouching
10 A: of, those grouchers

11 B: ((*whispers*)) grouching
12 A: are they still grouching?

13 B: ((*whispers*)) grouching grouching grouching
14 A: and do you grouch back at them?

15 B: ((*whispers*)) grouching grouching ((*coughs*))
16 A: or don't you (2)hm? (2)

17 B: ((*whispers*)) grouching grouching grouching
18 A: ((*soft voice*)) stop *that grouching stop that grouch*ing

19 B: ((*whispers*)) grouching
20 A: ((*soft voice*)) *do stop that grouch*ing (2)

21 B: ((*normal voice*)) what do you say
22 A: ((*normal voice*)) is it inside is it inside (2) yes?

23 B: ((*normal voice*)) they are grouching too much is not nice
24 A: ((*normal voice*)) uhuh *no*, certain-

25 B: ((*normal voice*)) food is alright
26 A ((*normal voice*))ly not! food is alright (1)yes(1)

27 B: ((*whispers*)) grouching too much
28 A: ((*normal voice*))what did you have for dinner to*day*

29 B: ((*whispers*))grouching
30 A: ((*normal voice*)) and they do grouch about the food, (3)

31 B: ((*whispers*)) grouching grouching
32 A: ((*normal voice*)) and do they listen (2) ((*soft voice*)*stop*

33 B: ((*whispers*)) grouch
34 A: that *grouch*ing (3) ((*normal voice*))hm? only about the food

35 B: ((*whispers*))grouching grouching

Something remarkable happens here with respect to the repetitions. A first tries to get access to the topic B initiates in line 1; after the evaluation *oh no you don't like that*, A defines that topic: Arnhem. The repeated questions about the possible topic:

line 4: how=what of Arnhem?
line 4: did you live in Arnhem
line 6: have you *been* in Arnhem?

are not answered by B; B does not fill the slots of the silences until after the last question, with the whispered *grouching too much grouching* (line 5).

B continues to whisper *grouching*, which is then treated as a next possible topic by A:

line 8:	but then *you*'re not grouching are you?
lines 8, 10:	what are they speaking of, those grouchers
line 12:	are they still grouching?
line 14:	and do you grouch back at them?
line 16:	or don't you

Perhaps because there are no silences as an answer to A's questions, A can ask more questions about 'grouching'; of course B does not really answer A, but the repeated 'grouching' does not lead to a change of topic for A either. It does change, however, the mood of A's utterances; in line 18, A initiates the imperative '*stop that grouching*' in a low voice, showing that:

(1) A concludes that B is involved in some other conversation, belonging to his own world;
(2) A tries to get access to B's 'conversation';
(3) A's flexibility of 'voice' with changes from a low voice for B's own conversation to a normal voice for the preferred conversation demonstrates the different types of conversation A is prepared to initiate on the level of interaction.
(4) A displays B's inaccessibility as a participant in the conversation preferred by A;

For a short moment A appears to be successful in getting access to B's availability for interaction:

line 22: A:	is it inside,
line 21: B:	what do you say?
line 22: A:	is it inside?( ) yes?
line 23: B:	they are grouching too much
line 24: A:	uhuh
line 23: B:	is not nice
line 24: A:	*no*, certainly not!
line 25: B:	food is alright
line 26: A:	food is alright. (1)yes (1) what did you have for dinner to*day*
line 29: B:	(*whispers*) grouching

In line 21, B demonstrates that for him the precondition of audibility was not fulfilled, implying that he was available for A as a participant in the conversation at that moment. Also, until line 29 he utters *grouching* in a normal voice, although of course that does not imply 'availability' in itself.

More importantly, it seems to me, in this small part of the conversation A and B are taking turns: a practical problem with this audiotape is that, in the parts where B is whispering and A is not, I am not quite sure whether B stops whispering while A is talking. If B continues whispering while A takes his turns, then B does not show any awareness of it: he does not prevent A from turn-taking, nor does he give A the turn during his rhythmic *grouching grouching*. In this part of the conversation, however, A and B could indeed be involved in the *shared* activity of turn-taking.

On the other hand, B's answer to A's question *is it inside?* is not necessarily a display of availability. In fact, A's question could be added to the small list of questions about the topic 'grouching' mentioned above, because this time A asks about the location of the 'grouching'. A returns to that topic, this time demonstrating more explicitly a frame-incongruence with B: asking *but you're not grouching, are you* (line 8) does not locate the 'grouchers' as possibly existing 'inside' B, while the question *is it inside?* (line 22) does. B's answer is not a specific reply to the question; B does not say that he has problems with grouchers that day or something like that, which could be interpreted as a phenomenon that is inaccessible for A *and* that B knows that. B's *they are grouching too much* reveals A's question as inaccessible for him. For B there does not seem to be a difference between 'Arnhem', 'grouching' and 'food' in accessibility for A.

For A, however, there is a difference between these topics. Compare how A handles the possible topics 'Arnhem' and 'food':

(1) B: they are grouching
A: oh no you don't like that
B: better be in Arnhem

A: *Arn*hem.how what of Arnhem

(2) B: they are grouching too much
A: uhuh
B: is not nice
A: *no*, certainly not!
B: food is alright
A: food is alright (1)yes(1) what did you have for dinner to*day*

A reacts at first with a sympathizer in both cases: in (1) with the evaluation of B's sad mood, in (2) with a minimal response. In (1) A repeats *Arnhem* (no reaction to the wish of B to be there) so the topic is chosen immediately. In (2) there is first a response cry (I don't think A has any other choice), but then after the IR *food is alright* there is the pattern I discussed on p. 314 before A asks a question about 'food'. So, in the second fragment there is more sympathizing on A's part as a preface to a topical question. What happened in between apparently urges A to use those sympathizers. They do not really work though: B starts whispering again, and consequently again presents A with the problem of getting access. No longer asking questions, A then intermingles—in the affirmative—all topics selected earlier: *and they do grouch about the food* (line 30); *only about the food* (line 34). A interchanges this with the repetition of the imperative *stop the grouching.*

None of A's strategies leads to access on the level of interaction. Throughout the conversation, A demonstrates that the precondition of availability was not fulfilled. A tries to get that precondition fulfilled by using sympathizing techniques and the imperative to get B out of his saddening involvement with the grouchers. B, being so intensely occupied, does not seem to notice A as a participant, except for *what do you say*, as in line 21, which recurs in the course of the conversation. What B shows is an intensive self-repetition and evaluation of his own words, e.g. *it is not nice* (line 22)—be it self-talk or hallucinations; that is not the point here—reported to A in a very sad voice. Indeed, it is not even certain that A is considered as a participant at all.

This type of talk by someone who is hardly aware of his partner, nor consequently of his partner's problem of access, is very striking. Usually, however, the precondition of availability is fulfilled—explicitly or implicitly—at the beginning of the conversation. If this is not the case, participants will indicate that they are temporarily not available. At the beginning of this paragraph I mentioned that the conversation from which the fragment discussed above stems is exceptional in my material. In other conversations there are shorter sections where access on the level of interaction is the problem; this conversation is exceptional at the point that, *throughout* the conversation, accessibility on the level of interaction is the problem of the nonschizophrenic participant.

Inaccessibility at the level of topic. Once the precondition of availability is fulfilled, there is no problem of accessibility for the overall activity of being conversation partners. However, the 'next' problem of accessibility can be getting access to the participant's frame. This problem of access can be demonstrated by showing that the precondition of proposition specification is not fulfilled. And when the partner does not fulfil that precondition, as happens in the next fragment, the use of the whole register of sympathizing techniques can display the struggle for access on that level.

In the next fragment B (who could be called psychotic here) says he is the emperor of China, and as an emperor had had chestnut trees planted. The fragment is not from the beginning of the conversation; immediately before this, B has told A where he had had chestnut trees planted, namely in Europe and all Mediterranean countries:

(6)

1 B: and—ehm I said I am Albert Peter Bernards
2 A: why exactly chestnut trees?
3 B: emperor of China! I order to plant them! in succession of(.)
4 A: yeah
5 B: Alexander the Great in succession of Napoleon in succession
6 A: *Hm*hm yes
7 B: of(.) Caesar all those all those gardens
8 A: I *see* those great generals
9 B: ordered to lay out gardens
10 A: *oo*h I see yeah (1) why exactly chestnut trees
11 B: ch*e*stnut trees, they're
12 A: is there something the matter with chestnuts?
13 B: delicious! delicious
14 A: well, *ye*s, I like them but I could think of
15 B: I do have other
16 A: something else as well, oranges, mandarins,
17 B: plantations but I, chestnut trees, how do I know,
18 A: I see hm. you like
19 B: (6)as far as in China planted chestnuts
20 A: chestnuts most (.)hm *ye*s, sure I can see that, yeah
21 B: and silk trees I am emperor of China
22 A: uhuh (.) what of China? *em*peror of China

In line 3 B says that he is the emperor of China, and as an emperor had had chestnut trees planted. A's minimal response *yeah* in line 4 has a dual function here: on the one hand it functions as a sympathizer, on the other it functions as an apparently tentative (line 22) acceptance of B's former proposition that he is indeed the emperor of China. Of course A must be well aware of the fact that it is impossible to live in a psychiatric hospital and be the emperor of China as well; so, in accepting, A accepts B's frame in which he, as someone living in the hospital, proposes himself as the emperor of China. That is to say: in accepting, A considers the matter as something which can be talked about, requiring some further questions to be answered before it might be accessible.

One of those questions, then, is *why exactly chestnut trees?*. The formulation is delicate in terms of frame difference: the question could be addressed to someone whose job it is to plant trees in a garden. B, disregarding this completely, continues, which apparently leads A to sympathizing as a preface to the repetition of the question:

2 A: why exactly chestnut trees
4 A: yeah
6 A: *Hm*hm
6 A: yes
8 A: I *see*
8 A: those great generals
10 A: *oh* I see, yeah(1) why exactly chestnut trees

This fragment contains a series of sympathizers: the minimal response *yeah* in line 4, another minimal response in line 6, a response cry in line 8, an IR in line 8 and, in lines 8–10 the completion of the small pattern mentioned above (pp. 314, 321): IR + *yeah* + (1).

The insertion of *oh*, marking a new element in the conversation (Heritage 1984) immediately followed by the response cry *I see*, may very well be due to the fact that the IR was not the right one:

B: in succession of! Alexander the Great
A: *Hm*hm
B: in succession of Napoleon
A: yes
B: in succession of (.) Caesar!
A: I *see*
B: all those all those gardens
→ A: those great generals
B: gave orders to lay out gardens
A: *oh*, I see, yeah (1) why exactly chestnut trees

Having asked the question *why exactly chestnut trees?* for the second time, A gets an answer:

10 A: why exactly chestnut trees,
11 B: chestnut trees
12 A: is there something the matter with chestnuts?

B's IR *chestnut trees* does not function as a continuer here: by stressing his reaction, B indicates that he interprets A's question as one he cannot answer, as an irrelevant one.

A then specifies the question, demonstrating frame incongruence more directly: it is quite unusual to ask someone whose job it is to plant trees in a garden, for instance, if 'there is something the matter with chestnuts'. A asks quite straightforwardly for a specification of a possible special, perhaps symbolic, meaning of 'chestnuts' for B, revealing his own frame of reference; the awareness of the fact that it is impossible that B should have done such a job. Here A demonstrates the problem of getting access.

Now that A has displayed the problem of accessibility, frame incongruence becomes more explicit as well:

12 A: is there something the matter with chestnuts?
13 B: delicious!
14 A: well, *yes*, I like them
13 B: delicious
14 A: but I could think of something else as well, oranges, mandarins
15 B: I do have other plantations
16 A: I see
15 B: but I, chestnut trees, how do I know
18 A: hm.you like chestnuts most(.) hm (6)

B's reaction *delicious* is his answer to A; he is prepared to *have other plantations*, but apparently he cannot do much with A's problem: *how do I know*. A's sympathizing (lines 14,16) does not get the precondition of proposition specification fulfilled for A.

After A's minimal response and the evaluation in l. 18, there is a very long silence, of six seconds, which also indicates the impossibility of continuing the topic. As soon as B takes the turn, the same pattern is repeated:

19 B: as far as in China
20 A: yes, sure I can see that, yeah
19 B: planted chestnuts and silk trees
22 A: uhuh (.) what of China?
21 B: I am emperor of China
22 A: *em*peror of China

A uses sympathizers—minimal responses, response cries (line 20). The minimal response in line 22 is a preface to the next question asking for proposition specification: *what of China?*. This question is contradicted by the response cry: *sure I can see that*, suggesting that it was apparently accessible to A that the chestnut trees were planted *as far as in China*. B, who has already announced himself as the emperor of China, repeats this (line 21). A's IR *emperor of China* can only function as sympathizer, and not as an instance of access to the topic. This repeated pattern of using sympathizers as a preface to questions about proposition specification demonstrates the problem of getting access at the level of topic.

Concluding remarks

The fragments discussed were all taken from the 'free' conversations, in which the job was to talk, not necessarily about a specific topic. So in fact the job was to keep the conversation going. Therefore the frequent use of the four techniques of sympathizing on which I have focused in this chapter could be considered as an artificiality resulting from this method. This, however, is by no means a unique case: it is what happens in any first contact. When potential participants in a conversation meet, they will try to get their conversation 'going', otherwise they cannot demonstrate that they are potential participants.

Especially in conversations without an agenda, the problem of access leads beyond the point where speakers usually give up. The task of the nonschizophrenic participants in these conversations is an extremely difficult one: to be a 'good' participant and to have a 'good' conversation they had to make frequent use of sympathizers as a preface to getting preconditions fulfilled: without these, there is no access. In many cases the frequency of this pattern did not solve the problem of access, but on the contrary made the problem more explicit; the sympathizing became less 'sincere' and more humouring. The free conversations turned out to be more difficult than the agenda conversations; that is to say, after the free conversations, it happened more frequently that the nonschizophrenic participant commented that it had been 'difficult'. Of course there are also fragments in these conversations where there is no demonstration of a problem of access. This may be due to the fact that the topic was 'known' to both participants in some way, or, to put it differently, that a topic discussed did not reveal a frame incongruence, although a specific proposition might need specification.

Moreover, the four techniques described are not only prefaces to getting preconditions fulfilled in order to get access, but they are the ones that could become 'humouring' and as such display a certain delicacy on the part of the speaker who wants to continue the conversation. In focusing on the techniques of the nonschizophrenic participants, I wanted to demonstrate that it is possible to formulate an important problem concerned with talking with schizophrenic speakers. This problem may be due to some 'language disorder' on the part of the schizophrenic participant, but concentrating only on *his* specific contributions in a conversation does not solve the whole problem. It is not so much that there is something specifically the matter with 'schizophrenic language', but that there is something 'schizophrenic' in talking with schizophrenic people.

Of course the four techniques of sympathizing are used in other conversations as well. Sympathizing is quite common in conversations among friends, for instance. but then it is a shared activity, in which there is some apparent reaction to the sympathizer, be it an expression of agreement or refusal (as in: *o my god, awful/are you kidding?*) (Goodwin, 1984). Since no specific reaction to sympathizers is used by the schizophrenic participants, they are obviously regarded as 'not the right' sympathizers or as no sympathizers at all. Since that which does *not* happen, i.e. a reaction to the sympathizer, can be interpreted as 'something should have happened', the inconclusiveness of the situation can even be due to the repetition of the sympathizers. The fact that the schizophrenic participants never use sympathizers in the function described above does not mean that they should have done so, in the sense that it would have been 'normal' to do so, for neglecting—which is what they do—is a very 'normal' strategy.

The overall problem of conversations with schizophrenic people is, rather, that the use of 'normal' techniques by schizophrenic participants poses so many problems to 'normal' participants.

Notes to Chapter 13

1 The research discussed in this chapter is supported by the Foundation for Linguistic Research, which is funded by ZWO, the Netherlands organisation for the advancement of pure research.
The author wishes to thank Erica Huls, Martha Komter, S. C. Dik, J. Th. P. M. Dröes, J. G. Goekoop and H. G. M. Rooymans for their valuable comments on this part of the research or on an earlier draft of this chapter.

2 The translation of original fragments is always a delicate and problematic matter, and always imprecise. The specific problems of the fragments discussed in this paper are the translation of the 'sympathizers' like *gee, yeah, yes*, etc. In fragment 6, the problem is that the Dutch word *kastanjes* means both 'chestnut trees' and 'chestnuts'. The most 'coherent' translation was chosen: *kastanjes* connected with 'planted' was translated to 'chestnut trees', and connected with 'delicious' to 'chestnuts'. The association in Dutch is less direct than in the translation.

References

Atkinson, J. M. and Heritage, J. C. (eds.) 1984: *Structures of Social Action*. Cambridge: Polity Press.

Carpenter, M. D. 1976: Sensitivity to syntactic structure: good versus poor premorbid schizophrenics. *Journal of Abnormal Psychology* 85(1).

Chaika, E. 1974: A linguist looks at schizophrenic language. *Brain and Language* 1.

Chapman, L. J., Chapman, J. and Miller, G. 1964: A theory of verbal behaviour in schizophrenia. In B. A. Maher (ed.), *Progress in Experimental Personality Research*, vol. 1.

Franck, D. M. L. 1979: *Grammatik und Konversation*. Unpublished dissertation, University of Amsterdam.

Fromkin, V. A. 1975: A linguist looks at 'A linguist looks at schizophrenic language'. *Brain and Language* 2.

Gerver, D. 1967: Linguistic rules and the perception and recall of speech by schizophrenic patients. *British Journal of Social and Clinical Psychology* 6.

Goffman, E. 1981: *Forms of Talk*. Oxford: Blackwell.

Goodwin, C. 1984: Prefaces to assessments. Contribution to the International and Multidisciplinary Conference on Interaction and Language Use, British Sociological Association of Language Study Group, Plymouth.

Heritage, J. C. 1984: A change of state token and aspects of its sequential placement. In J. M. Atkinson and J. C. Heritage (eds), *Structures of Social Action*. Cambridge: Polity Press.

Maher, B. A. (ed.) 1964: *Progress in Experimental Personality Research*, vol. 1. New York.

Pomerantz, A. 1978: Compliment responses: notes on the cooperation of multiple constraints. In J. Scheinkein, (ed.), *Studies in the Organization of Conversational Interaction*. New York: Academic.

Portnoy, S. 1973: A comparison of oral and written verbal behavior. In K. Salzinger and R. S. Feldman (ed.), *Studies in Verbal Behavior: An Empirical Approach*.

Rochester, S. R., Martin, J. R. and Thurston, S. 1977: Thought-process disorder in schizophrenia: the listener's task. *Brain and Language* 4.

Rochester, S. R. and Martin, J. R. 1979: *Crazy Talk: A Study of the Discourse of Schizophrenic Speakers*. New York: Plenum.

Rutter, D. R. 1979: The reconstruction of schizophrenic speech. *British Journal of Psychology* 134.

Salzinger, K., Portnoy, S., Pisioni, D. B. and Feldman, R. S. 1970: The immediacy hypothesis and response-produced stimuli in schizophrenic speech. *Journal of Abnormal Psychology* 76.

Salzinger, K. and Feldman, R. S. (eds.) 1973: *Studies in Verbal Behavior: An Empirical Approach*. New York:

Weijdema, W., Dik, S., Oehlen, M., Dubber, C. and de Blauw, A. 1982: *Strukturen in verbale interaktie*. Muiderberg: Continho.

Wykes, T. 1980: Editorial language and schizophrenia. *Psychological Medicine* 10.

Appendix 1 Symbols used in the transcription of conversational fragments

(These symbols are adapted from those which are commonly in use for conversational analysis.)

(1) a.A:what do you have with fish, did you do something with fish=
B: =invested!
b.B:(...)and then I will catch fish for the food=for the money

The = signs at the end of one speaker's utterance and at the beginning of the next speaker's indicates that there is no discernible interval between the first speaker finishing and the next starting, but that the next did not actually overlap. When this sign occurs between the words of one speaker, it similarly indicates no interval between these words.

(2) B: ((*whispers*)) grouching (2) ((*coughs*))
A: hm you like chestnuts most (.) hm

Double brackets indicates aspects of the conversation which are not verbalizations. Single brackets are used for silences. A short gap between turns or within a single speaker's turn (i.e. less than a second) is indicated by a dot inside brackets. A number inside brackets indicates, in seconds, the duration of a pause in speech.

(3) A: *Arn*hem. how=what of Arnhem? (2) did you live in Arnhem,

Intonation patterns are indicated as follows: a question-mark indicates upward intonation on the whole preceding word. Commas indicate upward intonation at the end of the word. A dot indicates a downward intonation. Italics are used to indicate stress on (part of) a word.

(4) → A: sure, sure, yeah

An arrow indicates a line to be discussed.

Appendix 2 Original fragments

(1)
1 B: terwijl ik geïnvesteerd had (zacht) 't was 6000 gulden
2 A: hoeveel?
3 B: 8000 gulden vis
4 A: *jee*tje zeg! (.) heb je wat met vis?
5 B: niks gekregen!
6 A: heb je wat met vis of zo, heb je wat met vis ge=
7 B: =geïnvesteerd!
8 A: ja,

(2)

1 B: ze willen mijn geld hebben
2 A: ja,
3 B: 'k moet toch kleren ook kopen,
4 A: tuurlijk tuurlijk, nee

(3)

1 B: nou, die negen jaar dat bedoel ik niet voor de genezing,
2 A: nee?
3 B: wat we n*u* doen
4 A: wat we n*u* doen(.) ja ja (1) toch ook weer voor de genezing (.) hm
5 B: nou, ook voor de genezing, maar heel v=heel *wat*
6 A: ja,
7 B: ((*lachend*)) d'had ik d'had ik nog wat nooit zoveel meegemaakt!
8 A: ((*lachend*)) goh! nou!
9 B: ((*laehend*)) eh-j*a*, nog nooit meegemaakt zoveel!
10 A: nee, nou dat is helemaal eh helemaal en goed teken hè?
11 B: ja, ik voel 't voel 't ook hè,
12 A: j*a*, je voelt 't ook.

(4)

1 B: en dan ga ik de wereldzeeën bevaren, dan ga ik vis vangen voor het
2 voe=voor 't geld, en verder-eh ogen (zacht) de ogen de kost geven
3 A: hoge?
4 B: ogen de kost geven
5 A: de *O*gen de kost geven, j*a* (1) ja (1) nou dat is mooi zeg, een mooi plan!

(5)

1 B: ze kankeren je kan beter in Arnhem zijn
2 A: oh bah daar hou je niet van

3 B: *Arn*hem. hoe=wat is er in Arnhem? (2) woonde je in Arnhem? (4) *kom*
4 A: je

5 B: ((*fluistert*)) kankeren kankeren kankeren
6 A: wel es in Arnhem? (2) maar *jij* kankert toch

7 B: ((*fluistert*)) kankeren teveel kankeren
8 A: niet hè wat zeggen ze allemaal,

9 B: ((*fluistert*)) kankeren kankeren kankeren ((*hoest*)) (2) kankeren
10 A: die kankeraars

11 B: ((*fluistert*)) kankeren
12 A: kankeren ze nou nog?

13 B: ((*fluistert*)) kankeren kankeren kankeren
14 A: en kanker je terug?

15 B: ((*fluistert*)) kankeren kankeren ((hoest))
16 A: of niet? (2) hm? (2)

17 B: ((*fluistert*)) kankeren kankeren kankeren
18 A: ((*zacht*)) hou *es op met dat gekanker*

19 B: ((*fluistert*)) kankeren
20 A: ((*zacht*)) *schei es uit met dat gekanker* (2)

21 B: ((*normaal*)) wat zegt u
22 A: ((*normaal*)) zit 't in je hier van binnen zit 't hier van binnen?

23 B: ((*normaal*)) ze kankeren teveel is niet leuk
24 A: ((*normaal*)) (2) ja? uhuh *nee* zeker niet!

25 B: ((*normaal*)) eten is goed
26 A: ((*normaal*)) eten is goed (1) ja (1)

27 B: ((*fluistert*)) kankeren teveel
28 A: ((*normaal*)) wat heb je van*daag* gegeten dan,

29 B: ((*fluistert*)) kankeren kankeren
30 A: ((*normaal*)) en toch maar kankeren over 't eten (3)

31 B: ((*fluistert*)) kankeren kankeren
32 A: ((*normaal*)) luisteren ze daar naar (2) ((zacht)) *schei*

33 B: ((*fluistert*)) kanker
34 A: es *uit* met dat ge*kank*er (3) ((*normaal*)) hm? alleen maar over 't eten

35 B: ((*fluistert*)) kankeren kankeren

(6)
1 B: en-ehm ik heb gezegd ik ben Albert Peter
2 A: waarom kast*an*jes eigenlijk

3 B: Bernards, keizer van China! Ik laat dat planten! in opvolging van (.)
4 A: ja

5 B: Alexander de Grote in opvolging van Napoleon! in opvolging
6 A: *hmm*hm ja.

7 B: van (.) Caesar al die al die tuinen tuinen laten
8 A: *ja*ja die grote veldheren

9	B:	aanleggen kast*an*jes
10	A:	*oooh*ja (1) waarom kastanjes eigenlijk? is d'r iets
11	B:	is toch lekker!
12	A:	met kastanjes? m*ja*, ik vind 't heerlijk, maar ja, 'k zou
13	B:	
14	A:	me ook iets anders kunnen voorstellen, sinaasappels of eh
15	B:	nou ik heb ook wel (.) andere aanplantingen maar 'k.
16	A:	mandarijnen, jaja
17	B:	kastanjes, weet ik veel precies
18	A:	hm. maar kastanjes bevalt 't best(.)hm
19	B:	tot in China kastanjes geplant en zijdebomen
20	A:	(6) *ja*-a, dat begrijp ik wel ja jaja(.)
21	B:	ik ben keizer van China
22	A:	wat heeft u met China? *kei*zer van China

14 Assertive speech acts in psychotic discourse

William Van Belle

Introduction[1]

Psychotic discourse is often associated with 'disturbed discourse'. However, over the last few decades, many studies of psychotic language and discourse have concluded that the observed disturbances or peculiarities in psychotic discourse are not found in the speech of all individuals who are diagnosed as psychotic. And, moreover, it is also a fact that these disturbances, if they occur at all in the utterances of a psychotic person, do not occur always, but rather infrequently (see Pavy 1968; Rochester and Martin 1979 for an overview of recent studies).

To explain my own position, I should say that I am interested in psychotic discourse not because I want to prove something about psychosis or psychotic discourse, but because I believe that by studying this discourse one can gain a better insight in what is called normal discourse.

In the first part of this chapter I intend to discuss some peculiarities of assertive speech acts in psychotic discourse. In the second part I will discuss these observations in the context of a general theory of communication and discourse.

The assertive speech act

To explain the problem of assertives I will start with Searle's theory of speech acts, some basic concepts of which I will briefly outline. In Searle's theory (1969), every utterance is seen as a speech act and is, as a result, to be analysed into two parts: the propositional content of the utterance and its illocutionary force. The illocutionary force indicates which speech act is performed by the utterance. I give some examples to clarify this fundamental statement of speech act theory:

(*1*) I promise to be on time
(*2*) I order you to clean the rooms
(*3*) Can you pass me the salt, please?
(*4*) The president opened the meeting

An essential part of the meanings of these sentences is that, when used, they conventionally perform a certain speech act: a promise (1), an order (2), a request (3), a statement (4). Which act is performed by a particular utterance, i.e. its illocutionary force, can be expressed by different means. In (1) and (2) the illocutionary force is expressed by a performative verb in the first person singular present tense (*I promise* versus *I order*), in (3) and (4) it is expressed by the sentence type and the intonation (interrogative versus declarative sentence). The meaning of a specific speech act is specified by a set of rules or conditions. Searle (1979) distinguishes five basic categories of speech acts: assertives, directives, commissives, expressives and declarations.

The category of assertives includes such speech acts as statements, descriptions, explanations, suggestions and hypotheses. They have the following characteristics in common—characteristics by which they are also distinguished from other speech act types:

(*1*) They commit the speaker to the truth of the expressed proposition. The degree of this commitment can vary considerably: there is clearly a difference between, for instance, 'putting something forward as a hypothesis' on the one hand and 'stating' or 'swearing' on the other. But in hypothesizing or in suggesting that something is the case, the truth of the propositional content is also involved. Searle summarizes this commitment to the truth of the expressed proposition in the following *preparatory condition*: 'the speaker must be in a position to provide evidence or reasons for the truth of the expressed proposition.' I think that such a formulation is fairly compatible with the concept that truth is intersubjectively determined. Such a concept implies that the evidence one can provide has to be acceptable for (at least some) other persons.

(2) The members of the assertive class of speech acts are also distinguished from other classes by the psychological state they express: the speaker *believes* the proposition expressed in the utterance—Searle calls this the *sincerity condition*. The belief the speaker commits himself to can also differ in degree.

Before discussing some examples of assertives in psychotic discourse, I will mention how I interpret these conditions or rules. The question is whether the psychological states or positions specified by the speech act rules are to be considered as real psychological states, or simply as conditions that can eventually not be fulfilled. I start from what seems to me a fundamental distinction, although it is not always recognized as such in speech act theory nor in linguistics in general: the distinction between the real psychological states of a person and the psychological states contained in the speech acts he utters or, more generally, the psychological states he *says* he has. In any case psychoanalysis has taught us that a person has no privileged, direct insight into his own intentions, beliefs, etc. and that therefore the ideas he has of himself cannot be considered as the only truth. Therefore, rather than the formulation 'real psychological state' I would use 'the psychological state a person thinks he has'.

Furthermore, it can also be observed that one can perform a speech act from a position one pretends to occupy. These observations are not meant to lead to the conclusion that communicating is nothing but deceiving the others. Communication is an agreement, a pact—although it is not concluded—that demands that the participants in it act as if they really mean and believe what they say, and that they moreover identify themselves with the psychological states required by what they say. Thus I will take it that in discourse it is usually implied that the conditions as specified, for instance, by Searle's speech act rules are satisfied. For instance, when I say to someone, *I promise to be on time*, I might not have any intention of keeping my promise, but by uttering that sentence it is nonetheless conversationally implied that I have that psychological state.

Assertives in psychotic discourse

I will discuss now the assertive speech act in some pieces of discourse by persons who were diagnosed as psychotic. The following texts are translations as close as possible to the Dutch originals. The Dutch texts can be found in the Appendix to this chapter.

Maria B

Maria B is a paranoid schizophrenic woman who has been living for many years in a psychiatric institute. Her discourse displays a delusion of persecution.

M: Paula said that Mrs Rita too much in my stomach ... that she made her suffer too much, she said.
T: That she made Paula suffer too much.
M: Yes, that's what she said.
T: Yes go on?
M: By putting into my stomach it was, you know it.
T: Paula, she suffered in fact because something was put into your stomach.
M: Yes, yes
T: You like Paula?
M: .... I am not asking for it.
T: You are not asking for it.
M: Yes, I also have liked her, she has also been good to me.
T: She is good to you.
M: She has been good to me, good and bad, I think then.
T: Both.
M: I think so then.
T: Are there other people who have been good to you? ... er, there is Paula.
M: She has done me much harm.
T: Who?
M: Paula.
T: I don't know about that.
M: Ah, you don't know that no...
T: Do you think so?
M: I don't know either but ... she has harmed me, they have said so.
T: They, who are they?
(...)
M: Yes a while ago I understood that they said so.

In this interview Maria B is saying again and again that different people have harmed her in various ways. And, as becomes apparent at the end of this fragment, Maria B's assertive speech acts in this dialogue do not display the implication that the reasons she has for asserting that others harmed her have to be intersubjectively acceptable. Truth is here not guaranteed by an intersubjective system, but by *they* (i.e. the voices).

We may also doubt whether Maria B believes what she is asserting. One of her statements is, in fact, *She has done me much harm. I do not know it. But they have said so*. This way of asserting is fairly typical for her. On the basis of other pieces from this dialogue, which are not reproduced here, I have constructed the following typical statement:

> (I think that) (I do not know) (but it is possible that) X has harmed me, they have said so

All those modifications of the assertion do occur together in some instances: *When I was sleeping, she did ... she and and someone else who was there ... that she was also at my bed, I don't know, but it is possible that*.

This way of modifying a statement indicates, I think, that one cannot use the term 'belief' to denote the psychological state of Maria B as regards what she is asserting. The French psychoanalyst Jacques Lacan has said that a psychotic does not really believe in the reality of his hallucinations, but that he is certain of it. It is a 'radical' certainty: the psychotic may admit that those hallucinations belong to another order than reality and even to a certain extent that they are not real; but such 'concessions' do not affect his certainty (Lacan 1981: 87–8).

Paul A

Paul A is a young man who at the time of this interview was staying in the section for young psychotic patients of a psychiatric institute. To understand the following communication he made to his therapist, one has to know that he had formerly built up for himself a system of 'rules' that governed his life.

> And it suddenly shot through my mind: damn well give up these rules. I suddenly took my decision: I'm giving up my rules [let fall]. Good! And there they lay. The following morning I awoke. Well, I have given up these rules. What am I to do now. Now I have got rid of my shield ('shield-weapon') eh. Now I have made again a very short rule and this one simply contains the following: I am a 'socially thinking' man who makes few problems out of things and who takes the thousand beautiful things out of life. (...) I feel already on the way to recovery through the following, I say it again: I am a man, a 'socially thinking' man. 'To think socially' that means to think of other people. To be a man that means to be really a man in the real sense of the word. To take the thousands of beautiful things out of life, yes that is self-explanatory. And of anything, seldom to make problems of anything.

I am a man, a socially thinking man ... has the character of a formula. Later on in the therapeutic interview Paul A repeats this rule twice in the same fixed form. As a speech act it has an ambiguous character. It is a rule he has set up for himself; hence it is on the one hand a kind of directive speech act, on the other a self-definition, an assertive act. He is himself very ambiguous about it: it is introduced as a rule, but sometimes it is no longer a rule, but reality. At a certain moment in the interview he expresses also a kind of disbelief in his self-definition:

> But there is something in me that does not give me the enthusiasm to say: ha, now I am at last a socially thinking man who takes the

thousand beautiful things out of the world and who makes problems, who seldom makes problems out of anything.

In Paul A's self-definition the dimensions of truth and belief are present, but because of its ambiguous character, the psychological state expressed in it is a combination of belief and desire. (This can, of course, be said of all self-definitions which are not simply informative.) As such it resembles a type of speech act called a 'declaration' by Searle. A declaration is a speech act where one brings a state of affairs into existence—or where one at least tries to do so—by declaring it to exist (Searle 1979: 16). By saying, for example, *I am ill* or *You are ill*, I describe a certain state of affairs and—usually—I am not making myself or the other ill by saying that. Declarations, on the contrary, attempt to get language to match the world. Examples are *pronouncing a couple man and wife*, *declaring war*. Normally, declarations involve the existence of an extra-linguistic institution (the Church, the law, the State, etc.) and to perform a declaration successfully speaker and hearer have to occupy special positions within this institution. Supernatural declarations—such as *Let there be light*, said by God—form an exception. I think that Paul A's self-definition can be compared to such a supernatural declaration, because it tries to bring into existence 'a specific kind of personality for himself' by repeating a stereotyped formula. Language is used here as if it had a magical power: a name or a sentence sufficiently often repeated can realize the thing or the state of affairs referred to.

Such a belief in the magical power of language is also to be found in the discourse of Alex C.

Alex C

Alex C is a young man about twenty years old, who was taken into a psychiatric institute in the delusional state of thinking he was Christ. At the time of this interview his delusion had largely disappeared.

A: (*has said he would like to become a priest or an actor*) I would like to choose between two things, either to become a priest and ... Yesterday my decision was almost taken. because after all you are nothing without your faith, at least I think so. Let people go on acting, I will watch it. All the world is a stage, you can not deny that, can you?
T: Even as a priest?
A: Mm. In fact I put it in a suitcase ... on that weekend 'Youth and inability' that I wanted to follow Jesus. In principle, a rude awakening I had from it, because otherwise I would not be here essentially, but otherwise since you cannot teach an old dog new tricks—and that is also a fact—nobody has to teach me new tricks, er I should rather choose the other one, for the

priesthood or the diaconate, because I think, well, thus possibly to live together with a woman or something, that one cannot have everything here and in the idea that afterwards that would probably be rewarded. I am also living near the water just like a friend of mine and yes I think he leads me to those cool waters, I think I will be just like that friend of mine, I am living also near the water in Velodrome Street, that is also near the sea. (...) That psychiatrist has also said that I emulate the image of my father very much and that I too would like to be like that, like God's ways are inscrutable. That is, well, I cannot leave behind my Catholic education, you can't do that, can you? You can't do that. Yes, and I find money, it may be interesting, but after all it does not make you happy. (...) So, am I longing for a woman or for a man. (...) It is (C), that is something between the cart and the horse and, on the other hand, it is (S), so we are wearing black trousers, so sexuality is, as regards our names, not so important.

T: Could you explain that?

A: My father is called (C), that is 'of the (C)', a (C) is hanging between the cart and the horse (...) and so, on the other hand, my mother is called (S), so we are wearing black trousers, so, basically sexuality is not so important because it has got black trousers around it. (...) If I consider carefully which teachers I used to have difficulties with, as regards the name it all fits together.

One can observe in this text that Alex C has a (certain) belief in the magical power of names. Sexuality is not so important for him—at least he says so—because of the name of his father and mother. This reminds us of the ancient belief that the name of a thing (here a person) contains the nature of the thing named. Because he lives in Velodrome Street, he thinks he resembles a friend of his and can live like him. In the next interview he gives the explanation for this idiosyncratic association and way of reasoning: that friend of his got married recently and he resembles his friend because he lives, like his friend, in the neighbourhood of water, viz. in Velodrome Street, which is a street that also exists in Blankenberge (a town on the Belgian coast). These examples are not isolated cases. At the end of the reproduced fragment he clearly expresses the belief that 'nomen est omen'.

A striking feature of this discourse is also the use of many proverbs, biblical quotations and common expressions: e.g. *you are nothing without your faith, all the world is a stage, I had a rude awakening from it, you cannot teach an old dog new tricks, you cannot have everything here, he leads me to those cool waters*. Some parts are virtually nothing but a succession of such expressions. These common phrases are alternated with idiosyncratic associations.

As for the assertive speech acts, it is not easy to say whether a commitment to the truth as an intersubjective system is implied here. One can observe that Alex C gives very idiosyncratic reasons for certain of his statements, but we certainly do not have such a resistance to common reasoning as in the case of Maria B. Moreover, there are also parts in the discourse of Alex C that display a way of reasoning that is intersubjectively acceptable. But, as concerns the expressed or implied belief, it is not at all clear whether, in the case of the common phrases used as assertive speech acts, a belief is expressed in the same way as what is usually understood as belief. The question is in which way or to what degree a subject is present in his own discourse (i.e. assumes responsibility for it), when he uses common expressions and biblical or other quotations. He has indeed always the possibility of saying: 'People (the bible or ...) say so, but I do not know.' This type of reaction to one's own discourse can be found in the discourse of Alex C. (See also the discourse of Maria B.)

'Normal' and psychotic discourse

In this last section I will try to interpret the elements of the above analysis into a comprehensive theory of speaking and discourse. The theory I propose is for a great part inspired by the psychoanalytical theory of Jacques Lacan.

The discourse of a person has an ambiguous character. On the one hand it is something individual, a selection and combination of words (or signifiers) by an individual to express his desires and thoughts, to boast and to deceive others, etc. To achieve that, he can make use of the existing stock of signifiers, he can make new signifiers by a combination of existing ones, and he can even try to make totally new words. But, on the other hand, if a person wants his discourse to be understood by others, he has to subject it more or less to the rules of discourse existing in the community, i.e. to the syntactic, semantic and pragmatic rules belonging to the existing universe of discourse.

This explanation has a triangular structure: (*1*) the subject and his discourse, (*2*) the other person(s) the subject is speaking to and his (their) discourse, and (*3*) the universe of discourse, which mediates the communication between the subject and the other(s). The triangularity of this relationship is to be stressed because the universe of discourse is not to be confused with the discourse of a particular person. The universe of discourse is a historically established whole, which is not homogeneous because it contains the possibilities of (social) differences between people. Everyone is subjected to this universe of discourse and is but a representative of it.

In this triangular structure the discourse of a subject can be situated between two extremes: (*a*) the total individual, idiosyncratic discourse, of which inextricable neologisms are an example, and (*b*) the total conformity of one's own discourse to a (particular) existing discourse. A typical example of the last position is the repetition of common phrases and formulas. In both extreme cases the third element of the triangle, the universe of discourse, is no longer present.

The relationship between a person and the others is not to be seen here as a relationship between two separately existing entities. According to psychoanalytical theory, one is constituted as a person (a subject) by one's relationships with other persons. As was mentioned above, this relationship is in the first place one of subjection to the existing universe of discourse, to the existing culture in general. In that way one receives a primary identity that is built up later on by the positions one can adopt and by the recognition one receives from others. What constitutes me as a subject, Lacan says, is my request to others to be recognized as a person (Lacan 1966: 299). This way of formulating the relationship between a particular person and the others does not imply that there is an opposition between the individual and the social. One's subjection to the universe of discourse is comparable to what Freud called 'die Bejahung' ('affirmation as a substitute for uniting') (Freud 1925: 239).

What is called 'normal discourse' takes place between the two mentioned extremes: total idiosyncracy and total conformity. The discourse of a subject can in a certain situation tend to one of the extreme poles, but in another situation it can take another position on the scale. Here we find word-play, strategy, rhetoric, and production of meaning in general.

In a discourse that is situated at one of the extreme poles, and in which there is no switch to another position, the production of meaning is blocked.

A word has no meaning on its own, but is a signifier that is meaningful by its difference from and its combination with other signifiers (i.e. by its paradigmatic and syntagmatic relationships). And, as has already been said, this selection and combination of signifiers has to be subjected to the rules of the universe of discourse. This means that meaning is intradiscursively and interdiscursively determined.

In both 'idiosyncracy' and in 'conformity', words or phrases are found that give the impression of having a particular meaning on their own, which cannot be explained in another way—or which need not be, in the case of the common expressions. Because their meaning is not paradigmatically and syntagmatically defined, those words and phrases no longer have the characteristics of signifiers.

What about the pieces of psychotic discourse discussed above? Since, in the discourse of Maria B, truth is not determined by the existing rules of the universe of discourse, but by an idiosyncratic system, the discourse is to be situated at the extreme pole of idiosyncracy or individuality. One may even doubt whether this universe of discourse still exists for Maria B: in many instances in her discourse it is in any case not recognized as such. Throughout the whole interview her discourse does not leave this extreme pole of idiosyncracy.

In the discourse of Paul A we have already observed the repetition of a stereotyped formula made up of some common phrases. For the speaker this formula has, so to speak, a fullness of meaning that cannot be explained by other words. If he explains the meaning of his 'rule', he does so in the same stereotyped phrases.

The discourse of Alex C regularly displays a switch from one pole to the other: on the one hand he uses stereotyped, common phrases that also give the impression of having a fullness of meaning that needs no explanation; on the other hand we find very idiosyncratic associations and ways of reasoning. And when these idiosyncracies are explained—usually as a response to a question of the therapist—the given explanation is usually no less idiosyncratic.

My discussion leads to the conclusion that in these three discourses the relationship to the universe of discourse, and consequently to other persons, is disturbed—or that there is at least a problem. This conclusion is not at all surprising, as it is completely compatible with most psychiatric and psychoanalytical literature on psychosis: one of the characteristics of psychosis is a disturbance in the relation between the subject and the outer world.

The theoretical framework I have proposed also gives some elements of an interpretation of the observed magical power of words. The first thing to note is that there is nothing strange about it that words can have a magical power. I may point here to the 'declarations' mentioned above. But also, in what is called 'normal discourse', words have a kind of magical power, because discourse contains a certain image of the speaker, and of the others with which they are supposed to identify themselves. But in normal discourse this image is not seen as reality; there is always a certain discrepancy between discourse and reality (the subject, the others) because language has a mediating effect on the relation of the subject to himself and to the outside world. That is a result of the fact that a word is not a term that refers immediately to a certain reality. The stock of words is not a nomenclature (de Saussure 1915: 97). A word or an utterance is a 'signifier' (a signifying element) the meaning of which is intra- and interdiscursively determined. In the above-mentioned extreme poles of idiosyncracy and conformity, words and utterances lose their mediating character since they no longer refer to the existing universe of discourse. In these cases words are used as if they had a particular meaning of their own. In other words, they are no longer used as 'signifiers'. As a result, the difference between the word and the thing named can be lost: 'saying makes it so.'

What Freud has called 'Organsprache' ('organ-speech') can in the same way be explained linguistically. Freud gives the following example:

> A patient of Tausk's, a girl who was brought to the clinic after a quarrel with her lover, complained that *her eyes were not right, they were twisted*. This she herself explained by bringing forward a series of reproaches against her lover in coherent language. 'She could not understand him at all, he looked different every time; he was a hypocrite, an eye-twister, he had twisted her eyes; now she had twisted eyes; they were not her eyes any more; now she saw the world with different eyes.' (Freud 1915: 197–8); (the German *Augen-verdreher* ('eye-twister') has the figurative meaning of 'deceiver')

The signifier *Augenverdreher* is not used here as an element which belongs to a whole network of signifiers, and which signifies by its intra- and interdiscursive relations. In this example, that word is signifying on its own and, as a result, it is possible that its 'acoustic image', and not its value in the network of signifiers, is the most important. Of course, such a use of signifiers can also be found in poetry and other types of discourse, but in the discourse mentioned by Freud one can no longer speak of 'word-play'.

For our observations about psychotic discourse there exist two opposed interpretations in psychiatric and psychoanalytical literature. In one interpretation, in which the idiosyncracies of psychotic discourse in particular are considered, (see, e.g., Delacampagne 1974: 160–75), these idiosyncracies are seen as a form of greater originality. The universe of discourse and its rules are considered as social constraints that have an impoverishing effect. According to the other interpretation (elements of which can be found in the writings of Lacan—but see also De Waelhens 1972) the relation of the psychotic to the others and to language is so fundamentally disturbed that one has to say that the psychotic is in fact outside language. His discourse is essentially composed of learned phrases.

Since I am neither a psychiatrist nor a psychoanalyst, I will not put forward a position in this matter. But as a linguist certainly influenced by psychoanalysis, I would respond to the first point of view by saying that it is doubtful whether an utterance has meaning at all if its meaning cannot be explained to others. As regards the second interpretation, I would say that one can often observe in psychotic discourse—except maybe in such severe cases as, for instance, the discourse of Maria B—that the psychotic tries to build up by his discourse a certain identity for himself. In the discourses discussed here, this is done by using common phrases, and as such these utterances are directed to others and contain a request for recognition by the hearer.

Note to Chapter 14

1 I should like to thank Jan Van Camp (Psychiatric Institute, Kortenberg, Belgium) for his critical comments, and to Kristin Davidse and Keith Carlon for correcting my English.

References

Delacampagne, C. 1974: 'L'écriture en folie. *Poétique* 5.

de Saussure, F. 1915: *Cours de linguistique générale*. Paris: Payot, 1915. Edition critique préparée par Tulio de Mauro, Paris: Payot 1972.

De Waelhens, A. 1972: *La psychose*. Brussels, Leuven and Paris: Nauwelaerts.

Freud, S. 1915: The unconscious. Reprinted in *The Standard Edition of the Complete Psychological Works of Sigmund Freud*, vol. 14. London: Hogarth Press and Institute of Psychoanalysis, 1957.

—1925: Negation. Reprinted in *The Standard Edition of the Complete Psychological Works of Sigmund Freud*, vol. 19. London: Hogarth Press and Institute of Psychoanalysis, 1961.

Lacan, J. 1966: *Ecrits*. Paris: Seuil.

—1981: *Les Psychoses le Séminaire de Jacques Lacan*, vol. 3, (1955–6). Paris: Seuil.

Pavy, D. 1968: Verbal behavior in schizophrenia: a review of recent studies. *Psychological Bulletin*, 70.

Rochester, M. and Martin, J. R. 1979: *Crazy Talk: A Study of the Discourse of Schizophrenic Speakers*. New York and London: Plenum.

Searle, J. 1969: *Speech Acts: An Essay in the Philosophy of Language*. Cambridge: Cambridge University Press.

—1979: A taxonomy of illocutionary acts. In J. Searle, *Expression and Meaning: Studies in the Theory of Speech Acts*. Cambridge: Cambridge University Press.

Appendix: Original Dutch texts

Maria B

M: Paula zei dat madame Rita te veel in mijn maag ... dat die te veel haar deed lijden zei ze.
T: Dat ze te veel Paula deed lijden.
M: Ja, dat zei ze.
T: Ja, en dan?
M: Door in mijn maag te doen was dat, weet ge het.
T: Paula die leed eigenlijk doordat in uw maag iets gedaan werd.
M: Ja, ja.
T: Ge hebt Paula graag?
M: ... ik vraag er niet naar.
T: Ge vraagt er niet naar.
M: Ja, ik heb ze graag gehad ook, ze is ook goed geweest voor mij.
T: Ze is goed voor u.
M: Ze is goed geweest voor mij, goed en slecht peins ik dan.
T: Alletwee.
M: Ja peins ik dan.
T: Zijn er nog mensen die goed geweest zijn voor u? ... éh, ge hebt Paula.
M: Die heeft me veel kwaad gedaan.
T: Wie?
M: Paula.
T: Dat weet ik niet.
M: Ah, ge weet dat niet nee ...
T: Denkt ge?
M: Ik weet het ook niet maar ... ze heeft me kwaad gedaan, hebben ze laten weten.
T: Ze wie zijn dat?
(...)
M: Ja, ik verstond daarstrak toch dat ze dat lieten weten.

Paul A

En ineens schoot me te binnen: laat verdomme die regels nu eens vallen. Ik nam ineens mijn besluit: ik laat mijn regels vallen. Bon! En daar lagen ze. De volgende dag werd ik wakker. Ja, ik heb die regels laten vallen. Ja, wat ga ik daar nu mee aanvangen. Nu heb ik mijn schildwapen kwijt hè. Nu heb ik terug ne hele korte regel in mekaar gestoken en die omvat gewoon het volgende: ik ben een sociaal denkende man die van weinig een probleem maakt en die de duizend mooie dingen uit het leven haalt. (...) Ik voel me al goed op weg om te genezen door het volgende, ik zeg het nogmaals: ik ben een man, een sociaal denkende man. Sociaal denken dat betekent aan de andere mensen denken. Man zijn dat betekent echt man zijn in de ware zin van het woord. De duizenden mooie dingen uit het leven halen, ja dat spreekt voor zichzelf èh. En van iets, zelden van iets een probleem maken dus.

Alex C

A: Ik zou dan nog tussen twee dingen willen kiezen, gewoon ofwel priester worden en ... Gisteren stond mijn besluit bijna vast. Omdat zonder uw geloof ben je toch ook niets, allé vind ik toch. Laat de mensen maar acteren, ik zal het maar afzien. Het leven is toch een schouwtoneel, daar kun je niet buiten èh?

T: Ook als priester?

A: Hm. Ik heb het eigenlijk in een valiesje gestoken ... op dat weekend 'Jeugd en onmacht' dat ik de weg van Jezus wilde volgen. In principe is het een kouwe reis waar ik van terug kwam, want anders zat ik hier niet in wezen, maar anderzijds vermits dat je geen ouwe aap toch geen smoelen moet leren trekken—en dat is ook een feit—niemand moet me leren smoelen trekken, euh zou ik dan liever voor het ander kiezen, voor het priester-zijn of voor het diaken-zijn omdat ik vind allè dus met een vrouw eventueel samenleven of zo, dat men toch niet alles heeft hier en in het gedacht dat dat waarschijnlijk beloond wordt achteraf. Ik woon toch ook aan het water net zoals een vriend van mij en ja ik denk hij voert me naar rustige wateren, ik denk dat ik net hetzelfde zal zijn als die vriend van mij, ik woon ook aan het water in de Velodromestraat dus, dat is ook aan de zee dus. (...) Die psychiater heeft ook gezegd dat ik het beeld van mijn vader erg nastreef en dat ik ook zo zou willen zijn, zo van Gods wegen zijn ondoorgrondelijk. Dat is allè ik kan mijn katholieke opvoeding toch niet achterlaten, dat kan je toch niet eh? dat kan je toch niet. Ja, en ik vind geld dat is wel heel interessant, maar het maakt toch niet gelukkig. (...) Dus tracht ik naar een vrouw of tracht ik naar een man. (...) 't Is (C), dat is tussen een kar en een paard en anderzijds is 't (S), dus we hebben een zwarte broek aan, dus sexualiteit is kwestie van onze naam niet zo belangrijk.

T: Leg dat eens even uit.

A: Mijn vader heet (C), dat is 'van het (C)', een (C) dat hangt tussen een kar en een paard (...) en dus anderzijds mijn moeder heet (S), dus we hebben een zwarte broek aan, dus in wezen die sexualiteit is niet zo belangrijk want der is een zwarte broek rond. (...) Als ik goed naga met welke leraars ik vroeger last heb gehad, kwestie van naam komt dat helemaal uit.

15 The language of schizophrenics as a reflection of meanings concealed by culture and the individual

Janusz Wróbel

Introduction

This chapter presents the results of research on the language of schizophrenics, focusing on its semantic level, with special emphasis on the relation between denotative and connotative meaning in schizophrenic language. The analysis is based on samples of oral and written accounts collected by the author among schizophrenics in Poland, and on similar examples from the psychiatric literature.

Conversations with schizophrenic subjects have shown that the word *father* is used and understood by them in a very specific way. The specific meanings of the word *father* among schizophrenics will be compared to those in standard Polish. Then an attempt will be presented to formalize the meanings in both languages through the use of the semic analyses of meaning (cf. Lyons 1977). In the following part of the chapter, the results of the confrontation of the schizophrenic meanings with those of standard Polish will be discussed. The concluding section presents an interpretation of results.

Fundamentals of the semantic approach

The basic principles of the method of semic analysis are as follows: (*1*) any meaning is composed of denotative and connotative semes;

(*2*) among these, primary and secondary meanings can be found;
(*3*) the primary denotative semes are to be found in the lexical meaning of the given word;
(*4*) the primary denotative semes have a distinctive character, i.e. even when only one seme is different, the meaning of the word changes;
(*5*) the secondary denotative semes stand in relation to the primary semes, often being their secondary phraseological variant;
(*6*) the denotative semes reflect dictionary meanings, while the connotative semes describe individual and personal meanings;
(*7*) the primary connotative semes illustrate the kinds of association which are recognized by the majority of the speakers of a given language;
(*8*) the denotative semes contain the meanings of words and consequently 'create' the lexical field of a particular word, while the connotative semes create the word's semantic field;
(*9*) in the order of semes, the denotative ones occupy the central position, while the connotative semes assume a peripheral one.

These statements can be viewed as the basic tools for the semantic analysis of any context. The system will be applied here for the analysis of standard usage as well as for schizophrenic usage.

The material

The schizophrenic material comes from interviews carried out by the author, from the author's personal contacts, his correspondence with schizophrenics in Poland, and from publications across the world.

The material concerning standard Polish has been derived from dictionaries by authors such as Karłowicz *et al.* (1898–1927) and Doroszewski (1958–69).

The meaning of 'father'

The denotative semes The dictionaries agree upon the following: 'father' is a man having a child (of his own) (Doroszewski). The secondary denotative semes can be found upon analysis of the different uses of the term. Karłowicz, Kryński and Niedzwiecki give the following meanings:

> 1. 'the one who begot somebody, parent', 2. 'creator, inventor, maker, source, origin, initiator, nestor, author, originator, founder', 3. 'ancestor, grandfather, great-grandfather, forefather, progenitor, patriarch', 4. 'the one whose role of father is due to taking care, foster father, protector, patron, superior, confessor, the Holy Father, city father', 5. 'holy fathers, Fathers of the Church, venerable ancient

fathers of the church, doctors of the church, apostolic fathers, the Fathers of the Church who communed with apostolic fathers', 6. the address given to the person of advanced age: 'Father, how much does the wood cost?', 'an elderly man' (especially of the peasantry or lower class).

Doroszewski offers the following meanings: 'a male of mammals or birds having descendants'. Some phraseological terms may be added here: the godfather, God the Father, Eternal Father, the Almighty, the omnipotent God, the Heavenly Father, adoptive father, 'the first man'.

All this adds to the following analysis of primary and secondary semes:

1	Primary semes	2	Secondary semes
1.1	a man having offspring	2.1	a man
1.2.	a man/offspring link through the fact of begetting	2.2	a link with someone or something due to the fact of being responsible for its origin or for initiating the subject.
1.3	caring for an offspring (of one's own), for its education and developing its character	2.3	continuation of one's own creation; developing, and caring for it

The primary semes are distinctive in that the absence of one of the semes causes a change in the meaning of this word. For example, if the term *child* is taken as the reference point, *mother* and *father* differ through the absence of seme 1.1 in the meaning of the *mother*; *stepfather* differs from *father* through the absence of semes 1.1 and 1.2; *adoptive father* lacks seme 1.2; and *father* differs from *unfit father* because the latter term does not contain seme 1.3, as can be seen from Table 15.1.

TABLE 15.1 *Different semes for five father-related words.*

Word	Semes	1.1	1.2	1.3
father		+	+	+
mother		–	+	+
stepfather		–	–	(–)
adoptive father		+	–	+
unfit father		+	+	–

Table 15.2 represents the positions of the primary and secondary denotative semes in the meaning of words constituting the lexical field of *father*.

TABLE 15.2 *Positions of primary and secondary denotative semes for the lexical field father.*

Word	Semes	1.1	2.1	1.2	2.2	1.3	2.3
godfather		+				+ or	+
Heavenly Father, Eternal Father, The Almighty, God the Father			+		+		+
adoptive father stepfather		+				(+)	
creator, inventor, maker, initiator, author, originator, founder			+		+		(+)
ancestor, forefather patriarch			+		+		
the Holy Father, the Pope			+				+
father confessor, priest			+				+
confessor, monk			+				
Father of the Church			+		+		+
city father			+				+
elderly man			+				
male having descendants of his own				+		+	

The connotative semes The connotative semes are found in the metaphoric uses of the word *father* (primary semes) or *fatherland* (secondary semes). The use of words results from attaching certain emotional meanings to them. In the case of the word *father*, phrases such as *to be a father to someone* 'to be someone's solicitous protector or educator; to care for someone'; *to father someone* 'to act as a substitute for the father', i.e. 'to have someone under father-like care; to look after someone in a father-like way'; *to love someone like a father* 'to love someone very much'.

There are also expressions such as *father's love/goodness/care/concern, paternal kiss/blessing/gentleness* (see Doroszewski 1958–69: 895; and Karłowicz *et al.* 1898–1927: 726). All the features mentioned above also exist in words originating from the word *father*, such as *fatherland* (home country) or *paternal*. According to Doroszewski, *paternal* means 'heartful, protecting and tender' and *paternally* means 'gently and caringly'. However, there are also expressions such as *father's will/power/prestige/authority/reprimand/anger/punishment/severity* (see Karłowicz *et al.* 1898–1927). Karłowicz *et al.* quote the swordsman's term of *paternal cut* which stands for 'a stroke with the flat of the sword on someone's bottom'.

In standard use the word *stepfather* has very strong negative connotations. Karłowicz states that *stepfatherly* means 'like a stepfather, strict, without a father's tolerance, uncaring, harsh, neglecting', illustrating this with quotations such as 'this stepfather's care was bearable'; 'Sir, take good care of the Republic, be a father, not a stepfather to us'. Further, Karłowicz quotes a Polish slang expression *ojczaszek* to describe a father or stepfather who does not care for his children, or who mistreats them. Whereas the expression *one's own father* brings positive associations with the word *father*, the expression *unfit father* contains negative ones. The word *unfit* means 'one who has become degenerate, one being worse than other family members, one who has lost the qualities typical of his family, one who is behaving improperly, immorally and unjustly. Consequently, the meanings of *father* and *stepfather* approximately correspond to the position of primary and secondary connotative semes of *father*, as in Table 15.3.

TABLE 15.3 *The connotative semes of father* (semantic field of *father* in standard Polish).

Father: somebody who for his child is:	
his/her own father	unfit father
loving	heartless
good	bad
caring	unconcerned
thoughtful	uncaring for the child
giving instructions and admonitions (*father's will*), even harsh and severe on occasions	being a ruthless tyrant (*father's power*); cruel
fair (his reprimands and punishments being just or even lenient)	unfair (ever-punitive, for whatever reason)

This list of theoretical possibilities derived from the dictionary does not imply that in everyday language use there are no other possibilities. Of course there cannot be any universal pattern for connotative meanings, since the latter include specific individuality which cannot be foreseen.

However, Table 15.3 can be used as a probabilistic model, albeit one used by a great number of speakers. Personal experiences, especially those of a strong emotional nature, may cause a transmission in the sequence of primary and secondary items in the framework of connotative meanings. Such a change, however, does not destroy the hierarchy of the arrangement of semes because the central position of the denotative semes remains firm. For the average speaker of standard Polish, an expression such as *Mr X's father* means 'a man whose son is Mr X'. On the basis of some schizophrenic examples which I will discuss later, one may find reasons for reconstituting a meaning 'Mr X's oppressor', i.e. a man who dominates Mr X.

The term 'father' in schizophrenic language

Ann Gruszecka (1924: 6, 7) points out in her work on emotional experiences in schizophrenia a case of a patient who found himself hospitalized shortly after experiencing a schizophrenic illumination. Because of this he was able to describe the circumstances responsible for this condition. The patient stated that:

> On April 1st, 1923, he received a message announcing his father's death. However, he did not go to the funeral, because he felt that his conscience kept telling him he should not go ... When asked why he had not gone to his father's funeral, the patient took much pain in explaining. He related that prior to receiving the cable regarding his father's death on April 1st, he went for a walk and saw some lightning rods broken. For him this meant that contact with his father was broken off because of his father's death, which was what he had desired because he considered his father an evil spirit. The breaking of the wires in the lightning rod, however, was the work of an evil spirit, for it was meant to kill him. This did not occur because he took special care of himself. This event was related in a letter from his brother from Bolshevia, [the slang name for the Soviet Union before World War II] who is very much like his father. The brother had sent him a letter before his father's funeral in order to shift his attention from his mother to the trip to Siberia, in order to force him to attend his father's funeral without further hesitation. At the place not far from where his father died, his own death awaited him at the agency of those evil spirits.

The patient experienced his father's death with a sense of relief because of his previous experiences with him. Even contact with the father's grave he considered dangerous. Consequently he dislikes his brother because 'he resembles his father'.

The account presented above suggests that the schizophrenic attitude towards the father is experienced in a specific way. The universality of this phenomenon is also reflected in the research work by Irigaray and Dubois (1968), who have investigated deviances in linguistic structures of family relationships, including those of schizophrenics. One of the examinations involved interpretation of the expression *like father, like son*, resulting in the following (Irigaray and Dubois 1966: 68):

(*1*) If a father has some serious defect, of course... it will influence his son, that is he will be affected in the opposite way, or that... no, I do not know what 'like father, like son' means.
(*2*) A father and a son resemble one another. A father is like his son.
(*3*) If a father, let's say, is good, that means that his son is bad. And it means that a father is like his son.
(*4*) Father and Guy (ego) are brothers.
(*5*) A father is a son. A son is a father.
(*6*) I am a father myself.

In examples 1 and 3, attention should be paid to the unusual usage of the participle *a* ('un') by French schizophrenics, who said *If a father has...* and *a father is like a son*. Similar expressions were observed for Polish subjects. Talking about pigmentation of his hands, G said:

(*7*) I do not know who gave me these marks, surely some father of mine.

Unusual here is the linking of the indefinite pronoun *some* with the noun *father*, which is felt to be a logical impossibility. Let us consider what this 'impossibility' is based upon. The answer can be found in the conflict between the specific features of the term *father* and the semantically indefinite features of the expression *some (father) of mine*. Further, there is also a conflict between the supposition contained in the use of the pronoun *some*, meaning 'one or many or anyone' and the unitary meaning of *my father*, referring to one definite designation.

The 'anyone-ness' of the father expressed by the use of the pronoun *some* shows the patient's indefinite attitude to his father. In order to prove this conclusion, let me quote another statement by G:

(*8*) Father me, he came, that Treniel, like a father, he was supposedly was my father, he taught me, first of all he taught me the Polish alphabet.

In an analysis of the statements quoted above (1–6), Irigaray and Dubois (1968: 68) say that the relationship of similarity, sonship and identification of son and father is either unknown, reversed or neutralized. A very interesting example of a neutralized relation of son to father appearing as the unity of ego with the person of father is noted by Frostig (1933, vol. 2: 196):

(*9*) A patient considering himself to be 'God the Father', 'a son' and 'St Joseph' monologizes as follows: 'They ordered me to be put into a net, because they were afraid of my father. They thought it was madness, but I am not the one to be feared—I am the one to be obeyed.'

The expressions *were afraid of my father* and *but I am not the one to be feared—I am the one to be obeyed* document the absence of differentiation in the patient's experience between ego and the father. One of the author's respondents, faced with a question: *Is your father alive?*, delivered the following answer:

(*10*) Father?... as a matter of fact I am the father.

Bielawski (1925: 274) noted a statement like the one above in one of his schizophrenic patients:

(*11*) He has three sons, the third one is he himself.

Still another example of this kind of identification comes from a poem on the subject of a monastery. The author is the same patient, G, already mentioned above:

(*12*) 'A monastery'
Everybody who was monastic
comes out it a real
father son of Jesus.

Irigaray and Dubois (1966: 68) noted the case of a patient considering his father's birthday to be his own (13). Confronted with the question of how the patient considered the persons listed below, the authors collected the following answers:

(*14*) *my father's brother* = my brother; Cain
(*15*) *my father's father* = my father; Abraham
(*16*) *the children of my father's brother* = my nephews
(*17*) *my father's wife* = my wife

The term *father* used by schizophrenics can often be related to expressions from the lexical field of authority:

(*18*) Jesus was also subordinated to a powerful father (God) and did not indulge in sexual live. (Kipphardt 1980: 191).

(*19*) It appears from what I have said that the power (father) serves strength the best. (Kipphardt 1980: 48)

The last two examples come from a book entitled *Aleksander März* by Kipphardt, a fictionalized documentary based on a selection of psychopathological texts compiled by Navratil (1971). The major portion of Navratil's book contains texts written by Alexander, one of his schizophrenic patients. Kipphardt often quotes this Alexander. Among others, he quotes a passage of Alexander's using the word *Abraham* (20) instead of *father* (Kipphardt 1980: 53). An identical expression was used by the schizophrenic in example 15. There is no doubt that both these schizophrenics referred to an episode in Abraham's life called Isaac's holocaust *The Holy Bible* (King James Version), *Genesis* 22, 1–10:

> And it came to pass after these things, that God did tempt Abraham, and said unto him, Abraham: and he said, behold, here I am. And he said, Take now thy son, thine only son Isaac, whom thou lovest, and get thee into the land of Mo-ri-ah; and offer him there for a burnt offering upon one of the mountains which I tell thee of. And Abraham, rose up early in the morning, and saddled his ass, and took two of his young men with him, and Isaac his son, and clave the wood for the burnt offering, and went unto the place of which God had told him. Then on the third day Abraham lifted up his eyes, and saw the place afar off. And Abraham said unto his young men, Abid ye here with the ass; and I and the lad will go yonder and worship, and come again to you. And Abraham took the wood of the burnt offering, and laid it upon Isaac his son; and he took the fire in his hand, and a knife; and they went both of them together. And Isaac spoke unto Abraham his father, and said, My father: and he said Here am I, my son. And he said, behold the fire and the wood: but where is the lamb for a burnt offering? And Abraham said, My son, God will provide himself a lamb for a burnt offering: so they went both of them together. And they came to the place which God had told him of; and Abraham built an altar there, and laid the wood in order, and bound Isaac his son, and laid him on the altar upon the wood. And Abraham stretched forth his hand, and took the knife to slay his son.

We must recall, that Isaac was not Abraham's only son. Abraham had another son with Agara, the slave. Because of Sarah's order, Abraham drove out Agara and his son by her, Ismael (*Genesis* 21, 14):

> And Abraham rose up early in the morning, and took bread, and a bottle of water,and gave it unto Ha-gar, putting it on her shoulder, and the child, and sent her away: and she departed, and wandered in the wilderness of Beer-she-ba.

The ethical expression for what Abraham did is that he was willing to murder Isaac: the religious expression is, that he was willing to

> sacrifice Isaac; but precisely in this contradiction consists the dread which can well make a man sleepless...

comments Kierkegaard (1982: 38), reflecting on the paradoxical nature of faith. Two qualifications depicting Abraham's action are available; but a schizophrenic evaluation does not consider the religious point of view, and is based on an emotional opposition to Abraham's intention. Both Abraham, as well as God sending Jesus to death, are used by schizophrenics as symbols of a powerful and cruel father. Schizophrenics, sensitive to injustice, often charge God with the fact that he let his son be crucified. Edgar Lee Masters (1948: 81–2) also made this charge in his *Spoon River Anthology*, in an epitaph for the madman Wendell P. Bloyd:

> They first charged me with disorderly conduct,
> There being no statute on blasphemy.
> Later they locked me up as insane (...)
> Therefore the Lord God sent Him forth from the garden of Eden.
> (The reason I believe God crucified His Own Son
> To get out of the wretched tangle is, because it sounds just like Him.)

Let us now attempt a formalized description of the meaning of *father* in schizophrenic language. Such a description will allow us to conceptualize the differences of meanings in the framework of the system.

Summary

Examples 1–20 above show that, in the statements by schizophrenics, the father does not meet the following requirements:

(1) a determinate, specific man (*some father*);
(2) responsible for the birth of a child (*a father is a son, a son is a father*);
(3) caring for a child (/father/ *serves the strength the best, would be glad to get rid of his son*).

Table 15.4 compares the occurrence of the primary denotative semes in the meaning of the word *father* in the standard language and in the statements by schizophrenics. It shows that, in the schizophrenic meaning of the word *father*, the primary denotative semes do not occur. As it appears from the examples quoted above, in the schizophrenic statements the word *father* is linked in various contexts with words from the lexical field of *authority/power*, especially with negative features associated with

TABLE 15.4 *Comparison between standard language and schizophrenic language primary denotative semes.*

	a specific, substantial man	who fathers a child	who cares for a child
standard language	+	+	+
language of schizophrenics	–	–	–

the schizophrenics, such as betrayal, misfortune, strength and menace. These features dominate among the connotative semes (see the semantic field *father* in the language of schizophrenics):

a father is the one who:
exercises an unlimited, ruthless power over a schizophrenic (son);
makes use of undue authority;
employs power;
causes misfortune to the schizophrenic (son);
threatens and humiliates the schizophrenic (son).

The above semes correspond to the secondary connotative semes of *father* in the standard language (see 'unfit', 'indifferent', 'negligent', 'being a ruthless tyrant', 'unjust' and 'cruel').

The lexical field of *father* is composed of words which name persons in authority, thus representing the negative aspects of authority. The lexical field of *father* in language of the schizophrenic is as follows:

boss, superior, teacher, master, priest, examining magistrate, chief of the company, doctor, hospital attendant, evil spirit, Abraham

As opposed to the standard language, in which the lexical field of *father* is created by words whose similarity of meaning is based on denotative semes, in schizophrenic statements the lexical field of *father* is created by words whose similarity of meaning is based on the connotative semes.

The mechanism of the change of meaning of *father* in schizophrenic statements in relation to the standard language is based on the absence of both the primary and secondary denotative semes and the primary connotative semes, as well as on the complete replacement of the semes mentioned above with the secondary connotative semes. The relation between the denotative and connotative semes in the standard language and in the language of schizophrenics is illustrated in Figure 15.1. In Figure 15.1, *(a)* illustrates the hierarchy of semes in a probable standard variant. *(b)* depicts a situation in which the secondary connotative semes eliminate the primary connotative semes, owing to strong negative associations. *(c)* shows a situation described in the schizophrenic statements in which the position of central denotative semes and the position of primary connotative semes is pre-empted by secondary connotative semes.

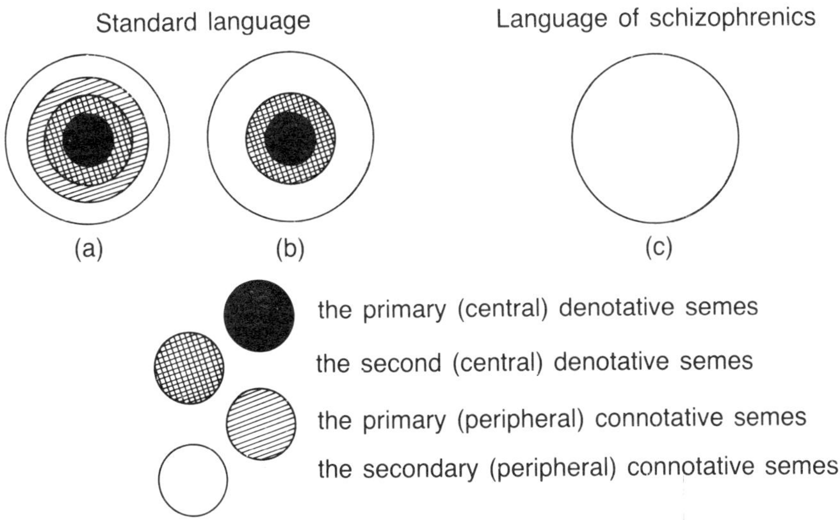

FIGURE 15.1 *Relation between denotative and connotative semes in standard language and schizophrenic language.*

Interpretation

Introduction

According to the authors quoted earlier in this chapter, the source of disturbance in the structure of relationships on the level of the ego/father/relationships lies in the schizophrenics' lack of experience of identification with the father. The same authors say that this identification is essential for the construction of the ego and for the whole structure of family relations. This instability is viewed as the cause of the disintegration of the whole structure of relationships which finds its expression in the overlapping of generations (Irigaray and Dubois 1966: 68).

Rosenbaum and Sonne (1979) adopt a similar position, stating that the source of the absence of reality among schizophrenics is the lack of stability of relation between the first and second person (I/you). This relation is thought by Rosenbaum and Sonne to be critical for the stabilization of ego identity. However, neither Irigaray and Dubois nor Rosenbaum and Sonne try to explain the reasons for the disturbance of the basic relational system of ego/father, the reasons causing schizophrenics' failure to experience identification with the father. It is likely that an answer to this question can be found in the examination of archetypal language features. According to a number of psychiatrists, the functioning of archetypes is more apparent among schizophrenics than among nonschizophrenics. Thus, for example, in a matriarchal society of Trobriand Islanders in which 'the child was of the same substancy as his/her mother (...) and there was no physical relation between father and child (Malinowski 1957: 5), the role of the father was marginal. Emotional contact between son and father is also difficult to develop in a patriarchal system where the father is absolute ruler of the family and bearer of *patria potestas*, or, as it may happen, tyrant as well (Malinowski 1981: 171).

Discussing the Oedipus myth, Fromm (1977) presents the thesis that hostility between father and son, a frequent motive in the Sophocles trilogy, should be considered an attack against the victorious patriarchal order, an attack led by the representatives of the defeated matriarchal system.

Specific usage of the term 'father' by schizophrenics in the light of Laplantine's cultural matrices

The symbolism of the person of father in schizophrenic language is multidimensional. The father complex has probably been best described by Alexander, who called it 'Abrahamism':

> (*21a*) What is Abrahamism? I was terrified to discover, one morning, that a man has not got just one father he can hardly put up with but that almost the whole world is composed of formal fathers. Every boss or superior postures as a father and takes advantages of the fear and humiliation caused by him. What seems to be to your disadvantage is in fact being done for your good. You will not lord it over your father but you will be obedient to him in every case. And then you will be able to understand him.

Alexander is of the opinion that a child is expected to worship, love and obey his father. As a matter of fact, the relationship between son and father is based on subordination, inferiority and severity. Father stands for power, authority and strength and not for the love of his son:

> (*21b*) This is what a teacher, a master, a priest, a magistrate, and a chief of the company do. And finally, here in Lohberg is what the beloved doctor Kofler, the senior hospital attendant and professor Fenerstein do. All of them personify the father who does his best and who is never allowed to be completely despised.

Also the father finds it easy to sacrifice his son, even by sending him to his death. It is only death that can make one capable of winning the father's affection. A son can be rewarded with the father's acceptance only if he ceases to be himself, identifies with the father, so that he himself becomes the father:

> (*21c*) Of course, it would be the best for the father to kill his son; just take a look at the examples of Abraham and of Jesus. Only the son who is reconciled with his own death may be resurrected in the father. Then he is just like him. It has never been my desire to become such as this (Kipphardt 1980: 204)

Thus the father's goal is to destroy the individuality of the son. Let us reconsider the following sentence appearing in example 21b: *all of them personify the father who does his best and who is never allowed to be completely despised*. Alexander, the author of this statement, points out the fact that the cultural patterns governing societies do not allow for hatred towards the father. Thc expression of such emotions meets with disapproval, and is considered bad behaviour. It is worth quoting here Laplantine's point of view (1973: 65–7), who treats psychiatric disorder as a conformity to the cultural patterns of bad behaviour, rejected by society. Laplantine states that there are two 'cultural matrices' functioning in every society. The primary matrix generally contains positive patterns. A favourable attitude towards dogs (frequently called *man's best friend*), observed in most European societies, may serve as an example here. Many languages have expressions equivalent to *as faithful as a dog*. However, there are also negative elements associated with the dog, e.g. *in weather like this you wouldn't turn out a dog*, *to go to the dogs*, *dogs of war*, *a dog's life*. This is the other side of the coin, and the secondary matrix.

It is not the case, however, that the primary matrix always contains the positive attitude, for there are considerable differences existing among various societies, even within one cultural sphere. Negative attitudes towards the dog, masked by Polish society in the secondary matrix, are revealed in the primary matrix in Bulgaria, sometimes assuming even a hostile attitude to the dog. It can be noted, interestingly enough, that this hostility is even institutionalized by Bulgarian law. Here is a piece of information reprinted in the columns of a Polish weekly *Zycie Literackie* (5 March 1982):

> *Zamedelsko Zname* has sharply criticized the extensive campaign of extermination of dogs, which includes not only the savage ones wandering all over farm-land but also those perfectly fit, the slaughter often being carried out in front of horrified masters and even children. The only exception is granted to animals vaccinated against all canine diseases. However, the vaccination certificates are not considered valid if not accompanied by a dog-owner's annual tax receipt. This tax recently hit the 300L level, three times a Lada-owner's road tax and four times the average monthly salary. In closing the story, the daily notes that in the Soviet Union where the dog is considered man's best friend, there is a Moscow-based Dog Lovers' Association, while Leningrad has opened a 'hotel' for pets whose owners have to leave town for a business trip or holiday.

Customary language usage, and especially the rules of language pragmatism, frequently cause the secondary matrix to be concealed, and manifestations of it are unacceptable. It is the same with the term *father*. Expression of negative emotions associated with *father* does not exist in the model of the primary matrix. Schizophrenia reveals that which is concealed: dislike and fear.

> Each language represents a different equation between manifestations and silences. Each people leaves some things unsaid in order to be able to say others. Because *everything* would be unsayable. Hence the immense difficulty of translation: translation is a matter of saying in language precisely what that language tends to pass over in silence. (Ortega y Gasset 1982: 246)

The schizophrenics' silence, of their own choice, is well known. Here the situation is reversed. The schizophrenic uses his language to express things the common language tends to be silent about. It is no easy task to tell people things they do not want to know or to speak about.

Guiraud (1975: 104) uses the term 'image' to describe the primary matrix:

> The ideas of *image, message* and *manipulation* of public opinion by means of an understanding of its 'deep motivation' are keys to

> contemporary culture spreading from America to Europe. It has moved from the domain of advertising and has invaded politics and social relations. Stars, politicians and little by little everyone else has an 'image' which is patiently constructed and carefully maintained.

In the light of Laplantine's cultural matrices, one may assume that the primary and secondary connotative semes are a reflection of a meaning matrix: the primary, i.e. the socially acceptable one, and the secondary, i.e. the socially unacceptable one. Laplantine (1973: 65) considers the mechanism of revealing the secondary matrix as a characteristic feature in psychosis, and states that schizophrenia:

> is never pure nonsense ... it is countersense or, more precisely, a different sense from the one which the given society defines as the primary sense.

This is the reason why madness can be called abnormality—because the disease deviates from the cultural norm shared by the majority of society.

References

Bielawski, O. 1925: Schizofrenia. *Nowiny Psychiatryczne* 4.

Doroszewski, W. (ed.) 1958–69: *Słownik jezyka polskiego,* vols. 1–9. Warsaw: PWN.

Fromm, E. 1977: *Zapomniany jezyk.* Warsaw: PIW.

Frostig, J. 1933. *Psychjatrja,* vols. 1 and 2. Lwów: Zakład Ossolińskich.

Gruszecka, A. 1924: Stosunek myślenia do przezywania psychotycznego w pewnych przypadkach schizofrenii. *PTPN. Prace Komisji Lekarskiej* 2 (6). Poznań.

Guiraud, P. 1975: *Semiologia.* Warsaw: WP.

Irigaray, L. and Dubois, J. 1966: Les structures linguistiques de la parenté et leurs perturbations dans les cas de démence et de schizophrénie. *Cahiers de lexicologie* 8.

Karłowicz, J., Kryński, A. and Niedźwiedzki, W. (eds.) 1898–1927: *Słownik jezyka polskiego,* vols. 1–8. Warsaw: WP.

Kierkegaard, S. 1982: *Bojaźń i drzenie.* Warsaw: PWN.

Kipphardt, H. 1980: *Aleksander März.* Warsaw: PIW.

Laplantine, F. 1973: *L'Ethnopsychiatrie.* Psychothèque, Paris: Editions Universitaires.

Lee Masters, E. 1948: *Spoon River Anthology.* New York: Millar.

Lyons, J. 1977: *Semantics*, vol. 1. Cambridge: Cambridge University Press.

Malinowski, B. 1957: *Zycie seksualne dzikich w północno-zachodniej Melanezji.* Warsaw: PWN.

— 1981: *Rodzicielstwo jako podstawa struktury społecznej.* In A. K. Paluch, *Malinowski.* Warsaw: WP.

Navratil, L. 1971: *a und b leuchten im Klee—Psychopathologische Texte.* Munich:

Carl Hauser.
Ortega y Gasset, J. 1982: *Bunt mas i inne pisma socjologiczne*. Warsaw: PWN.
Rosenbaum, B. and Sonne, H. 1979: *Det er et bånd der taler: Analysis of Language and Body in Psychosis*. Copenhagen: Gyldendal.

16 Over-inclusion and cognitive disturbances in schizophrenic communication: An empirical study

Karl-Ernst Bühler and Hildegard Vogt

Introduction

The aim of the study reported in this chapter was the investigation of cognitive disturbances of schizophrenic patients, especially the 'over-inclusive thinking' suggested by Cameron (1938a,b; 1939a; 1939b; 1944). According to this thesis, the schizophrenic show a fuzzy concept formation, that is, they consider irrelevant as well as relevant aspects and elements. It is a disturbance of cognitive organization and integration induced by a defect of selection and elimination of information. The thinking is imprecise because the concepts may overlap.

This defect is brought to light by object-sorting tests (Payne 1962; Weckowicz and Blewett 1959; Chapman and Taylor 1957). However, in these tests the three representational modes of the coding of external events postulated by Bruner (1964) are not differentiated—that is, the enactive mode, the iconic mode and the verbal mode. To avoid this shortcoming, the use of colours as stimuli is suitable, because the coding process is mainly accomplished by the verbal mode and not by the enactive mode, as in the sorting tests, nor by the iconic mode. This was employed in the test used by Kelter *et al.* (1977), who investigated the verbal ability of aphasics by senseless visual structures which could be represented iconically as well as verbally because of secondary processes of Gestalt formation, so that the two representational modes contaminate each other. To isolate the verbal representational mode is very important for the investigation of schizophrenic concept formation, because the verbal ability due to the illness is only minimally reduced (see Payne 1961), and so a specific verbal influence can be neglected if it is not tested as such.

The organization of sensory data as a part of the concept formation is made evident by the verbal representation and their verbal labelling; therefore the concept formation, as well as its disturbance in schizophrenics, can be experimentally examined by our procedure. To achieve this end, a range of verbal representation with simple referents is necessary; these simple referents must be definable unequivocally by objective measures of their physical properties. This is the case in verbal descriptions of simple sensory perceptions, concerning for example temperature, taste, hearing, seeing—in sum, the 'language of experience' according to Lenneberg (1967). The range of colours, with its simple structural organization, is appropriate for testing the language of experience, because every colour shows a specific position in this continuous spectrum and can be discriminated very precisely.

Method

To test the alternating effects of perception, of concept formation and of language, Brown and Lenneberg (1954) have developed a specific experimental design using colours as stimuli. The verbal coding of the colours is operationally defined as codability, and scored *(1)* as the mean length of colour descriptions, called 'brevity of description' (especially the number of words and syllables), *(2)* the mean time of reaction in coding (RZK), and *(3)* the agreement of the subjects in respect to the specific descriptions (BU). Nonverbal cognition is measured as preciseness of recognition (WE). Lantz and Stefflre (1964) have introduced another measure of codability called communication accuracy (KG) which should be (in contrast to the other scores) independent of the specific arrangement of the colours. Therefore, besides the coders who described the colours verbally, a group of decoders is required who decode the verbal descriptions. The variable 'communication accuracy' is a social phenomenon, whereas the preciseness of recognition of the colours is exclusively an intrapersonal process. The communication of the colours is dependent on the verbal productivity as well as on the creativity, because the description of the colours does not follow rigid conventions.

Stimuli

In order to avoid the confusion of the three representative modes—enactive, iconic and verbal—the subjects were shown 48 colours from the HKS sample[1] (see Kast and Ehinger) which was also used by Hepting and Solle (1973) in their research with sane subjects. Therefore a comparison of the two studies is possible. Another advantage of the HKS sample is that it is smaller than the 85 colours of the Farnsworth-Munsell set and the 120 Munsell colour array used by Brown and Lenneberg (1954) and by Lantz and Stefflre (1964), so they do not exaggerate the motivation and the cooperation of the patients.

First the patients were shown all the colours for three minutes to give them a holistic impression of the stimuli to come. Then all subjects, schizophrenics as well as controls, were required to carry out the recognition task, ordered with different degrees of complexity. According to the degree of complexity, one colour or a sample of colours was shown to them. Afterwards they had to recognize the shown colours out of a changing pattern of 48 colours. To avoid unusual situations for the patients, the colours were not shown in a tachystoscope, but simply on tables with a white background, illuminated by daylight. After this procedure, one group of the subjects had to code all 24 colours (the other 24 colours were used only in the recognition task), and the other group had to decode the codes made by the coders.

Subjects

The group of schizophrenic patients consisted of 24 women and 24 men, 12 coders and 12 decoders in each group. They were compared with healthy subjects. The four groups—the schizophrenic coders and decoders as well as their normal comparison group—were matched in age, sex, education, professional training, verbal intelligence, and socioeconomic status of the parents.

The patients were treated in the psychiatric state hospitals in Lohr/Main, in Werneck, in Lengerich, and in the psychiatric clinic of the University of Würzburg. The diagnosis of schizophrenia was confirmed by means of the records, applying the Research Diagnostic Criteria (Taylor and Abrams 1975; Strauss and Gift 1977). The following conditions had to be fulfilled: *(1)* repeated hospital treatment, *(2)* delusions, hallucinations and thought disorders in the patient's history, *(3)* exclusion of a schizo-affective psychosis, *(4)* no alcoholism and drug abuse, *(5)* onset of the illness before the age of forty, and *(6)* lack of neurological disturbances. Mentally subnormal persons were excluded (i.e. those with a verbal IQ below 85) to avoid any additional influence of lack of intelligence on the concept formation.

Performance of the test (following Hepting and Solle 1973)

Recognition task The subjects had to recognize colours out of 48 colours according to recognition task 1 (one colour after five seconds of waiting), recognition task 2 (four colours after five seconds of waiting), and recognition task 3 (four colours after thirty seconds of waiting).

Coding and decoding The coders had to describe 24 colours one after the other, in such a way that other persons could recognize the colours from those descriptions. The decoders had to find the colours under several conditions: DK1, using the codes of the matched partner; DK2, using the codes of a coder out of the comparable group of intelligence; and DK3, using the codes of a coder selected by chance. The conditions DK4 to DK6 were examined only by the controls decoding the codes of the control coders: DK4 using the codes of the matched partner; DK5 using the codes of a coder out of the comparable group of intelligence of the controls; and DK6 using the codes of a coder out of the randomly selected control group. The schizophrenic decoders used only the codes of the schizophrenic patients (DK1–3), whereas normal subjects used the codes of the schizophrenic (DK1–3) as well as the codes of the sane coders (DK4–6: DK4 of the matched partner; DK5 of the comparable intelligence group; DK6 of a random partner by chance).

Results

Comparison of the codability and the recognition between schizophrenics and nonschizophrenics

Measures of codability The intrapersonal variability of coding is defined as the number of different codes of the 24 colours used by one specific subject. This additional measure was introduced by us because it shows the differentiation of the coding, and thus the tendency towards 'overinclusion'.

The brevity of description is the mean number of syllables as well as of words used by a person for the description of the colours. The time of reaction in coding (RZK) is to be seen as the mean of the duration from the beginning of the presentation of the stimuli until the beginning of the verbalization. The communication accuracy (KG) is measured by the number of correctly decoded colours out of the 24 colours under six different conditions (DK1–6). The number of the correctly recognized colours is the measure of preciseness of recognition.

Hepting and Solle (1973) found differences between men and women in an increased 'brevity of description' and a smaller reaction time in men, and this was also the case in our investigation (see Table 16.1, p. 368).

This sex-specific variation was eliminated in our investigation of schizophrenia by an analysis of covariance mediated by a multiple regression. After that procedure we found differences in all measures of codability and the conditions of recognition 1 and 2 (see Table 16.2) with lower scores for the schizophrenics. Salzinger *et al.* (1966) also described a higher stereotypy in schizophrenic speech especially increased repetition of words which showed itself in type/token-ratio.

Correlations between codability and recognition

The measures of codability, of the conditions of recognition, and of the time of reaction (measured according to the procedures of Brown and Lenneberg (1954) and Lantz and Stafflre (1964)) were correlated with each other. For both groups, schizophrenics and controls, the correlations were differently significant for different variables; but as the correlations were computed for each group separately, these differences have no significance within the scope of this chapter.

Discussion of the results

This section discusses only those results which differentiate between the schizophrenic and the non-schizophrenic. First to be considered is the question whether the results show disturbances in the concept formation of schizophrenics and if so, what effects these have on communication.

The measures of codability— variability, brevity of description, and time of reaction in coding—indicate differences. The schizophrenics showed decreased variability, lowered time of reaction, and a fewer number of syllables and words. This may be caused by a disorganized structuring of complex stimuli and a lack in the differentiation of predicates. One predicate is used for different shades of colours, and therefore

TABLE 16.1 *U-tests of significance.*

	Women			Men			Men and women		
	M-H	M-S	SIG	M-H	M-S	SIG	M-H	M-S	SIG
variability	23.17	22.25	—	22.92	19.75	**	23.04	21.00	**
syallable number	4.92	3.57	—	7.77	2.95	**	6.34	3.26	**
word number	2.59	1.85	—	4.38	1.38	**	3.48	1.61	**
RZK	6.30	4.58	—	8.16	6.16	*	7.23	5.37	**
DK1	0.46	0.47	—	0.49	0.39	*	0.48	0.43	—
DK2	0.41	0.36	—	0.43	0.43	—	0.42	0.40	—
DK3	0.43	0.45	—	0.48	0.44	—	0.46	0.45	—
DK-sum	0.43	0.42	—	0.47	0.42	*	0.45	0.42	—
WE1	0.66	0.50	*	0.66	0.50	*	0.66	0.50	***
WE2	0.40	0.33	—	0.37	0.31	—	0.38	0.32	—
WE3	0.42	0.42	—	0.35	0.28	—	0.38	0.34	—
RZ-DK1	3.45	3.28	—	2.72	3.94	*	3.08	3.61	—
RZ-DK2	3.00	3.13	—	2.70	3.48	—	2.85	3.30	—
RZ-DK3	2.70	2.92	—	2.13	3.86	*	2.42	3.39	*
RZ-DK-sum	3.08	3.15	—	2.55	3.82	*	2.79	3.44	—
RZ-WE1	4.04	5.81	—	3.60	6.25	**	3.81	6.06	**
RZ-WE2	2.96	4.71	—	4.88	5.44	—	3.84	5.05	—
RZ-WE3	5.82	4.76	—	6.00	7.29	—	5.92	6.14	—

Key to Tables 16.1 and 16.2:
DK1-3 = decoding conditions 1–3; H = healthy; M = mean; RKZ = reaction time; RZ-DK1-3 = reaction time of decoding conditions 1–3; RZ-WE 1–3 = reaction time of recognition conditions 1–3; S = schizophrenics; SIG = significance (* = 5%; ** = 1%; *** = 0.001%); WE 1–3 = recognition conditions 1–3

TABLE 16.2 *Analysis of covariance.*

	Mean corrected		
	H	S	SIG
variability	23.73	20.31	**
syllable number	5.79	3.82	**
word number	3.15	1.94	**
RZK	6.37	6.23	*
DK1	0.49	0.42	**
DK2	0.39	0.42	—
DK3	0.45	0.45	—
WE1	0.66	0.50	**
WE2	0.39	0.31	*
WE3	0.39	0.33	—
RZ-DK1	3.10	3.59	**
RZ-DK2	2.83	3.32	*
RZ-DK3	2.32	3.49	**
RZ-WE1	3.81	6.05	**
RZ-WE2	3.66	5.23	—
RZ-WE3	5.76	6.30	—

the intrapersonal variability is diminished. Also, the reduced numbers of syllables and words indicate a conceptual simplicity. As the time of reaction is a sign of the difficulty of a problem, as it is shortened for the schizophrenic coding, it is probable that the patients cannot recognize the complexity of the task. All these results indicate 'over-inclusion', simplification and insufficient cognitive differentiation. Another argument is the impaired intrapersonal communication indicated by the reduced recognition of schizophrenics in conditions 1 and 2, and the positive correlation of condition of recognition 3 (WE3) with the number of words. The short predicates seem to be over-inclusive for the schizophrenics and therefore not suitable for recognition. The decreased variability, i.e. the increased stereotypicality, contradicts the hypothesis of higher creativity in schizophrenics (see Hasenfus and Magaro 1976; Treece 1956), because a presupposition for creativity is cognitive flexibility (see Mednick 1962; Getzels and Jackson 1962; Torrance 1963) and there is no indication of this in the schizophrenic group.

Of the utmost importance for the disturbed concept formation is its effect on interpersonal communication. The latter is testable by our experimental design. Comparing the results of decoding by the Wilcoxon test (see Hays 1973), there is no difference between the decoding of schizophrenic codes by sane subjects and the decoding of sane codes by sane subjects. But the schizophrenic subjects obtain poor results in decoding the schizophrenic codes. We hypothesize that the disturbed communication of schizophrenics is caused mainly by lack of understanding rather than by impaired verbal expressibility.

We would conclude by saying that the results of our investigation support the hypothesis of disturbed concept formation in the sense of 'over-inclusion'.

Note to Chapter 16

1 HKS refers to a system of colours produced by the firm of Kast & Ehinger in Stuttgart.

References

Brown, R. W. and Lenneberg, E. H. 1954: A study in language and cognition. *Journal of Abnormal and Social Psychology* 49.

Bruner, J. S. 1964: The course of cognitive growth. *American Psychologist* 19.

Cameron, N. 1938a: A study of thinking in senile deterioration and schizophrenic disorganisation. *American Journal of Psychology* 51.

— 1938b: Reasoning, regression and communication in schizophrenics. *Psychological Monographs* 50(1).

— 1939a: Schizophrenic thinking in a problem-solving situation. *Journal of Mental Science* 85.

— 1939b: Deterioration and regression in schizophrenic thinking. *Journal of Abnormal and Social Psychology* 34.

— 1944: Experimental analysis of schizophrenic thinking. In J. S. Kasanin (ed.), *Language and Thought in Schizophrenia*. Berkeley: University of California Press.

Chapman, C. J. and Taylor, J. A. 1957: Breath and deviate concepts used by schizophrenics. *Journal of Abnormal and Social Psychology* 54.

Getzels, J. W. and Jackson, P. W. 1962: *Creativity and Intelligence*. London: Wiley.

Hasenfus, N. and Magaro, P. 1976: Creativity and schizophrenia. *British Journal of Psychiatry* 129.

Hays, W. L. 1973: *Statistics for the Social Sciences*. New York: Holt, Rinehart & Winston.

Hepting, U. and Solle, R. 1973: Über geschlechtsspezifische Unterschiede verbaler Farbkodierung. *Archiv für Psychologie* 125.

Kelter, S. *et al.* 1977: Verbal coding and visual memory in aphasics. *Neuropsychologia* 15.

Lantz, De L. and Stefflre, V. 1964: Language and cognition revisited. *Journal of Abnormal and Social Psychology* 69.

Lenneberg, E. H. 1967: *Biological Foundations of Language*. New York: Wiley.

Mednick, S. A. 1962: The associative basis of the creative process. *Psychological Review* 69.

Payne, R. W. 1961: Cognitive abnormalities. In H. J. Eysenck (ed.), *Handbook of Abnormal Psychology*. New York:

— 1962: An object-classification test as a measure of overinclusive thinking in schizophrenic patients. *British Journal of Social and Clinical Psychology* 1.

Salzinger, K. *et al.* 1966: Verbal behavior in schizophrenics and some comments toward a theory of schizophrenia. In P. H. Hoch and J. Zubin (eds.), *Psychopathology of Schizophrenia*. New York: Grune & Stratton.

Strauss, J. S. and Gift, T. E. 1977: Choosing an approach for diagnosing schizophrenia. *Archive of General Psychiatry* 34.

Taylor, M. A. and Abrams, R. 1975: A critique of the St Louis psychiatric research criteria for schizophrenia. *American Journal of Psychiatry* 132.

Torrance, E. P. 1963: Developing creative thinking through school experience. In S. J. Parnes and H. F. Harding, (eds.), *A Source Book of Creative Thinking*. New York: Scribner.

Treece, H. 1956: *Dylan Thomas*. London: Benn.

Weckowicz, T. E. and Blewett, D. B. 1959: Size constancy and abstract thinking in schizophrenic patients. *Journal of Mental Science* 105.

Notes on contributors

Susanne Bleiberg Seperson received her PhD from the Graduate School and University Center of the City University of New York in 1981. She is currently Associate Professor of Sociology at Dowling College, Oakdale, New York. Her current interests include sociolinguistics, the sociology of mental illness and applied sociology.

Gerd Buchkremer is Senior Consultant Psychiatrist in the psychiatric department of the University and Medical School at Münster, FRG. He has done research work on methods of nicotine-weaning, and is now particularly interested in the therapeutic prevention of relapses of schizophrenia, and in the treatment of the schizophrenic patient's family members.

Karl-Ernst Bühler, MD, psychologist, psychotherapist, psychiatrist, is Assistant Professor of Psychotherapy and Psychosomatic Medicine at the University of Würtzberg. His fields of study include medicine, psychology and philosophy. He has carried out research in the fields of psychiatry, psychotherapy and psychosomatic medicine, and has published several articles and chapters in books.

Brigitte De Decker studied Dutch and English at the Vrije Universiteit of Brussels (VUB). She is currently working as a researcher for the National Science Foundation of Belgium. She is preparing a doctoral dissertation on language and schizophrenia.

Hans Rudi Fischer has studied psychology, linguistics, philosophy and child psychiatry. He wrote a dissertation on Wittgenstein's philosophy of psychology. He has published on Wittgenstein's philosophy, psychoanalysis and philosophy of language, meditation and psychotherapy, and the concept of rule in psychopathology. His scientific interests include the philosophy of language, language and schizophrenia, psychotherapy (family therapy), scientific problems of psychology and psychiatry.

Helmut Gruber studied psychology, applied linguistics, pedagogics and german philosophy at the University of Vienna, and is at present working on a doctoral dissertation 'Evaluation and Standardization of a Projective Sentence-Supplement Test for Children'. His main areas of interest are discourse analysis, models of cognitive text planning and therapeutic discourse.

Marie-Louise Kaesermann was trained as a psychologist at the University of Berne, Switzerland. After her dissertation on 'Language Acquisition and Interaction' in 1978, she stayed at the Max Planck Institute for Psycholinguistics in Nijmegen for two and a half years. In 1980 she started working at the research department of the psychiatric clinic of Bernese University, Switzerland. There she began basic research on the verbal behaviour of psychotic (especially schizophrenic) people. Her main interest is in a functional view of verbal and nonverbal communication, and she tries to apply psychological as well as psycholinguistic methodology to problems of psychopathology.

Karin Kichler studied linguistics and psychology at the University of Vienna. Her main interests are social psychology, sociolinguistics and discourse analysis. She is currently working on a doctoral dissertation about the image of women in radio advertisements.

Johanna Lalouschek studied linguistics and psychology. She is currently working on a project studying doctor–patient communication and is writing a doctoral dissertation about TV discussions.

Peter Nowak studied linguistics, and took part in a language therapy project for mongoloid children in 1982. His interests include discourse analysis, psycholinguistics and client-centred therapy.

Günter Peuser studied German and romance philology at Göttingen, Madrid and Freiburg from 1956 to 1961. From 1961 to 1970, he was Assistant Professor of Romance Philology at Freiburg, and published on syntactic problems of Spanish and French. From 1970 to 1980, he was clinical linguist at the Rhenanian Provincial Hospital at Bonn. Since 1981, he has been Professor of Applied Linguistics and Patholinguistics at the University of Cologne; he has published on aphasia, and a volume of the monographical series 'Patholinguistica' and 'Logotherapia'. He is a member of the editorial board of the *British Journal of Communication Disorders*.

Klaus Schonauer studied medicine, linguistics, psychology and sociology in Münster. He has worked on speech phenomena of schizophrenic psychosis and on medical semiotics.

Agnes Speck and Sabine Stitz are scientific collaborators on a project on therapeutic discourse at the Freie Universität Berlin begun in 1983.

William Van Belle is Associate Professor at the Department of Linguistics of the University of Louvain. He has published several articles on general linguistics, psychoanalysis, and discourse analysis. His current research concerns rhetorical and argumentative structures in political and psychotic discourse.

Diek van Bijsterveld studied general linguistics and language philosophy. At the moment she carries out research on conversations with schizophrenic people at the University of Leiden (ZWO, Department of Psychiatry, Psychiatrisch Ziekenhuis Endegeest, Endegeesterweg 2–5, Oegstgeest). Her chapter in this volume is part of that research. She formerly published under the name Wenckebach-van Bijsterveld.

Peter Van de Craen studied Dutch, English and neurolinguistics at the Vrije Universiteit of Brussels (VUB). His PhD thesis on social linguistics tried to develop a hermeneutic way in looking at language phenomena. He is currently lecturer at the University of Brussels. His main interests include sociolinguistics, the study of urban multilingualism, language and education, and deviant language behaviour.

Hildegard Vogt studied medicine and specialized in psychiatry and medical psychology. She wrote an experimentally orientated thesis concerning linguistic and cognitive disturbances of schizophrenics, advised by K.-E. Bühler. Part of her contribution to the volume results from this work.

Stephan Von Block studied romance languages, linguistics and pedagogy. Since 1978 he has worked at the University of Bonn. He is mainly interested in psycholinguistics, first language acquisition, aphasia, and communication problems of schizophrenic people.

Ruth Wodak received her PhD in 1974 from the University of Vienna, where, since 1983, she has been Professor of Applied Linguistics, Sociolinguistics and Psycholinguistics. She is the author of numerous articles and several books, of which the most important are *Das Sprachverhalten von Angeklagten bei Gericht* (1975); *Das Wort in der Gruppe* (1981; English translation, *Language Behavior in Groups*, 1985); *Hilflose Nähe? Mütter and Töchter erzahlen* (1984); and *The Language of Love and Guilt,* with Muriel Schulz (1984). She published under the name Leodolter until 1976, and subsequently under the names of Wodak-Leodolter and Wodak.

Janusz Wróbel was born in Cieszyn, Poland. Since 1978 he has been working at the Polonia Institute of the Jagiellonian University, Krakow, Poland. He has studied problems of Polonia (Poles abroad). Psycholinguistics is his main research interest. The subject of his PhD dissertation was the semantics and pragmatics of the language of schizophrenics, and he is the author of a number of works in this field. He is currently an exchange professor in the Slavic Department, Wayne State University, Detroit.

Chapter abstracts

Chapter 1

This chapter covers some aspects of a broad study of therapeutic discourse in an open group of suicidal patients in the crisis intervention centre of Vienna. It concentrates on the therapeutic effect, and on the possibilities of 'measuring' the success (or lack of success) of therapy with the help of text-linguistic, sociolinguistic, and psycholinguistic methods. First, the methods and models being used up to now in the study of therapeutic discourse are examined. Secondly, my own (three-level) model is elaborated. Three layers of meaning are differentiated in an interdisciplinary approach. Each text has therefore to be analysed on several levels simultaneously. Two texts from the same patient describing the same problem are analysed in a qualitative way, illustrating the methodology, the model of meaning and the interdisciplinary approach, as well as the means of objectifying the therapeutic effect. The textual macrostructure (in relation to other categories) is the most important indicator. This approach is relevant for the theory of psychotherapy, for theories of text-planning as well as for therapeutic practice.

Dieser Aufsatz behandelt einen Aspekt einer größeren Studie zur therapeutischen Kommunikation von Suizidgefährdten in einem Kriseninterventionszentrum, Wien (siehe Wodak 1981) Die 'Gruppentherapeutische Problemdarstellung' (monologische Präsentation *des* zentralen Problems durch den Patienten) einer Patientin wird qualitativ untersucht, u.z.w. im Grad höchster Involviertheit und ein Jahr später, als sie das Problem 'im Griff hat'. Der *therapeutische Effekt* kann also objektiviert werden, anhand textlinguistischer Methoden (der Texttyp u.a. ändert sich signifikant, gemäß der 'Soziopsychologischen Theorie der Textplanung'; außerdem sind natürlich textinhärente Faktoren betroffen, wie auch der Gefühlsausdruck, Abwehrmechanismen usw.) Die genaue qualitative Analyse illustriert auch das 'Drei-Ebenen-Modell', das speziell für therapeutische Kommunikation, zur Erfassung des komplexen Prozesses und der vielschichtigen Bedeutungen, entworfen wurde. Dieser Ansatz ist für die Theorie der Textplanung und Textproduktion, für die Methodendiskussion innerhalb der Psychotherapie, für die Überprüfbarkeit therapeutischer Behandlungen und für die therapeutische Praxis relevant.

Chapter 2

The aim of this investigation is to describe the linguistic means of persuasion in psychotherapy. How does the therapist persuade the client to adapt to the therapist's view of the world? In addition, the detailed linguistic analysis of the client's reactions can show the quality of the effect that therapy has on the client. A discourse analysis of this kind can also be the basis for further comparison of different forms of therapy. Two sections of a text from a therapy session are qualitatively analysed while considering four levels of meaning: the manifest colloquial structure of the therapeutic interventions, the latent intentions of the therapist, the manifest reactions of the client (the interactive dimension), and the latent meaning of the client's remarks.

Suggestive Psychotherapie in ihrer Komplexheit als vielschichtige Kommunikationssituation zu erfassen, ist Ziel dieser Arbeit. Da der Therapeut in der suggestiven Psychotherapie mit latenten Bedeutungen und Intentionen arbeitet, die dem Klienten nicht bewußt werden sollen, wurde ein 'Mehr-Ebenen-Modell' zur Analyse dieses Diskurses angewandt. Zwei Textstellen wurden jeweils auf den folgenden vier Ebenen analysiert:
1 die manifesten Interventionen des Therapeuten;
2 die latenten Intentionen des Therapeuten;
3 die manifesten Reaktionen des Klienten (interaktive Dimension);
4 die latenten Bedeutungen der Klientenreaktionen;
Mittels dieses differenzierten psycholinguistischen Analyseansatzes kann die komplexe Struktur indirekter Suggestion und ihre Wirkung auf den Klienten genau analysiert und aufgezeigt werden.

Chapter 3

Confrontation, used as an activity to encourage psychic change, is examined from an ethnomethodological and conversational point of view. A paradigm and a grammatical model of confrontation are developed, and the activity is analysed by focusing on its essential features. Reality confrontation requires at its minimum: (1) an implicit or explicit disagreement between the two speaker-hearers, (2) a punch line arrived at in a non-direct way, (3) in the form of a rhetorical question which points out a basic inconsistency. The data is based on transcripts of audiotaped psychotherapy sessions. Examples of completed and incompleted confrontations, as well as variations, were analysed.

In diesem artikel wird der Begriff Konfrontation als ein Mittel um psychische Veränderung zustande zu bringen aus einem ethnomethodologischen und Konversationsanalytischen Standpunkt untersucht. Ein Paradigma und ein grammatisches Konfrontationsmodell werden entwickelt und die wichtigsten Kennzeichen davon werden untersucht. Die Konfrontation mit der Wirklichkeit beinhaltet zumindest: (1) einem impliziten oder expliziten Meinungsunterschied zwischen der zwei Sprechern/Zuhörern, (2) einen 'punch line' in der Form eine rhetorische Frage. Das material kommt von Transkriptionen von auf Tonband aufgenommene Therapiesessionen. Beispiele von völlständigen oder unvollständigen Konfrontationen und Variationen davon werden analysiert.

Chapter 4

This chapter analyses the therapy beginnings of thirty-one clients, being treated by four therapists, systematically in the light of the question: how do both participants in therapeutic discourse make it clear to each other that they find themselves in a specific discourse situation with one another? First, we will consider, in more general terms, how institutional frames and a definition of the situation, which is to be worked out by the participants, can be linked together in discourse. Secondly (after a short discussion of the specific therapeutic concepts) the different methods of initiating (bound to the specific concepts) which are used by the participants will be described.

1 Behavioural therapy: the patients and the therapist work out together interactional routines of conversational *openings*; this corresponds to the 'normal form pattern' for initiating 'commencements' of discourse.
2 Client-centred therapy: the clarification of therapy beginnings takes place explicitly: in the form of a therapeutic instruction, the beginning is made visible.
3 Depth-psychology-orientated therapy: the opening is realized by a question formulated in common everyday terms, such as *How are you doing*?—it stresses thus the 'constitution of normality' in the therapeutic setting.

By this study we can show that the therapeutic situation is both frame constitutive and (in its particularity) worked out by the participants or made clear by one to the other.

In diesem Beitrag werden die Therapiestunden(anfänge) von 31 Patienten bei drei Therapeuten systematisch unter der Fragestellung untersucht: Wie verdeutlichen sich die Teilnehmer therapeutischer (Einzel-)Gespräche, daß sie sich in einem spezifischen Gespräch miteinander befinden? Zum einen werden allgemeine Vorüberlegungen darüber angestellt, wie im Gespräch institutionelle Gebundenheit mit der von den Aktanten zu erarbeitenden Situationsdefinition verbunden ist. Zum anderen werden (nach einer kurzen Diskussion der jeweiligen Therapiekonzepte) die je nach Konzept verschiedenen Methoden des 'Anfangens', die von den Teilnehmern verwendet werden, dargestellt.

1 Gesprächstherapie: Die Verdeutlichung des Therapiebeginns geschieht explizit: in Form einer therapeutischen Instruktion wird hier sichtbar das 'Anfangen' verdeutlicht.
2 Tiefenpsychologisch orientierte Therapie: Die Eröffnung wird durch die alltagsweltlich vertraute Formulierung 'wie geht es Ihnen' realisiert und ist damit betont 'normalitätskonstituierend'.
3 Verhaltenstherapie: Die Patienten und der Therapeut entwickeln Interaktionsroutinen bei der Eröffnung des Gesprächs; dies korrespondiert mit in 'Normal-form' abgewickelten Stundenanfängen.

Es kann durch die Untersuchung gezeigt werden, daß die therapeutische Situation sowohl rahmensetzend wirkt, als auch das Verständnis der Besonderheit der Situation von den Teilnehmern erarbeitet bzw. Sich gegenseitig verdeutlicht wird.

Chapter 5

In this analysis of group therapy sessions, we show that such a session can be divided into three stages: 'outset', 'describing the problem' and 'ending'. Particularly, we try to find out the structure of the 'outset' stage, and to describe and classify the phenomena appearing there, based on the methods of qualitative discourse analysis. Our main interest was to pinpoint the transition from 'outset' to 'describing the problem' by the use of linguistic criteria. The stage of outset can be further divided: 'start' means the moment the therapist enters the room; 'begin' stands for the actual outset of the session, the moment the stage of 'describing the problem' starts. The period between 'start' and 'begin' we call 'outset', in which we include all utterances which could lead to a 'begin' if not inhibited by the other participants.

In unserer Analyse therapeutischer Gruppensitzungen konnten wir zeigen, daß sich ein Therapiegespräch in die Phasen 'Anfang', 'Problemdarstellung' und 'Ende' gliedern läßt. Unser spezielles Interesse galt der Struktur der Anfangsphase undden dort auftretenden sprachlichen Phänomenen. Mittels linguistischer Kriterien gelang es uns, den Übergang von der Anfangsphase zur Phase des eigentlichen therapeutischen Gesprächs, den Problemdarstellungen zu erfassen. Die Anfangsphase einer therapeutischen Sitzung läßt sich somit weiter unterteilen: mit 'Start' bezeichen wir den Moment, in dem der Therapeut den Raum betritt; mit 'Beginn' den Anfang des eigentlichen therapeutischen Gesprächs. Den Zeitraum zwischen 'Start' und 'Beginn' nennen wir 'Anfang'. Darunter fallen alle Äußerungen, die zu einem 'Beginn', also einer Problemdarstellung führen könnten, von den anderen Teilnehmern aber durch bestimmte Strategien verhindert werden.

Chapter 6

This chapter discusses the differences in the planning and design of texts in normal and neurotic adolescents, male and female. Hypotheses and categories are developed for the analysis of a thirteen-item projective sentence supplement test, which was carried out by twelve-year-olds, based on the sociopsycholinguistic theory of textplanning. The results show significant differences between normal and neurotic adolescents concerning semantic-syntactic complexity and variance of content of the answers. Qualitative analysis of two text samples shows additional differences between the two groups in respect to surface structure and cognitive text planning. These differences are also discussed within the theoretical framework of SPTT.

In Dieser Arbeit werden die Unterschiede in der Textplanung und Gestaltung bei normalen und neurotischen Jugendlichen dargestellt. Ausgehend von der sozio-psycholinguistischen Theorie der Textplanung werden Hypothesen und Kategorien zur Analyse eines 13 Items umfassenden projektiven Satzergänzungstests, der den 12-jährigen vorgelegt wurde, entwickelt. Die quantitativen Resultate zeigen signifikante Unterschiede in der semantisch-syntaktischen Komplexität und der inhaltlichen Streuung zwischen der normalen und der neurotischen Stichprobe. Die qualitative Analyse zweier Beispieltexte zeigt zusätzliche Unterschiede in der oberflächensyntaktischen Ausgestaltung und der kognitiven Textplanung zwischen normalen und gestörten Jugendlichen. Diese Unterschiede werden ebenfalls im theoretischen Rahmen der SPTT erörtert.

Chapter 7

This chapter proposes an analysis of the phenomena of schizophrenia which is orientated to the late philosophy of Wittgenstein. The speech-interactive aspect of deviant behaviour is stressed, and psychosis is interpreted as an expression of a form of family life. Wittgenstein's conception of 'language game' as a social practice stresses the interconnection of language and action, with particular regard to the acquisition of language. Since Fromm-Reichmann's publication (1948) about the schizophrenogenic mother, the family as a socializing agent was emphasized by psychiatric investigations. This provides the opportunity to introduce Wittgenstein's concepts of 'language game' and 'grammar' as a means of research. The author shows that the language games of schizophrenic families have an epistemology of their own, which may be analysed by linguistic criteria and reduced to an intersubjectively introduced grammar as a 'form of representation' as Wittgenstein sees it. This specific grammar moulds not only the perception of reality describable by language but also the patterns of action and interaction. According to Wittgenstein, grammar is an expression of forms of life; and therefore I postulate a symmetry of grammar and forms of life. In abnormal cases this symmetry is distorted or even destroyed. The 'divided self' which is, according to Laing, specific for schizophrenic persons shows that 'schizophrenic forms of life' correspond to an antinomic grammar which gives the abnormal individual an inevitably contradictory reality. Schizophrenia is conceived as a form of life, and therefore fundamentally as an object of interpretation in psychology and psychotherapy.

Der Autor versucht im vorliegenden Aufsatz Wittgensteins Begriffe der 'Grammatik' und des 'Sprachspiels' für eine kommunikationstheoretisch orientierte Schizophrenieforschung fruchtbar zu machen. An einem Beispiel wird deutlich gemacht, daß dem 'schizophrenen Sprachspiel' eine entsprechende Lebensform korrespondiert. Für den Normalfall wird eine Symmetrie zwischen Grammatik und Lebensform postuliert. Die operationalen und perspektivischen Komponenten der Grammatik als Form der Organisation und Darstellung von Wirklichkeit werden herausgearbeitet. Die postulierte Symmetrie zwischen Grammatik und Lebensform ist im pathologischen Falle gestört. An einem Beispiel macht die vorgeschlagene Analyse deutlich, daß die Perspektive des 'schizophrenen Sprachspiels' insoweit gestört ist, als die für die Sprachspiele über psychische Zustände fundamentale kriterienlose Selbszuschreibung kriteriell wird. Der Schizophene ist damit wehrlos den Zuschreibungen anderer ausgeliefert. Das Subjekt hat eine antinomische Grammatik internalisiert, die es in einer widersprüchlichen Welt gefangen hält.

Chapter 8

Double-binds are interpreted by Watzlawick *et al.* as 'paradoxical injunctions'. They are basically concerned with complex injunctions, containing unsolvable semantic contradictions. Due to a close and vital interpersonal relationship, the receiver of the message can neither comment on the paradoxical situation nor escape from it. According to the frequency of the 'paradoxical injunction', the reaction to this form of communication may correspond to the clinical picture obtaining in cases of neurotic or schizophrenic disturbances. This chapter deals with 'paradoxical injunctions' in 'everyday and in scientific language'. First of all, presuppositions of terminology are clarified ('everyday language', 'language of science', etc.). In the practical section, 'paradoxical injunctions' are discussed in different contexts. Examples of pedagogics are dealt with as being representative of the 'language of science'. For 'everyday language', magazine columns containing psychological advice are examined. Furthermore, the possible connections between 'paradoxical injunctions' and the development of stuttering are examined.

Doppelbindungen werden von Watzlawick *et al.* als 'paradoxe Handlungsaufforderungen' interpretiert. Es handelt sich im wesentlichen um komplexe Aufforderungen, die unlösbare semantische Widersprüche bergen. Aufgrund einer engen und lebenswichtigen zwischenmenschlichen Beziehung kann die paradoxe Situation jedoch von dem Empfänger der Botschaft weder kommentiert werden, noch kann er sich der Situation durch Flucht entziehen. Je nach Häufigkeit der 'paradoxen Handlungsaufforderung' kann die *Reaktion* auf diese Form der Kommunikation dem klinischen Bild neurotischer und schizophrener Störungen entsprechen. Der vorliegende Beitrag untersucht 'paradoxe Handlungsaufforderungen' in der 'Sprache des Alltags und der Wissenschaft'. Zunächst werden Voraussetzungen terminologischer Art geklärt ('alltagssprache', 'Sprache der Wissenschaft', etc.). Im praktischen Teil werden 'paradoxe Handlungsaufforderungen' in verschiedenen Kontexten besprochen. Stellvertretend für die 'Wissenschaftssprache' werden Beispiele aus der Erziehungswissenschaft herangezogen. Im Bereich der 'Alltagssprache' werden Beratungsrubriken in Illustrierten untersucht. Außerdem wird die *mögliche* Rolle 'paradoxer Handlungsaufforderungen' in der Entstehung des Stotterns erörtert.

Chapter 9

By comparing two types of deviant speech, this chapter aims to demonstrate that contrastive analysis is a useful method of patholinguistic research, provided that a relatively well-known phenomenon (jargonaphasia) is compared with a less well-known phenomenon (schizophasia). The contrastive analysis of individual cases of jargonaphasia and schizophasia yields the following main results.

The schizophasic speaker deliberately changes from normal to a very special type of deviant speech which is characterized by semantic neologisms. This deliberate change of register is denied to the jargonaphasic whose deviant speech is characterized by semantic paraphasias and phonemic neologisms.

The analysis of provoked speech, i.e. confrontation naming and sentence comprehension, points to another striking difference between jargonaphasia and schizophasia: the linguistic competence of the jargonaphasic is severely disturbed, whereas sentence comprehension and word finding in the schizophrenic speaker are intact. (Occasional ruptures of syntactic cohesion have to be ascribed to a momentary breakdown of psycholinguistic competence, i.e. of memory and concentration.)

Aphasic and schizophasic jargon have different communicative functions: whereas the jargon of the aphasic is reduced to the only function of establishing and maintaining social contact, schizophasic jargon can be used for persuasion and self-assertion.

As the schizophasic utterances of the schizophrenic speaker are triggered by an interlocutor begging for more information, schizophasia can be interpreted as a reaction to communicative stress.

A model describing the different steps of word-formation explains neologistic jargon by the disinhibition of phonemic, morphological and semantic processes which are blocked in normal speakers. But this disinhibition produces different results: the linguistic faculties of the schizophrenic are (temporarily) increased, whereas the utterances of the aphasic are (more or less permanently) reduced to a meaningless gibberish.

In diesem Aufsatz wird der Versuch unternommen, durch die kontrastive Analyse jeweils eines Falles von Jargonaphasie und Schizophasie die Differentialdiagnose beider Störungen auf gesicherte Kriterien zu stützen und gleichzeitig durch die Konfrontation mit der patholinguistisch besser untersuchten Jargonaphasie das Bild der Schizophasie zu erhellen. Neben dem Registerwechsel zwischen normalem und abweichendem Sprachgebrauch erweist sich die Verwendung von semantischen Neologismen als wichtigstes differentialdiagnostisches Kriterium der Schizophasie. Im

Gegensatz dazu ist die Spontansprache des Jargonaphatikers durch die Verwendung von semantischen Paraphasien und phonematischen Neologismen gekennzeichnet. Zusätzliche differentialdiagnostische Kriterien liefern provozierte Sprachleistungen, d.h.: Wortfindung (Bildbenennung) und Sprachverständnis (Drei-Figuren-Test), die beim Aphatiker gestört, beim Schizophrenen jedoch intakt sind.

Im Gegensatz zu dem auf die phatische Funktion reduzierten Jargon des Aphatikers dienen die schizophatischen Äußerungen der Selbstdarstellung und Überredung des Kommunikationspartners. Da sie durch insistierende Gesprächspartner ausgelöst werden, können sie als Reaktion auf kommunikative Streß gedeutet werden. Indem die schizophatischen Passagen die private Weltsicht des Patienten mehr oder weniger verschlüsselt kundtun, bieten sie der Psychotherapie wesentliche Aufschlüsse.

Anhand eines Modells der Wortproduktion werden die phonematischen Neologismen des Jargonaphatikers und die semantischen Neologismen des Schizophrenen als pathologische Enthemmung von normalerweise blockierten phonematischen bzw. semantischen und morphologischen Prozessen gedeutet. Diese Enthemmung wirkt sich jedoch sehr unterschiedlich aus: Im Gegensatz zum Aphatiker, dessen Kommunikationsleistung dadurch verringert wird, kommt es beim Schizophrenen zu einer vorübergehenden Steigerung seiner sprachlichen Fähigkeiten.

Chapter 10

This chapter presents a new way of looking at the schizophrenic syndrome, combining the communicative and the lateralization hypotheses. Communication with schizophrenic people shows many violations of conversational maxims as defined by Grice. It is hypothesized that, at least in some schizophrenics, their specific way of communicating may be a reflection of the hemisphericity hypothesis, which states that in many right-handed schizophrenic people the left hemisphere is overactivated. This hypothesis is discussed by means of a case study. It is concluded that this approach is promising with respect to the development of an interpersonal theory of schizophrenese, as suggested by Sullivan.

In diesem artikel werden wir uns Schizofrenie auf eine neue Weise ansehen. Wir werden die sog. Kommunikationshypothese in Verband mit der Lateralisationshypothese bringen. Kommunkation mit schizofrenen Menschen weist zahlreiche Abweichungen auf von der Maximentheorie von Grice. Die vorgebrachte These ist, dass, zumindest bei einer gewissen Anzahl von schizofrenen Menschen, diese spezifische Art von Kommunikation eine Reflektion von der Hemisphärhypothese ist. Die Hemisphärhypothese behauptet, dass die linke Hemisphäre vieler rechtshändiger schizofrener Menschen überaktiviert ist. Anhand einer 'case study' werden wir diese Annahme diskutieren. Die Konklusion ist, dass, nach Sullivan, diese Näherung wertvoll ist in Bezug auf die Entwicklung einer interpersönlichen Theorie van Schizofrenie.

Chapter 11

Seventy texts, which had been produced in standardized contexts by schizophrenic and nonschizophrenic speakers, were empirically analysed in order to investigate the speakers' different ways of text constitution in spontaneous speech. For this purpose we used the taxonomy of 'cohesive ties'—developed by Halliday and Hasan—which enabled us to some extent to describe the semantic and lexicogrammatical 'inner coherence' of a spoken text by using a rather nomothetical procedure. In the texts of our nonparanoid schizophrenic speakers we found significantly fewer 'cohesive ties' than in those texts which had been produced by nonschizophrenic speakers. As a result of an additional longitudinal analysis, we found in the texts of the schizophrenic subject group after attendance at a three-month psychotherapy programme an increased amount of 'cohesion'. It had been a central aim of this programme to support the schizophrenic patient's faculties of coping with stress, both on a social and on a more cognitive level. The statistical results of our study are discussed mainly in connection with some specific cognitive symptoms of the schizophrenic psychosis.

70 spontansprachliche und in standardisierten Kontexten zustandegekommene Texte schizophrener und nichtschizophrener Sprecher wurden empirisch daraufhin untersucht, welche Strategien die Sprecher verwenden, um ihrer Äußerung Stringenz und inneren Zusammenhang zu geben. Dabei wurde die von Halliday und Hasan erarbeitete Typologie 'kohäsiver Verknüpfungen' verwendet, die es ermöglicht, die semantische und lexikogrammatische Geschlossenheit eines sprachlichen Textes quantitativ zu beschreiben. In den Texten der untersuchten nicht akut psychotischen schizophrenen Sprecher waren die Sätze durch signifikant weniger kohäsive Verknüpfungen miteinander verbunden als in den Texten der Vergleichsgruppe. In einer zusätzlichen Längsschnittuntersuchung konnte gezeigt werden, daß in beiden schizophrenen Probandengruppen das Ausmaß der 'Kohäsivität' bei der spontansprachlichen Textproduktion

größer wurde, nachdem sie an einem dreimonatigen Psychotherapieprogramm teilgenommen hatten. Ziel dieses Programms war die Verbesserung sozial-kognitiver Fertigkeiten im Umgang mit Stressoren. Die Ergebnisse der textstatistischen Untersuchung werden vor allem im Zusammenhang mit der spezifisch kognitiven Symptomatik der schizophrenen Psychose diskutiert.

Chapter 12

Against the background of a psychopathologically anchored definition of schizophrenics' difficulties with speaking, and of a communication model which allows the specification of some characteristic aspects, an instrument for the description of deviances which occur in dialogues between a schizophrenic patient and a psychiatrist has been developed. The recognition of types of deviances within the given model depends on an assumed structure of the task to be solved when answering questions, or when reacting to communicative demands/requests. This structure allows the forecasting of reactions which are conformous, as well as identifying and describing differentially the reactions which have to be considered as nonconformous with a set of given expectations. The main result of this work so far is that it is possible to develop an instrument which combines formal and functional criteria by which the total set of dialogue sequences can be categorized.

Die *Beschreibung* der relevanten Phänomene ist Grundlage einer angemessenen *Erklärung* der Sprechauffälligkeiten von Schizophrenen. Um systematisch beschreiben zu können, bedarf es einer Festlegung dessen, was am verbalen Verhalten von Schizophrenen gestört erscheint; auch aus psychopathologischer Sicht ist dies eher das kommunikative Verhalten als die Sprache selbst; und es muss festgelegt werden, wie Auffälligkeiten grundsätzlich erfasst werden können: das relevante Verhalten muss mit einem expliziten Standard verglichen und in seiner allfälligen Abweichung erfasst werden. Ein einfaches Kommunikationsmodell für eine minimale Dialogsequenz Sprecher A—Sprecher B (hier: die Schizophrene)—Sprecher A, in welchem die Äusserungen aufgrund *formaler* Merkmale bestimmten *funktionalen* Kategorien zugeordnet sind, wird als Standard expliziert. Auf diesem Hintergrund ist es möglich, erwartungskonformes Verhalten vorherzusagen und mit tatsächlich auftretendem Verhalten zu vergleichen, und Typen von nicht-erwartungskonformem Verhalten können als Auffälligkeiten definiert werden. Beschreibt man konkretes Dialogmaterial (7 Interviews eines erfahrenen Psychiaters mit einem chronisch schizophrenen Patienten) mit Hilfe dieses Instrumentariums, so lassen sich 5 Typen von kommunikativen Auffälligkeiten unterscheiden; inwieweit diese für Schizophrene typisch sind, kann im Rahmen dieser Einzelfall-Studie allerdings nicht entschieden werden.

Chapter 13

The central problem addressed by this chapter is 'accessibility'. Before one can have a conversation at all, one has to get access to the chosen participant: one has to announce an intended conversation one way or other. This is a call for access on the level of interaction. Once the access on the level of interaction is settled, speakers have to get access on the level of topic—to each of the propositions which compose the topic. The vehicle for getting access is coherence; if speakers' utterances are not coherent, however, the possibility of restoring coherence is less problematic than the persistent problem of getting access, once it is clear that there *is* a problem of access. To get access, several preconditions have to be fulfilled: to get access to the interaction, one has to be available for the interaction. To get access to a topic, one has to specify sufficiently the propositions which compose the topic. I focus here on four techniques which the nonschizophrenic participants use in order to fulfil the preconditions which are apparently necessary to continue the conversation. The very problem of access is displayed in the frequent use of those techniques. A conversation then can turn into a ritual dance, irrespective of what the theme or intentions of the partners are. 'Making' the conversation, keeping it going, can become the issue on the surface, instead of remaining on a deeper level of what a conversation is about, as is usually the case.

Das Hauptproblem dieses Vortrages ist 'Zugänglichkeit', sowohl auf dem Gebiet der zwischenmenschlichen Interaktion als auch auf dem Gesprächsthemas. Kohärenz muss diese Zugänglichkeit vermitteln. Wenn man daher das Problem definiert als eines des Zuganges zur schizophrenen Sprache, dann bleibt das Ringen um den richtigen Zugang das zentrale und persistierende Problem, auch wenn die schizophrenen Äusserungen nicht kohärent sind: diese Inkohärenzen lassen sich nämlich beheben. Für diese Zugang müssen einige Vorbedingungen erfüllt sein: um die zwischenmenschliche Interaktion in den Griff zu bekommen muss man als Gesprächspartner nicht nur 'körperlich' anwesend sein. Um das Gesprächsthema zu verstehen, muss man konkrete Angaben über die im Gespräch aufgestellten Behauptungen bekommen können. Ich werde vier gesprächstechniken belichten, die dem nicht schizophrenen Gesprächsteilnehmer zur Verfügung stehen, um diese Vorbedingungen zu erfüllen.

Das eigentliche Problem des Zuganges zur schizophrenen Sprache liegt in der richtigen Dosierung dieser gesprächstechnischen Möglichkeiten, trotz ihres häufigen Gebrauches.

Chapter 14

In 'normal' discourse, it is implied by assertive speech acts that the speaker commits himself to some degree to telling the truth, and that he also believes in what he is saying. Because truth is intersubjectively determined, the speaker is also supposed to have some evidence for the truth of what he has said. This chapter presents some examples of psychotic discourse that do not display these implications, or in which they are at least problematic. In some cases the assertive speech act acquires also a magical power: 'saying makes it so'. Such a 'belief' in the magical power of language can also be found in the use of proper names in psychotic discourse. These observations are interpreted in a general theory of discourse that is to a great extent inspired by the psychoanalytical theory of Jacques Lacan. If the discourse of a person is to be understood by others, it has to subject itself to the existing rules of language use. In that way, discourse can be situated between two extremes: total idiosyncracy and total conformity. In psychotic discourse these two extremes can be found. It is argued that, in total idiosyncracy and in total conformity, the signifying character of language elements is affected.

Im 'normalen' Diskurs implizieren assertive Sprechakte, dass sich der Sprecher mehr oder weniger dazu verbindet, die Wahrheit zu sagen, und dass er glaubt, was er behauptet. Da Wahrheit eine intersubjektive Gegebenheit ist, wird vom Sprecher vorausgesetzt, dass er die Wahrheit dessen, was er sagt, beweisen kann. Er werden Beispiele pyschotischer Diskurse besprochen, in denen diese Implikationen nicht vorhanden sind, oder in denen sie wenigstens ein Problem darstellen. In einigen Fällen erhält der assertive Sprechakt auch eine magische Kraft: 'Wenn man von etwas behauptet, dass es so oder so ist, wird es auch so.' Diese Beobachtungen werden im Rahmen einer allgemeinen Theorie des Diskurses interpretiert, die durch die psychoanalytische Theorie von Jacques Lacan inspiriert wurde. Der Diskurs des Subjektes muss sich den herrschenden Regeln des Sprachgebrauchs unterwerfen, um durch andere verstanden werden zu können; er spielt sich somit zwischen zwei Äussersten ab: zwischen vollkommener Idiosynkrasie und vollkommener Konformierung. Diese beiden Äussersten können im psychotischen Diskurs angetroffen werden. In diesen Äussersten sind die sprachlichen Elemente als Signifikanten gefährdet.

Chapter 15

This chapter analyses the language acts of schizophrenics, both oral and written, recorded by the author or cited from world psychiatric literature, where the term *father* is understood in a deviant way, when compared with Polish standard usage. In describing meanings, the author resorts to the seme method, differentiating denotative and connotative semes, which he in turn divides into primary and secondary semes. The primary denotative semes are derived from dictionary meanings. The chapter presents the following conclusions:

1 Denotative semes of the term *father* in the schizophrenic understanding do not occur
2 In the language of schizophrenics, there occur only secondary connotative semes (negative image of the father), instead of the primary and secondary denotative semes, as well as the primary connotative semes which occur in standard usage.
3 A schizophrenic changes the meaning of *father* from positive to negative. Thus, the secondary semiotic archetype of *father* (Laplantine), usually concealed by customary language usage, is made manifest. This archetype is shameful and socially unacceptable, and according to it, *father* has absolute authority over the son, and resorts to the use of physical strength, threatens and humiliates the son, etc.

Dieser Aufsatz analysiert die sprachlichen Akte von Schizophrenen im mündlichen wie im schriftlichen Gebrauch, beobachtet vom Autor oder zitiert aus der psychiatrischen Literatur, wo der Begriff *Vater*—im Vergleich zum normalen Sprachgebrauch im Polnischen—eine abweichende Bedeutung hat. Um Bedeutungen zu beschreiben, macht der Autor Gebrauch von Semen. Er unterscheidet denotative und konnotative Seme, die jeweils als primäre oder sekundäre eingestuft werden können. Die primären denotativen Seme lassen sich aus den Wörterbucheintragungen ableiten.

1 Denotative Seme des Begriffs *Vater* lassen sich in der schizophrenen Bedeutung des Wortes nicht feststellen.
2 In der Sprache von Schizophrenen treten nur sekundäre konnotative Seme auf (das negative Bild des Vaters) statt der primären und sekundären denotativen als auch der primären konnotativen Seme, wie sie im normalen Sprachgebrauch vorkommen.
3 Bei einem Schizophrenen wandelt sich der positive *Vater*-Begriff ins Negative. Denn der Vater hat die absolute Macht über den Sohn, er wird mit physischer Gewalt assoziiert, er bedroht und erniedrigt den Sohn usw. In dieser Weise manifestiert sich der sekundäre Archetypus

des *Vater*-Begriffs, ein negativer Inhalt, der im normalen Sprachgebrauch nur unterschwellig vorhanden ist, weil er sozial nicht akzeptabel ist.

Chapter 16

This chapter presents an investigation into disturbances of cognition in schizophrenics, especially overinclusive thinking. The patients, and a normal control group, were shown a set of colours in an experiment designed to test verbal representation of colours, organization of sensory data and conceptualization. Differences were found in the following measures of codability: less variability, shorter descriptions, and a shorter reaction time of coding in schizophrenics—all symptoms of overinclusive thinking. The lower variability of coding, and the absence of increase in communicability, contradicts the suggestion of higher creativity in the patients. The concept of overinclusive thinking is endorsed by the data presented.

Bei vorliegender Studie wurden Kognitionsstörungen Schizophrener hinsichtlich des 'overinclusiven' Denkens untersucht. Dazu wurden einer Gruppe von Patienten und einer parallelisierten Kontrollgruppe Gesunder Farbtafeln vorgelegt, wodurch die sprachliche Repräsentation und Benennung die Organisation sensorischer Daten (ein Teilbereich der Begriffsbildung) offenkundig macht. Unterschiede ergaben sich in folgenden Kodabilitätsmaßen: geringere Variabilität und Kürze der Beschreibung, sowie kürzere Reaktionszeiten bei der Kodierung von Schizophrenen, beides Hinweise auf mangelndes Erfassen der Komplexität mit verminderter Differenzierung der Bezeichnungen (Folge des 'overinclusiven' Denkens). Als ein weiterer Beleg dafür sei die bei Schizophrenen verminderte intrapersonale Kommunikation genannt. Auch die größere Stereotypie widerspricht der Annahme einer höheren Kreativität von Schizophrenen, denn bei einem größeren Erfindungsreichtum in der Formulierung von Bezeichnungen wäre eine bessere Kommunikation von Farbwahrnehmungen zu erwarten.

Index